Comprehensive Overview of Foot and Ankle Trauma - Diagnosis, Treatment, Sequels and Rehabilitation

Edited by Khaled Elawady

Published in London, United Kingdom

Comprehensive Overview of Foot and Ankle Trauma - Diagnosis, Treatment, Sequels and Rehabilitation
http://dx.doi.org/10.5772/intechopen.1007240
Edited by Khaled Elawady

Contributors
Ahmed Khalil, Ahmed Mohamed Abd-alkhalek, Ahmed Sayed Elshamy, Anandarajagopal Kalusalingam, Ashok Marudanayagam, Chadapully Kolumbu Ismail Sajeeth, Chiara Cicuto, Christopher Lenz, Federico Ricci, Franco Bassetto, Gayathri Anbumani Alamelu, Giorgio Pietramaggiori, Giovanni Frezza, Jamal Al-Asiri, Khaled Elawady, Luigi Corso, Maryam Alsaffar, Mohammed Ahmed Abd Elfattah, Munier Hossain, Murtada Khajah, Nijil Vasukutty, Rohit Rambani, S. M. Fazeela Mahaboob Begum, Saja Scherer, Saravanakumar Parameswaran, Satheesh Babu Natarajan, Sedeek M. Mosaid, Suriyakala Perumal Chandran, Wael Abdelkarim Aldahshan

First published in London, United Kingdom, 2025 by IntechOpen
IntechOpen is the global imprint of INTECHOPEN LIMITED, registered in England and Wales, registration number: 11086078, 167-169 Great Portland Street, London, W1W 5PF, United Kingdom

For EU product safety concerns: IN TECH d.o.o., Prolaz Marije Krucifikse Kozulić 3, 51000 Rijeka, Croatia, info@intechopen.com or visit our website at intechopen.com.

British Library Cataloguing-in-Publication Data
A catalogue record for this book is available from the British Library

Comprehensive Overview of Foot and Ankle Trauma - Diagnosis, Treatment, Sequels and Rehabilitation
Edited by Khaled Elawady
p. cm.
Print ISBN 978-1-83635-037-8
Online ISBN 978-1-83635-036-1
eBook (PDF) ISBN 978-1-83635-038-5

If disposing of this product, please recycle the paper responsibly.

Meet the editor

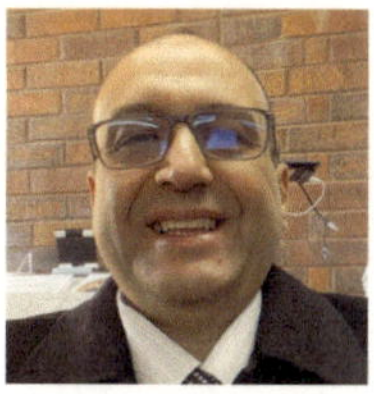

Dr. Khaled Elawady has been a Consultant in Trauma and Orthopedics at United Lincolnshire Teaching Hospitals since 2024, with notable prior locum and fellowship appointments across the UK, including Manchester, Nottingham, Alder Hey (Liverpool), and Brighton, among others. His specialist clinical interests include Major Trauma (adults and children), Arthroplasty (hip and knee replacements), Limb Reconstruction, Pediatric Orthopaedics, Foot and Ankle Surgery, Neurorehabilitation and Compartment Syndrome. Dr. Khaled has published several peer-reviewed journal articles, book chapters, including work on compartment syndrome, and posters at national and international congresses. Moreover, he is an active educator and lecturer in the School of Medicine.

Contents

Preface

The human foot and ankle, a marvel of evolutionary engineering, bears the immense responsibility of supporting our body weight, facilitating locomotion, and adapting to diverse terrains. However, precisely due to their pivotal role and intricate structure, they are exceptionally vulnerable to a broad spectrum of traumatic injuries. From a simple sprain to devastating fractures and dislocations, foot and ankle trauma presents a constant challenge to clinicians, demanding a profound understanding of anatomy, biomechanics, and the dynamic interplay of forces.

For too long, the comprehensive management of foot and ankle trauma has been fragmented across various specialties, often leading to disparate approaches and suboptimal outcomes. While excellent resources exist for specific aspects of diagnosis, surgical intervention, or rehabilitation, a singular, integrated volume that addresses the entire journey from injury to recovery, including the often-overlooked long-term sequels, has remained elusive. This book, *Comprehensive Overview of Foot and Ankle Trauma – Diagnosis, Treatment, Sequels and Rehabilitation*, endeavors to fill that critical void.

We aim to provide a definitive and up-to-date reference for orthopedic surgeons, emergency physicians, physical therapists, podiatrists, athletic trainers, and all healthcare professionals involved in the care of patients with foot and ankle injuries. We have meticulously curated contributions from leading experts in their respective fields, ensuring a multidisciplinary perspective that reflects the complexity of these injuries and the necessity of a collaborative approach to their management.

The journey within these pages begins with a thorough exploration of the anatomical and biomechanical foundations of the foot and ankle, crucial for understanding both injury mechanisms and treatment rationale. Subsequent chapters delve into the nuances of diagnostic imaging, encompassing the latest advancements in radiography, CT, MRI, and ultrasound, and emphasizing their role in accurate injury characterization. A significant portion of the book is dedicated to detailed discussions of various injury types, from common soft tissue injuries to complex fractures and dislocations, outlining evidence-based treatment algorithms, both conservative and surgical.

A unique and crucial aspect of this book is its dedicated focus on the “Sequels” of foot and ankle trauma. We recognize that successful acute management is only the first step. Many patients experience persistent pain, stiffness, instability, arthritis, or other long-term complications that significantly impact their quality of life. Understanding and addressing these sequels is paramount for holistic patient care. Finally, the book culminates with a comprehensive overview of rehabilitation strategies, emphasizing the critical role of individualized, progressive programs in restoring function, preventing recurrence, and optimizing patient outcomes.

We extend our sincere gratitude to all the contributing authors for their expertise, dedication, and tireless efforts in making this ambitious project a reality. Their commitment to advancing knowledge in this field is truly commendable. We also wish to thank our families and colleagues for their unwavering support throughout this endeavour.

Dr. Khaled Elawady
Department of Trauma and Orthopaedics,
United Lincolnshire Teaching Hospitals,
Lincoln, UK

Chapter 1

Perspective Chapter: The Principles of Ankle and Foot Post-Trauma Rehabilitation

Maryam Alsaffar and Murtada Khajah

Abstract

The ankle and foot are very complex structures of the musculoskeletal system. Any trauma to the ankle and foot complex might lead to a major disturbance in the gait dynamic, which may lead to disability. In order to avoid such problems, a proper rehabilitation program should be followed. In this chapter, an overview of the ankle and foot will be examined to have a better understanding of the impact of injuries on the joint, and the rehabilitation principles to follow post-injury for the desired recovery.

Keywords: ankle, foot, trauma, rehabilitation, recovery

1. Introduction

The foot and ankle joint is considered to be one of the most complex structures of the musculoskeletal system. It is supported with a strong ligamentous structure that aids in stabilizing the joints and acts as force transmitter between the lower extremities and the ground, because of that these joints are handling an elevated level of compression and shear forces during gait and weight bearing. Due to this structural and functional complexity, the ankle joint is more prone to injuries. It was reported in the literature that 22% of sport-related injuries presented to the emergency room were ankle injuries [1, 2].

Some of the injuries involving this region include lateral ankle sprains, which are considered the most common injury [2], along with all types of fractures of the tibia, fibula, tarsal's, metatarsals, and phalanges. Additionally, ankle injuries can result in post-surgical deformities and complications [3].

Having said that, patients with injuries or post-surgeries conditions should be managed with a proper rehabilitation program. A rehabilitation plan should be based on an understanding of the complexity of the joint structure, the impact of injuries, and post-surgical complications affecting the joint function. Given the intricacy of the ankle and foot joints, injuries in this area can significantly impact joint stability, mobility and the forces transmitted from the lower limb. Understanding the complexity of the ankle and foot joint in regards of the structure, biomechanics, and functional demands is key to developing individualized rehabilitation programs [4].

IntechOpen

The purpose of this chapter is to provide an explicit understanding of the ankle and foot, enabling healthcare providers to identify and address the crucial elements of assessment and management for post-traumatic foot and ankle conditions.

2. Anatomy and biomechanics of the ankle and foot

To understand and manage any joint, we should first study its structure. Therefore to understand the foot and ankle, the first element is to explore their anatomy. Although the joint occupies a small area of the body, it holds a great amount of weight and force transition. Its freedom of movement is critical to meet the functional capabilities of the joint [5].

2.1 Anatomy

The ankle joint is a highly specialized synovial hinge joint that connects the lower limb to the foot. It allows the complex function of transferring the weight of the body and maintains balance while walking, running, and jumping. The talocrural joint, which is another name for the ankle joint, is formed by the connection of the lower limb bones, the tibia and fibula with the talus, supported by a strong set of ligaments. This structural arrangement gives the joint a great level of stability, as the talus is secured by the medial malleolus of the distal of tibia and the lateral malleolus of the distal of the fibula as shown in **Figure 1**. The ankle joints allow dorsiflexion and planterflexion, which are primary movements during gait **Figures 1** and **2** [5–8].

The ankle's stability is further supported by a strong ligamentous structure as in **Figure 2**, and these ligaments include: medial ligament also known as the deltoid ligament, and the lateral ligaments that consist of the anterior talofibular ligament (ATFL), the calcaneofibular ligament (CFL), and the posterior talofibular ligament (PTFL).

The deltoid ligament that has a triangular structure is a strong ligament that prevents excessive eversion of the foot. In the other hand, the ATFL, CFL, and PTFL work together to prevent excessive inversion [9].

The tibia and the fibula as well connected by a fibrous joint are called the syndesmosis. This joint is strengthened by two ligaments: the anterior inferior tibiofibular ligament (AITFL) and the posterior inferior tibiofibular ligament (PITFL), which provide an extra support and stability [9].

The ankle joint is lined by synovial membrane, which produces synovial fluid to lubricate and nourish the articulation cartilage of the joint. The cartilage enables smooth movement and absorbs impact. In addition to the ligaments, the joint is surrounded by tendons that provide movement and promote support; these tendons include the Achilles tendon, which connects the calf muscles to the calcaneus and plays role in plantar flexion. Other tendons including the posterior and anterior tendons of the tibialis muscle control the fine movements and help in maintaining the foot arch.

The ankle joint is highly supplied by blood vessels from branches of the anterior and posterior tibial, and the fibular arteries to insure sufficient delivery of nutrients [7, 9]. Moreover, it innervated with nerve supply prances from the deep perineal, tibial, and sural nerves, and these nerves facilitate movement and transmit sensory impulses like pain, and proprioception to the brain [5].

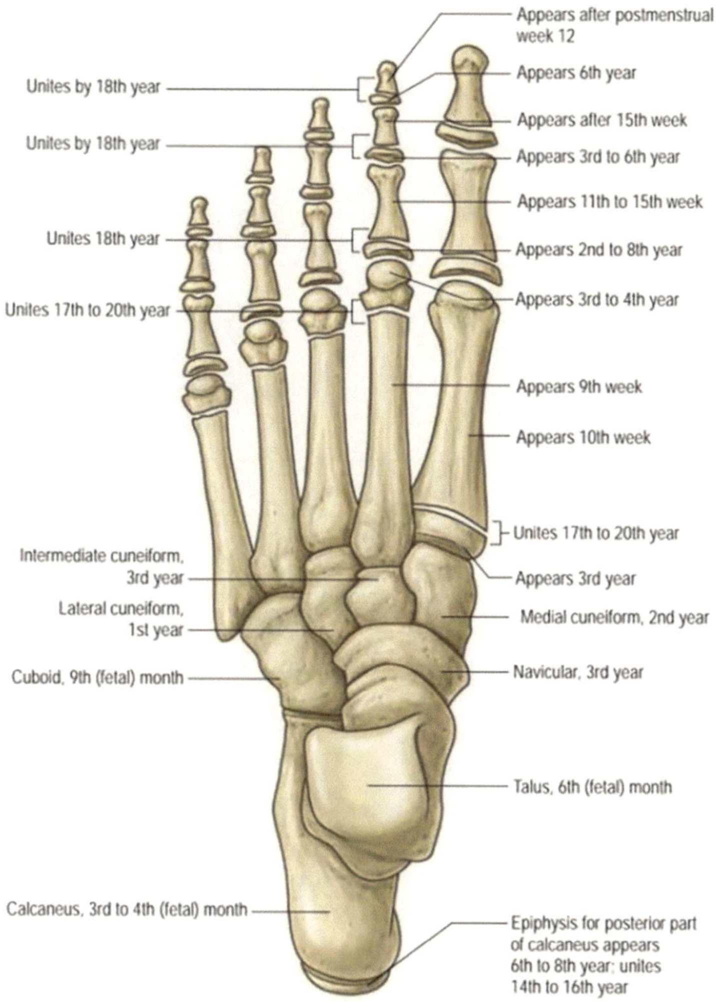

Figure 1.
The bone structure of ankle and foot [6].

Support and mobility are provided by several muscles divided into groups depending on their location and function. The anterior muscle group includes tibialis anterior, extensor hallucis longus, and extensor digitorum longus, which primarily facilitates dorsiflexion and toe extension. The posterior group, the gastrocnemius, and soleus muscles originate from the calf and attaches to the heel *via* the Achilles tendon (TA), enabling plantar flexion of the ankle [7].

In addition to that, a group of deep muscles are found posteriorly such as tibialis posterior, flexor digitorum longus, and flexor hallucis longus, and these muscles, which could be found on the medial aspect of the foot, aid with plantar flexion and foot inversion, providing arch support. Adding to that, a lateral group that includes the peroneus longus and brevis facilitate eversion and stabilize the ankle in weight-bearing activity. This group support balance foot posture, a group of smaller intrinsic muscles which found medial to the foot. All these muscles work together in coordination to provide adaptation and dynamic support [9].

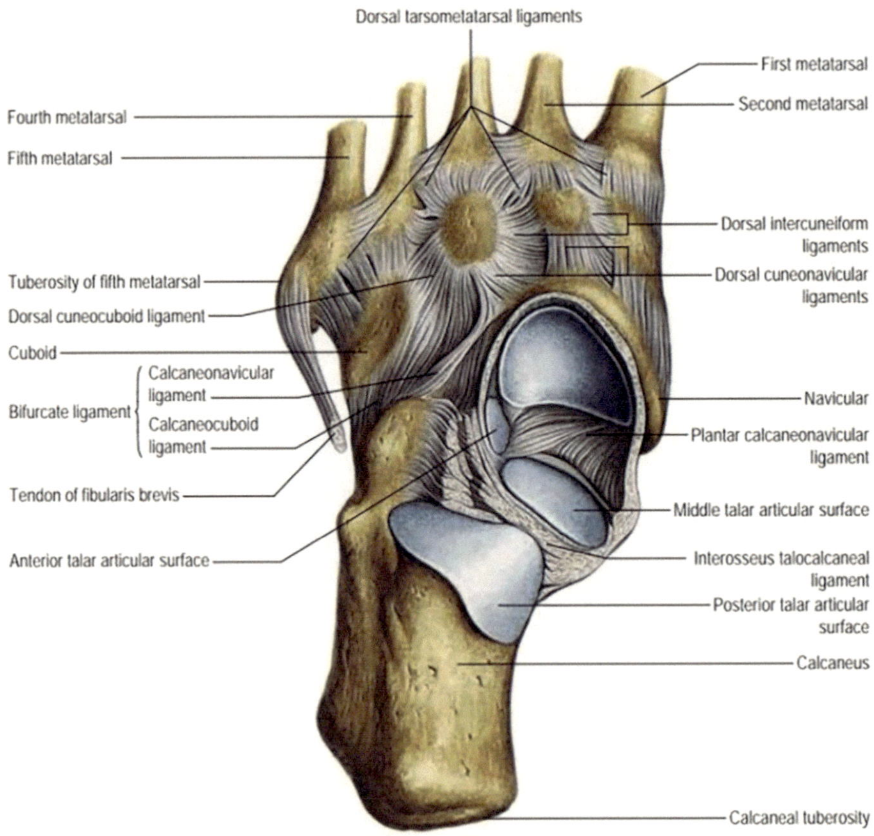

Figure 2.
Ligaments of the ankle and foot [6].

This anatomical structure allows the joint to effectively function and perform under the daily activity stress, and having said that, any disturbance to this structure may lead to impairment of the daily activities and quality of life.

2.2 The joint plain and freedom of movement

The ankle joint, as mentioned earlier, is a hinge joint that facilitates movement in the Sagittal plane and has one degree of freedom. This degree of freedom is very important in controlling propulsion and absorption of forces during gait, running, and jumping. It allows two movements that are dorsiflexion with a range that may extend up to 20 degrees and plantiflexion which may reach to approximately to 50 degrees as shown in **Figure 3**. The range varies depending on joint flexibility and overall health [11].

Although the talocrural joint is the primary moving joint, the ankle complex functions as a unit allows for additional movement because of it interaction with other joints, such as the subtalar and transverse tarsal joints. The subtalar that could be referred as talocalcaneal joint permits movements in the frontal plane including inversion end eversion. These movements are very important in adjusting the foot while walking on any uneven surface and maintaining balance. Inversion of the foot

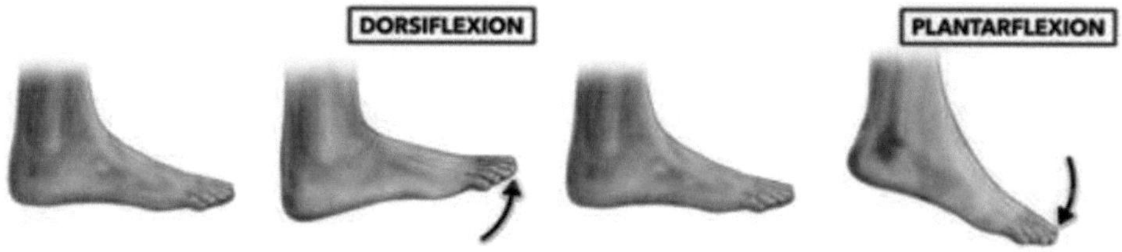

Figure 3.
Movements of the ankle joint [10].

tilts the sole of inward toward the midline, which ranges around 20–30 degrees, while eversion that involves tilting the sole of the foot outward is rather limited to approximately 5–10 degrees [9, 11].

The ankle complex has a lesser degree of movement in axial rotation such as adduction and abduction, and the available movements happening at the transverse plane mainly involve the subtalar and transverse tarsal joints. Despite the fact that the talocrural joint itself does not impact the rotation directly, the slight foot twisting facilitated by the ankle's anatomical interaction allows for multidirectional adjustments improving mobility and adaptability [1, 9, 11].

The interaction between these movements reinforces the functional versatility of the joint **Figure 3**. The talocrural joint works as the primary stabilizer in the sagittal plane; meanwhile, in hand the subtalar and other related joints provide dynamic adaptability across the frontal and transverse planes. To ensure the joint meeting the demands of all daily and complex activities depends on the interaction of these movements together. Because of that understanding, the plane of movement and degree of freedom are crucial for planning the rehabilitation programs, as it plays a key role in restoring and enhancing the ankle function and ability.

2.3 The biomechanics

Biomechanical system of the ankle and foot is important to induce adaptation to weight bearing and ground reaction forces by enduring the pressure and transferring of forces while walking, see **Figures 4** and **5** [12].

To have a better understanding of the ankle biomechanics it can be divided into: static stability and dynamic stability. Both of them are essential for maintaining good function during movement and rest.

2.3.1 Static stability

Static stability refers to the structural and passive forces on the ankle and foot to maintain balance and support while at rest or in situation where external forces are applied, such as standing on one leg or on uneven surface. This type stability relies on the alignment of the bones, integrity of ligaments, and the support of connective tissues such as the plantar fascia. A major contributing factor of the static stability is the medial longitudinal arch, which plays a major role in distributing weight and maintaining balance. Moreover, ligaments such as the deltoid ligament on the medial aspect of the ankle and the lateral ligament complex, together with ATFL, resist excessive inversion and eversion to help prevent sprains and dislocations of the ankle joint [13, 14].

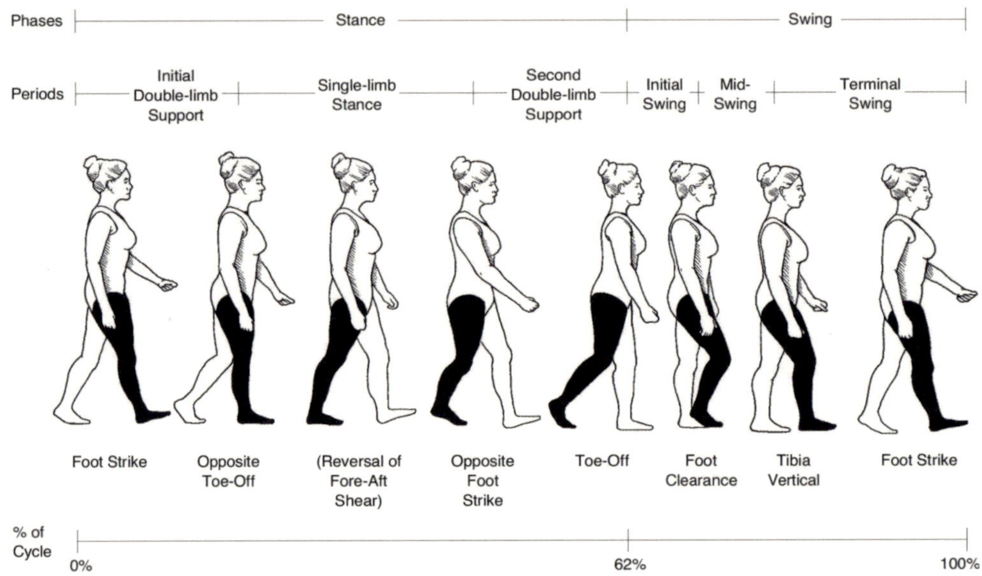

Figure 4.
Normal gait pattern [12].

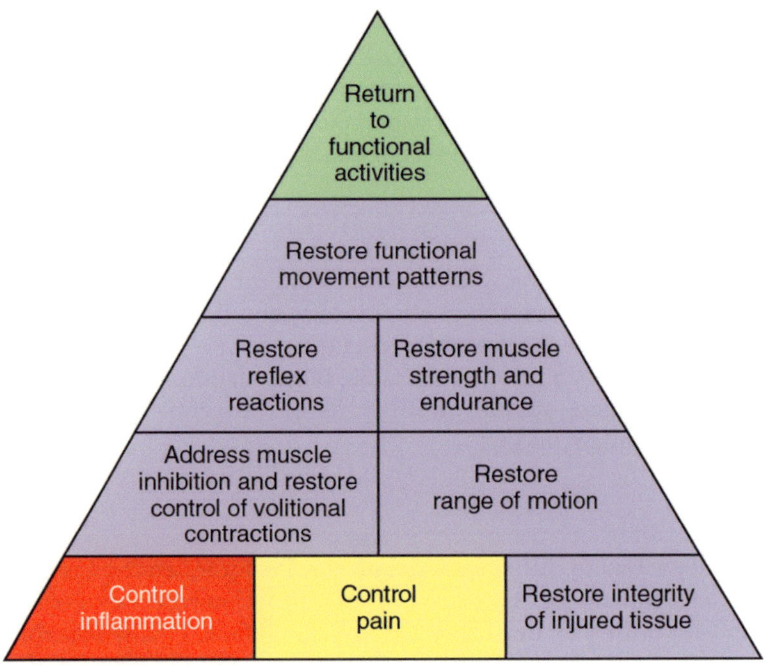

Figure 5.
The modified rehabilitation pyramid [4].

2.3.2 Dynamic stability

Dynamic stability of the ankle and foot refers to the ability of the complex to respond and adapt to changes in load and surface changing during movement to ensure balance and control. It is mainly the responsibility of the ligaments supporting the joint and the muscular forces that stabilize the articulation structures in the joint. Walking on uneven surfaces while trying to maintain balance is an example of dynamic stability [14].

2.3.3 Integration between static and dynamic stabilities

The ankle and foot are biomechanical wonder that integrate both the complexity of the structure and the ability to adapt to the function related. Alongside weight bearing, and shock-absorbing capabilities, they enable propulsion for generation of fundamental human movements. From biomechanical prospective, proper assessment and management of the ankle stability, whether static or dynamic, are critical for rehabilitation programs and injury prevention. For example, a weak or injured ATFL can compromise static stability, increasing the risk of recurrent ankle sprains. Likewise, weakened perineal muscles or delayed neuromuscular responses may impair the ability to adapt to sudden changes in the surface or load, resulting in instability or overuse injuries such as tendinopathies. Moreover, imbalance or misdistribution between static or dynamic stability can significantly affect over all ankle functions such as flat foot. The loss of the medial arch support impacts both static and dynamic stabilities, leading to alternation in gait pattern and causing an increased level of strain on the plantar fascia and TA.

Optimal ankle and foot function depends on having a synchronized interaction between dynamic and static stabilities. For instance, during jumping and landing, the static stabilizer gives the baseline of support; at the same time, the dynamic stabilizer works to adapt to the forces generated by the movement and tries to maintain balance. While the foot in landing, the medial arch will work as shock absorber by deforming slightly with the plantar fascia and the other ligaments to prevent excessive collapse. While transition into propulsion occurs, the components of dynamic stability take over by activating muscles and tendons to create controlled movements and restore energy for next step [13, 14]. This interaction is very important to maintain balance on uneven or unpredictable surfaces, in case rapid adjustment in muscle activation is needed to prevent falls.

Rehabilitation and management of ankle and foot injuries and prevention strategies need to take into account these three aspects (anatomy, *joint plane* and *freedom of* movement, and biomechanics). A comprehensive evaluation that involves all the tools is needed to identify and understand the problems, enabling medical caregiver to provide appropriate treatment and management.

3. Ankle and foot post-trauma rehabilitation

The rehabilitation of the ankle and foot complex relies on basic principles, with the main focus on returning to normal levels of activity before the injury occurred. Functional limitations are the first to considered by Magee et al. [4]. This functional limitation has a significant impact by pain, reducing range of motion, muscle strength, and endurance, which can contribute to poor balance and proprioception. To ensure effective rehabilitation a well-rounded assessment should be done followed by a proper management plan to recover fully and prevent future injuries.

3.1 Assessments tools of the ankle and foot

As one of the most complex joints in the body, the ankle joint is particularly vulnerable to impairments and disturbances. A wide range of tools are available for evaluation, including pain scales, range of motion tools, muscle strength assessment, endurance and balance measures, and imaging studies. Moreover, we have tools that are patient self-reported such as foot and ankle ability measures (FAAM) and the ankle and hind foot scale (AOFAS). These tools can help identifying issues and evaluate symptoms, which help therapists to determine the best rehabilitation program [14–19]. However, understanding the underlying cause of the symptoms requires good observational skills, allowing therapists to differentiate between symptoms and their associated causes effectively.

Both postures, static analysis and functional (movement) analysis are essential in determining the problem and creating an effective rehabilitation program.

3.1.1 Subjective assessment

Subjective assessment is essent (Box **1**) for physiotherapists, as it evaluates and processes patient information, providing crucial information for clinical decision making.

History taking, which is a key component of subjective assessment, helps in understanding the mechanism of injury. For example, understanding whether an injury resulted from a fall, a ligament tear, or a twisted ankle can help in providing important clues to the involved structure. Identifying whether the injury is acute or due to overuse repetitive stress such as running course, the injury can also offer valuable hint to the underlying cause [20].

Moreover, subjective assessment can identify whether previous injuries are related to the current condition. For example, whether repetitive ankle sprains are common and may indicate chronic ankle instability.

Pain is the main drive to seek professional help in most cases, so it is very important to understand the description and behavior of it to guide in correlating the symptoms cause and help in differentiation of the responsible structure. For example, tingling and numbness in the foot may indicate nerve involvement like tarsal tunnel syndrome. When assessing pain one should evaluate location of the pain, quality and intensity, and behavior [21, 22]. Visual analog scale is an example of an easy patient-reported pain outcome measure that is commonly used in the clinic [23].

Taking into consideration patient goals are very important, it helps in setting the rehabilitation process, by including the patient in decision making. This can help in adherence and improvement of the patient condition.

3.1.2 Objective assessment

A variety of objective assessment tools are available to evaluate patients to provide more insight joint physical impairments and deficits, and they are used for guild treatment and monitoring patient's progression. These tools include the evaluation of strength, range of motion (ROM), stability, functional performance, and overall foot mechanics (**Box 2**).

Subjective assessment:

1. Patient history
2. Pain assessment
3. Patient goals

Box 1.
Subjective assessment tools.

Objective assessment:

1. Muscle strength
2. Range of motion
3. Stability
4. Functional performance
5. Foot mechanics

Box 2.
Objective assessment tools.

Diagnostic imaging such as X-ray, MRI, and CT scans can give a detailed imaging to roll out bone fractures and soft tissue injuries post-trauma, and they are crucial to prevent tissue harm and to begin the process of rehabilitation [4].

Ankle and foot swelling is the first symptom post-trauma, it is a natural response from circular system where fluid and white blood cells are accumulated to the injured area. Swelling can be measured using tape measurement around the ankle; for example, The Figer of Eight method or by using volumetric measurement by submerging the foot in water and measuring the displaced volume are used to quantify edema or swelling [24].

Having full range of motion (ROM) is necessary in achieve a balanced gait, and any reduction in joint angle will have a direct effect on the function of the ankle joint. ROM is measured by using goniometry which is the common tool to use in the clinic, and measures joint angles of all movements pre- and post-treatment to evaluate the effectiveness of the rehabilitation program [4, 20, 25].

Another way to measure ankle dorsiflexion flexion is by weight-bearing lunge test (WBLT), limitation in the angle of ankle dorsiflexion may lead to gait abnormalities or movement compensation.

After ankle and foot injury especially in sprain injury, the most affected structures are the ligaments; therefore, ligament integrity tests are highly recommended to roll out the involvement of the ligaments.

The most used tests are Anterior Drawer Test, Tatar Tilt Test, and External Rotation Test. Anterior Drawer Test that mainly assesses the integrity of the anterior talofibular ligament (ATFL) found that excessive forward translation of the talus suggests positive results. Tatar Tilt Test evaluates the calcaneofibular ligaments (CFL), considered to be positive if there was an increase in inversion compared to the other ankle, while External Rotation Test helps in identifying syndesmotic injuries such as high ankle sprains [17, 24, 25].

Manual Muscle Testing (MMT) is used as an outcome measure to evaluate muscle ability to generate power, which has five-grading system starting from (0) as no muscle activation is detected to (5), where muscles can resist against maximum manual force [26].

Despite controversy of the validity and reliability of this tool, MMT is a commonly practice in the clinic due to the straightforward application; moreover, it could test several aspects of neuromuscular control [27, 28].

Other muscle testing tools are available such as Handheld Dynamometry that provides more objective muscle strength reading that MMT.

Balance and proprioceptive assessment of the ankle joint is a major evaluating outcome; it is the key elements in preventing future injuries to the joint.

Static balance can be evaluated by using Single-Leg Balance Test [29], while Star Excursion Balance Test [30] can evaluate dynamic balance. This test evaluates the ankle functional stability by reaching in multiple directions while standing in one leg.

Due to the fact that the aim of the lower limbs to serve the purpose of weight bearing and locomotion, gait analysis, as in **Figure 4**, is the most important assessment after ankle injuries. It provides thorough insight into the biomechanics and functional recovery of the patient. After an injury and due to prolonged limping or immobilization, the gait pattern may be affected, which leads to compensations in the gait pattern.

When assessing gait by visual observation, we need to find any ankle and foot deformities or deviations. Gait analysis helps in finding alteration in gait patterns, such as movement compensations or imbalance in weight distribution. On the other hand, gait analysis monitors recovery and progression, as it allows tracking of improvement over time. This process helps in setting clear goals and customizing rehabilitation plans for each patient. Adding to that by evaluating gait to detect and correct movement, the risk of further complications affecting other joints can be prevented [12].

Visual observation is the main physical therapy tool of evaluating and assessing gait, because of that a complete understanding of the normal gait pattern is needed.

Pressure Plate analysis is another tool that could be used to provide detailed data on plantar pressure distribution and timing during gait [31].

Other tests that could be included in the assessment of the ankle and foot are Functional performance tests such as Single-Limb Hop Test (to evaluate functional stability and balance), and foot posture and alignment tests that may include Foot Posture Index (FPI-6) that has six score to evaluate foot alignment. Navicular Drop Test is another test to evaluate medial arch collapse by measuring the difference in height with and without weight bearing [18, 24, 32].

Adding to all the mentioned assessment tools, the patients self-reported outcome measures (PROMs) that correlate with a valid and reliable assessment tool in the clinical filed. PROMs are believed to provide direct insight into patient's perspectives of their health, functional abilities, and quality of life [33].

There are many PROMs that can be used for ankle and foot patients depending on their complain and the clinical judgment of the therapist, and they could include Foot and Ankle Ability Measure (FAAM) that helps in tracking functional activity of daily living and sport [34] or Lower Extremity Functional Scale (LEFS) that assesses overall lower limb function [35].

Other nonspecific joint outcome measures include tools such as Berg Balance Scale (BBS) that evaluates balance and fall risk in adults and SF-12, which is the short form of Health Survey, it is a self-report outcome to assess the impact of health on people quality of life [36].

All these tools and outcomes could be used as an initial assessment to monitor patient progression and to evaluate the effectiveness of the rehabilitation program. The discussion of which tools to use depends on the patient's condition and symptoms, along with the therapist's clinical judgment. Planning an effective treatment plan is highly correlated with the ability to associate findings from these tools and critical clinical thinking of the therapist to find out comparable signs and underlying problems addressing them in the rehabilitation program.

4. Developing rehabilitation program

After the ankle and foot injury, the joint complex losses the ability to drive and support the gait circle; therefore, a proper rehabilitation program should be introduced considering both early mobility and injured tissue protection. This will allow promote healing and recovery of the neuromuscular system, which helps in preventing the recurrence of injuries or symptoms such as overuse injuries, is quite common in the ankle and foot complex. For this reason, therapist should use the skill of good judgment after assessing the patient to develop a tailored program that meets the patient complains and needs [4].

There are many different rehabilitation methods that can be followed when treating patients with post-ankle and foot injuries. Meanwhile, the principles of these techniques usually are the same. This section we will address the phases of post-injury rehabilitation and introduce rehabilitation principles that aid in promoting recovery and stability. Additionally, some of the protocols that are usually used post-surgeries will be mentioned later.

4.1 Rehabilitation principles and injury phases: a

The ankle and foot have an overly complex structure that involves the interaction between many structures, the severity of the injuries and the underlying structure, determining the phases of rehabilitation. To design a proper rehabilitation program that is relevant to injured tissue, the types of injuries include the following:

1. Injuries that do not involve disturbance of any tissue.

2. Injuries that involve soft tissue impairment.

3. Injuries that involve bone fractures.

Each type of these injury has a deferent bath of rehabilitation depending on the severity and the management (surgical, conservative) needed to resolve it; for example, T.A. Repair has a protocol that needs to be followed step by step based on the surgical procedure performed [37].

Before delving into each type of injury, the general principles of rehabilitation should be explained to make them comprehensible and easy to follow while developing the rehabilitation plan. According to the literature, one way to understand the healing process after injuries is by following the rehabilitation pyramid, which is modified by Hertel J and Deneger as shown in **Figure 5**. This paradigm is used to outline the framework for recovery for patients after injury. It focuses on regaining function and control to return to normal activity, and preventing further injury by following a systematic approach, with each phase depending on the phase before it [4, 38, 39].

As it could be seen in Figure, the base of the pyramid focused on first phase post-injury, where the aim of rehabilitation is to control inflammation and pain and restoring of injured tissue integrity. This is important as a foundation of building an effective recovery program. The aim of this phase is reducing pain and inflammation by using the RICE principle which is, rest, ice, compression, and elevation, with the prescription medication that helps in controlling pain and inflammation [4, 40, 41]. Adding to that, introducing muscle activation techniques in this level is crucial to prevent muscular weakness and atrophy. Joint immobilization can be achieved using braces, casts, or walking boots advised in on the need to provide a suitable environment for the damaged tissues to heal. Preventing weight bearing or reducing its impact is also important to ensure the protection of the tissues and the joint environment, aiding the recovery process [4, 42].

Moving to the top of the pyramid from the left side focuses on neuromuscular control; meanwhile, the right side is focused on restoration of movement; both sides aim to reach to the top of the pyramid, which returns to functional activity simultaneously.

Neuromuscular control is divided into three levels; the first level focuses on restoring the control of voluntary movement and muscle inhibition, followed by the second step that involves the control of reflex reaction. Meanwhile on the other side as it is shown in the paradigm, the first level is to restore a range of motions, followed by working on muscle strength and endurance. Working on these levels would facilitate stepping up the next level where the left and the right sides of the pyramid join to restore the functional movement pattern that is the third level of neuromuscular control [4, 43].

This system would allow therapists to develop and design rehabilitation programs for each patient's individual injuries and symptoms. Evidence suggests that by involving the progression of neuromuscular control throughout the rehabilitation system, patients allow to achieve study recovery.

4.1.1 Neuromuscular control techniques

Neuromuscular control involves joint movement and stability by integrating sensory feedback, proprioception, and motor response. The control is due to the interaction between the nervous system and the muscle groups, producing a smooth and precise movements. Maintaining dynamic balance and adapting to environment are crucial [4].

Rehabilitation techniques that help with developing the neuromuscular control may include the following:

1. Proprioception training.

Proprioception training is a critical element of ankle and foot rehabilitation. It focuses on enhancing the body's ability to sense joint position, which helps with preventing re-injuries by improving balance, coordination, and stability. Dynamic activities as well rely on proprioception input to maintain stability specifically during the rapid movement [44, 45]. Adding to that, a study by Rosen et al. shows a reduction in the symptoms of chronic ankle instability after proprioception training and an improvement in the functional outcomes [46–48].

2. Strengthening exercises

Muscle strengthening plays a fundamental role in the rehabilitation process. Following any injury to the ankle, the surrounding muscles often weaken affecting the joint function, compromising stability, disrupting biomechanics, and increasing the risk of chronic joint instability. Muscle strengthening enhances joint function by improving stability and shock absorption, while helping correct biomechanics imbalances and preventing re-injuries.

Strengthening exercises may include isometric exercises, weight loading, and concentric and eccentric exercises, as adding them to the rehabilitation plan helps to train muscle control and acts as shock absorbers during gait and running [4].

3. Open and closed kinetic exercises

Open kinetic exercises are also used as strength exercises in the rehabilitation plan. Open kinetic exercises involve movement where the distal part of the limb is free in space, while the proximal part remains stationary, focusing on isolated muscle activation.

Closed kinetic exercises involve the distal part of the limb being fixed (e.g., on the floor) while the proximal part moves. These exercises mimic functional weight-bearing activities, such as walking and stepping, enhancing functional strength and encouraging co-contraction of surrounding muscles to promote joint support [49].

4. Dynamic movements

Dynamic movements play a role in ankle and foot rehabilitation. They are as important as proprioception and strengthening training because they all help to achieve the same goals. Literature suggests that dynamic movements enhance functional outcomes, reduce the risk of repetitive injuries, and improve neuromuscular control [44, 45, 50].

5. Feedback mechanisms

Feedback mechanisms, whether intrinsic (from the body) or extrinsic (from an external source), help the patients perform exercises correctly and adapt to the biomechanics demands during rehabilitation. Examples of intrinsic feedback include balance exercises where the feedback is driven from sensory information within the body, such as joint positioning or muscle tension.

On the other hand, extrinsic feedback comes from external source, such as verbal advice from a therapist or visual feedback using mirrors to correct body alignment.

In addition to that, augmented feedback by using auditory or visual alert from a platform to deliberate external cues to facilitate intrinsic feedback could be used to improve exercise performance [4, 51, 52].

4.1.2 Range of motion and muscle strengthening techniques

To regain full joint performance, the joint should be clear and able to move freely without restriction. When the ROM is reduced due to joint articulation problem or muscle and soft tissue issues, it should be addressed and managed to restore function and prevent re-injuries. Techniques to improve ROM include active and passive movement exercises, manual joint mobilization, and muscle energy techniques.

For example, manual joint mobilization is one way to improve ROM of ankle planner-flexion or Doris-flexion; in addition, it influences pain reduction [53, 54].

Beyond ROM improving muscle strength and endurance should be addressed in the rehabilitation program to ensure full recovery. Muscle strength helps support joint stability, enhance movement efficiency, and prevent compensatory movement patterns. Strength also improves endurance, which is the ability in sustaining repeatable contractions over time. It is particularly important in daily activities such as prolonged standing and running. In addition to that, it improves shock absorption, protects the joint, and facilitates return to sport activities. Examples of strengthen exercises may include the following (**Box 3**):

Strengthening exercises:

- Isometric
- Isotonic
- Functional
- Endurance

Box 3.
Types of muscle strength types.

Isometric (static) exercises for early-stage rehabilitation followed by progression to, and isotonic exercises where they have more results when performed at low intensity but high repetition. Functional exercises that involve resistance and increase repetition like stepping or walking on toes may be used. Moreover, endurance exercises might include high repetition, low-load exercises, and dynamic activities, such as treadmill walking or light jogging [4, 55, 56]. All these exercises could involve concentric or eccentric muscle activation depending on the patient's need [57].

After understanding the basic principles of rehabilitation techniques and the rehabilitation pyramid, a treatment plan should be established for each level of injury depending on the severity of the problem and the patient's main concerns.

These could range from minor injuries like ankle sprains or bruising to shear conditions requiring surgical procedures.

In this section, some of the main diagnoses or injuries will be analyzed, along with an example of a rehabilitation program.

5. Examples of ankle trauma rehabilitation protocol

5.1 Lateral ankle sprain

Lateral ankle sprain is the most common injury of the ankle. It is usually treated in the emergency room but often not followed up in clinics, which means patients usually have no chance for proper recovery and rehabilitation [58]. An example of post-ankle sprain rehabilitation could include several phases like:

1. Acute phase (0–7 days)

The goal of this phase is to reduce pain and swelling associated with the injury. This can be established by protecting and stabilizing the joint by using weight-bearing braces if the pain is severe or tape if the pain is tolerable. It was indicated in the articles [59] that bracing or taping can reduce the risk of re-injury in sports by up to 50% if introduced during the first phase of the injury.

Cryotherapy is recommended to reduce pain and swelling as well, which could be combined with compression and evaluation (RICE principals) to obtain better results.

During this phase, early mobilization is highly recommended, pain-free range of motion exercises such as ankle circumduction, and active plantar flexion and dorsiflexion should be included to prevent joint stiffness and promote circulation [41].

Strength exercises in this phase should be guided by the patient pain level, and it is advisable to begin with isomeric strengthening exercises. For example, pressing the foot into resistance with a towel or wall, all movements of the ankle are involved.

DOI: http://dx.doi.org/10.5772/intechopen.1009529

2. Subacute phase (1–3 weeks)

The aim of the phase is to restore ROM, muscle strength, and proprioception while gradually introducing weight bearing depending on the patent's tolerance. Theraband resistance exercises to increase muscle strength and endurance in this phase, both concentric and eccentric muscle contractions, should be performed in this phase.

Balance exercises such as standing on one leg and using balance board are important during this phase to activate proprioception system of the ankle and foot [45].

In some patients, the joint ROM might be compromised, if so of manual therapy techniques could be performed to help with increasing ROM of the joint. Furthermore, some of the low-impact functional exercises such as swimming and cycling are recommended to improve overall performance and maintain fitness [60].

3. Strengthening Phase (3–6 weeks)

The primary goals of this phase include enhancing muscle strength, neuromuscular control, and functional stability. This phase focuses on the following:

- Increasing resistance in exercises such as heel rise, step up, and down, with theraband strengthening.

- Dynamic balance techniques are introduced for gait training exercises to improve endurance and gait stability.

- Functional movement, and plyometric training such as jumping and landing drills could be included to fulfill the phase aim.

4. Return to normal lifestyle and sport phase (6–12 weeks)

In this phase, the therapist needs to advance the level of exercises depending on the patient's goals and level of activity pre-injury. The aim of this phase is to restore full function, agility, and prevent re-injuries.

After completing this phase, patients should have full recovery and be ready to resume their normal level of activity with less chance of re injury.

5.2 Bone fractures

Bone fractures of the ankle and foot are quite common injuries. These fractures can range from simple stress fractures to complete displaced or non-displaced fractures. Regardless the type of the fracture, or whatever the reduction management is (conservative or operative), rehabilitation for post-fracture patients usually follows the same bath, focusing on restoring mobility, strength, and joint function [42, 61].

1. Immobilization phase (0–6 weeks)

The ankle will be stabilized with a cast, brace, or boot to stabilize the ankle, to allow bone heeling. Usually, patient would be recommended to use walking devices with non-weight-bearing gait pattern at the beginning of this phase. Some studies suggest that early weight bearing in stable fractures improves the recovery process without increasing the level of complications [62].

2. Mobilization phase (6–12 weeks)

In this phase of rehabilitation, a gradual ROM restoration and prevention of stiffness are crucial to prevent chronic joint stiffness. Active exercises, along with isometric strengthening techniques, should apply along with functional exercises such as gradual weight bearing and stepping exercises to enhance flexibility stability and function.

3. Strengthening phase (+12 weeks)

This phase aims to build up muscle strength, improve balance, and enhance endurance proprioception to ease the way to full recovery. This can be achieved by introducing resistance exercises, proprioceptive training, and functional exercises such as cycling.

4. Returning to normal level of activity (4–6 months)

The purpose of this stage is to reach to the full recovery and returning to the full functional capacity of the body, by introducing high-intensity exercises and specific strengthening programs tailored to the patients' needs and goals, are introduced. The gradual progression of exercises helps in preventing and reducing the risk of re-injuries [41].

5.3 Post Tendo-Achilles repair

The Tendo-Achilles, also known as the triceps surae, is considered the largest and strongest tendon in the human body. It connects the calf muscles (the aponeuroses of the gastrocnemius and soleus), and plantar is muscles to the calcaneus bone. Post-surgery patients need to follow a protocol to prevent the risk of injury to repaired tendon. The therapist and the surgeon should work together as a team to insure a full and healthy recovery [63, 64]. Phases of T.A. Rehabilitation include the following:

1. Immobilization Phase (0–2 weeks)

The aim of this phase is to protect the repaired tendon, and to minimize swelling. It is recommended to:

- Use posterior splint or flexible boot that allows 20 to 30 degrees of plantar flexion. As the literature suggests, early weight bearing with flexible immobilization achieves better outcomes [64].

- Non-weight bearing with crutches to reduce the load on the operated tendon.

2. Early mobilization Phase (2–6 weeks)

This phase focuses on restoring ROM and preventing stiffness. Early gentle mobilization exercises are recommended to avoid stiffness.

- Use functional boot with adjustable planter flexion angles.

- Start partial weight bearing with the boot (as patient tolerated).

- Avoid over stretching exercises to protect the tendon integrity [64].

3. Strengthening Phase (6–12 weeks)

The aim of this phase is to improve muscle strength and endurance, preparing patients to restoring full functional ability.

- Start gradual full weight bearing out of the boots.

- Isometric strengthening exercises of the ankle muscles.

- Progress to concentric and eccentric exercises, such as heel raises on both feet and then progresses to single leg.

Eccentric exercises help in improving tendons elasticity and strength that reduces the risk of re-injury [57, 65].

4. Functional Phase

Restoring of proprioception, balance, and functional performance are the aim of this phase.

- Advanced strengthening exercises are introduced and neuromuscular training to protect the tendon.

- Proprioceptive training to improve balance, for example, exercises on uneven surfaces.

- Incorporating functional training to improve neuromuscular control and readiness to sports. TA loading exercises with resistance are recommended to enhance tendon integrity [63].

5. Return to sport Phase

Final phase is sport specific to guide athletes returning to sport safely a proper rehabilitation program that tailored to the patient and sport should be followed [66].

- High-intensity functional exercises.

- Gradual introduction to sport-specific exercises under supervision.

These are examples of management strategies of post-injury and operative ankle and foot; other injuries would have a similar path, which mainly depends on the critical thinking and good judgment of the therapist to move from one rehabilitation phase and progressing to the next. Considering the other joints of the lower limb is also important, exercises of the knee and the hip joints may be included as early as possible to maintain their strength and prepare them for the procession of the rehabilitation phases.

6. Conclusion

The ankle and foot are an extraordinarily complex structures that bear a significant amount of stress and load to perform their functions and maintain stability and balance of the body. As consequence, they have a high incidence of injury. Although the rehabilitation of the ankle and foot complex can be challenging, a thorough out understanding of anatomy, joints, freedom of movement, and biomechanics will help therapists to build the suitable rehabilitation plans that align the patient needs and goals.

In addition, therapists should be aware of the fundamental strategies for physical therapy assessments to identify the associated problems and challenges. This awareness is important to design the effective patient management plans.

Following the rehabilitation principles stages is crucial to ensure healthy recovery throughout the rehabilitation process.

Abbreviations

ATFL	anterior talo-fibular ligament
CFL	calcaneo-fibular ligament
PTFL	posterior talo-fibular ligament
AITFL	anterior inferior tibiofibular ligament
PLTFL	posterior inferior tibiofibular ligament
TA	Tendo-Achilles
MMT	manual muscle testing
ROM	range of motion
PROMS	patient self-reported outcome measures

Author details

Maryam Alsaffar*† and Murtada Khajah†
Al-Razi Hospital, Ministry of Health, Sulibekhat, Kuwait

*Address all correspondence to: hm.rahd@gmail.com

† These authors contributed equally.

References

[1] Brockett CL, Chapman GJ. Biomechanics of the ankle. Orthopaedics and Traumatology. 2016;**30**(3):232-238

[2] Lin CWC, Hiller CE, de Bie RA. Evidence-based treatment for ankle injuries: A clinical perspective. Journal of Manual & Manipulative Therapy. 2010;**18**(1):22-28

[3] Fong DTP, Hong Y, Chan LK, Yung PSH, Chan KM. A systematic review on ankle injury and ankle sprain in sports. Sports Medicine. 2007;**37**:73-94

[4] Magee DJ, Zachazewski JE, Quillen WS, Manske RC. Pathology and Intervention in Musculoskeletal Rehabilitation (Vol. 3). Elsevier Health Sciences. Missouri: Southeastern Louisiana University 2016 Sample Performance Comments; 2015 Available from: http://www.southeastern.edu/admin/hr/eeandmngrinfo/managerinformation/pprcomments.html; [Accessed: November 3, 2016]

[5] Neumann DA. Kinesiology of the Musculoskeletal System-E-Book: Kinesiology of the Musculoskeletal System-E-Book. Missouri: Elsevier Health Sciences; 2016

[6] Standring S, editor. Gray's Anatomy E-Book: Gray's Anatomy E-Book. Missouri: Elsevier Health Sciences; 2021

[7] Drake RL, Vogl AW, Mitchell AW. Gray's Anatomy for Students Flash Cards: Gray's Anatomy for Students Flash Cards E-Book. Missouri: Elsevier Health Sciences; 2019

[8] Moore KL, Dalley AF. Clinically Oriented Anatomy. 8th ed. Wolters Kluwer India Pvt Ltd.; 2018

[9] Dawe EJ, Davis J. (vi) anatomy and biomechanics of the foot and ankle. Orthopaedics and Traumatology. 2011;**25**(4):279-286

[10] Understanding Athletic Achilles Injuries: Causes, Prevention, and Avanced Treatments. OrthoCarolina. 2025. Available from: https://www.orthocarolina.com/orthopedic-news/understanding-athletic-achilles-injuries-causes-prevention-and-advanced-treatments

[11] Castro MD. Ankle biomechanics. Foot and Ankle Clinics. 2002;7(4):679-693. DOI: 10.1037/h0042344

[12] Chambers HG, Sutherland DH. A practical guide to gait analysis. JAAOS-Journal of the American Academy of Orthopaedic Surgeons. 2002;**10**(3):222-231

[13] Belinha J, Campos JCR, Fonseca E, Silva MHF, Marques MA, Costa MFG, et al. Advances and Current Trends in Biomechanics. Portugal: CRC Press; 2021

[14] Donatelli R. Normal biomechanics of the foot and ankle. Journal of Orthopaedic & Sports Physical Therapy. 1985;**7**(3):91-95

[15] Nelson EC, Eftimovska E, Lind C, Hager A, Wasson JH, Lindblad S. Patient reported outcome measures in practice. BMJ. 2015;**350**:1-3

[16] Basch E, Deal AM, Kris MG, Scher HI, Hudis CA, Sabbatini P, et al. Symptom monitoring with patient-reported outcomes during routine cancer treatment: A randomized controlled trial. Journal of Clinical Oncology. 2016;**34**(6):557-565

[17] Hertel J. Functional anatomy, pathomechanics, and pathophysiology

of lateral ankle instability. Journal of Athletic Training. 2002;**37**(4):364

[18] Manske R, Reiman M. Functional performance testing for power and return to sports. Sports Health. 2013;**5**(3):244-250

[19] Ayeni A, Afolabi E. 2012 teachers' instructional task performance students' learning outcomes in Nigerian secondary schools. International Journal of Research Studies in Educational Technology. 2012;**1**(1):33-42. Available from: http://www.consortiacademia.org/

[20] Higgs J, Jones MA, Loftus S, Christensen N. Clinical Reasoning in the Health Professions E-Book: Clinical Reasoning in the Health Professions E-Book. Missouri: Elsevier Health Sciences; 2008

[21] Mathews KA. Pain assessment and general approach to management. Veterinary Clinics: Small Animal Practice. 2000;**30**(4):729-755

[22] Pinto FCF, Gomes SC, Letichevsky AC. The synthesis of the National High School Exam: Theoretical proposals and outcomes (in Portuguese). O ENEM em sntese: Propostas Tericas e Desdobramentos. Ensaio. 2003;**11**(40):261-281

[23] Klein R, Fontanive N. A new way to evaluate writing skills in high-school composition exams (in Portuguese). Uma nova maneira de avaliar as competłncias escritoras na redao do ENEM. Ensaio. 2009;**17**(65):585-598. Available from: http://www.scielo.br/pdf/ensaio/v17n65/v17n65a2.pdf [Accessed: November 16, 2016]

[24] Physiotherapy-Pediatric. Foot and Ankle Assessment. n.d. Available from: physio-pediatric.co

[25] Hertel J. Functional instability following lateral ankle sprain. Sports Medicine. 2000;**29**:361-371

[26] Ciesla N, Dinglas V, Fan E, Kho M, Kuramoto J, Needham D. Manual muscle testing: A method of measuring extremity muscle strength applied to critically ill patients. Journal of Visualized Experiments: JoVE. 2011;**50**:2632

[27] Conable KM, Rosner AL. A narrative review of manual muscle testing and implications for muscle testing research. Journal of Chiropractic Medicine. 2011;**10**(3):157-165

[28] Bohannon RW. Reliability of manual muscle testing: A systematic review. Isokinetics and Exercise Science. 2018;**26**(4):245-252

[29] Marcori AJ, Monteiro PH, Oliveira JA, Doumas M, Teixeira LA. Single leg balance training: A systematic review. Perceptual and Motor Skills. 2022;**129**(2):232-252

[30] Picot B, Terrier R, Forestier N, Fourchet F, McKeon PO. The star excursion balance test: An update review and practical guidelines. International Journal of Athletic Therapy and Training. 2021;**26**(6):285-293

[31] Santuz A, Ekizos A, Arampatzis A. A pressure plate-based method for the automatic assessment of foot strike patterns during running. Annals of Biomedical Engineering. 2016;**44**:1646-1655

[32] Bolgla LA, Keskula DR. Reliability of lower extremity functional performance tests. Journal of Orthopaedic & Sports Physical Therapy. 1997;**26**(3):138-142

[33] Meadows KA. Patient-reported outcome measures: An overview.

British Journal of Community Nursing. 2011;**16**(3):146-151

[34] Carcia CR, Martin RL, Drouin JM. Validity of the foot and ankle ability measure in athletes with chronic ankle instability. Journal of Athletic Training. 2008;**43**(2):179-183

[35] Lin CWC, Moseley AM, Refshauge KM, Bundy AC. The lower extremity functional scale has good clinimetric properties in people with ankle fracture. Physical Therapy. 2009;**89**(6):580-588

[36] Jenkinson C, Layte R, Jenkinson D, Lawrence K, Petersen S, Paice C, et al. A shorter form health survey: Can the SF-12 replicate results from the SF-36 in longitudinal studies? Journal of Public Health. 1997;**19**(2):179-186

[37] Lightsey HM, Noback PC, Caldwell JME, Trofa DP, Greisberg JK, Vosseller JT. Online physical therapy protocol quality, variability, and availability in Achilles tendon repair. Foot & Ankle Specialist. 2019;**12**(1):16-24

[38] Stark TW. Introduction of a pyramid guiding process for general musculoskeletal physical rehabilitation. Chiropractic & Osteopathy. 2006;**14**:1-6

[39] Steelman PJ, Groth G, Taras JS. Individualized rehabilitation program for flexor tendon repair: From pyramid to algorithm. Operative Techniques in Orthopaedics. 2007;**17**(2):148-154

[40] Fischer DC, Sckell A, Garkisch A, Dresing K, Eisenhauer A, Valentini L, et al. Treatment of perioperative swelling by rest, ice, compression, and elevation (RICE) without and with additional application of negative pressure (RICE+) in patients with a unilateral ankle fracture: Study protocol for a monocentric, evaluator-blinded randomized controlled pilot trial. Pilot and Feasibility Studies. 2021;**7**:1-9

[41] Van Den Bekerom MP, Struijs PA, Blankevoort L, Welling L, Van Dijk CN, Kerkhoffs GM. What is the evidence for rest, ice, compression, and elevation therapy in the treatment of ankle sprains in adults? Journal of Athletic Training. 2012;**47**(4):435-443

[42] Moseley AM, Beckenkamp PR, Haas M, Herbert RD, Lin CWC, EXACT Team. Rehabilitation after immobilization for ankle fracture: The EXACT randomized clinical trial. JAMA. 2015;**314**(13):1376-1385

[43] Pfile KR, Gribble PA, Buskirk GE, Meserth SM, Pietrosimone BG. Sustained improvements in dynamic balance and landing mechanics after a 6-week neuromuscular training program in college women's basketball players. Journal of Sport Rehabilitation. 2016;**25**(3):233-240

[44] Hupperets MD, Verhagen EA, Van Mechelen W. Effect of unsupervised home based proprioceptive training on recurrences of ankle sprain: Randomised controlled trial. BMJ. 2009;**339**:1-6

[45] McKeon PO, Hertel J. Systematic review of postural control and lateral ankle instability, part I: Can deficits be detected with instrumented testing? Journal of Athletic Training. 2008;**43**(3):293-304

[46] Rosen A, Swanik C, Thomas S, Glutting J, Knight C, Kaminski TW. Differences in lateral drop jumps from an unknown height among individuals with functional ankle instability. Journal of Athletic Training. 2013;**48**(6):773-781

[47] Eils E, Schroeter R, Schröder M, Gerss J, Rosenbaum D. Multistation proprioceptive exercise program

prevents ankle injuries in basketball. Medicine & Science in Sports & Exercise. 2010;**42**(11):2098-2105

[48] Rivera MJ, Winkelmann ZK, Powden CJ, Games KE. Proprioceptive training for the prevention of ankle sprains: An evidence-based review. Journal of Athletic Training. 2017;**52**(11):1065-1067

[49] Kwon YJ, Park SJ, Jefferson J, Kim K. The effect of open and closed kinetic chain exercises on dynamic balance ability of normal healthy adults. Journal of Physical Therapy Science. 2013;**25**(6):671-674

[50] Hertel J, Braham RA, Hale SA, Olmsted-Kramer LC. Simplifying the star excursion balance test: Analyses of subjects with and without chronic ankle instability. Journal of Orthopaedic & Sports Physical Therapy. 2006;**36**(3):131-137

[51] Sykes K. Electromyographic feedback and neuromuscular education. British Journal of Sports Medicine. 1975;**9**(4):175

[52] Wagemans J, Bleakley C, Taeymans J, Schurz AP, Kuppens K, Baur H, et al. Exercise-based rehabilitation reduces reinjury following acute lateral ankle sprain: A systematic review update with meta-analysis. PLoS One. 2022;**17**(2):e0262023

[53] Calixtre LB, Moreira RFC, Franchini GH, Alburquerque-Sendín F, Oliveira AB. Manual therapy for the management of pain and limited range of motion in subjects with signs and symptoms of temporomandibular disorder: A systematic review of randomised controlled trials. Journal of Oral Rehabilitation. 2015;**42**(11):847-861

[54] Weerasekara I, Osmotherly P, Snodgrass S, Marquez J, de Zoete R, Rivett DA. Clinical benefits of joint mobilization on ankle sprains: A systematic review and meta-analysis. Archives of Physical Medicine and Rehabilitation. 2018;**99**(7):1395-1412

[55] Anwer S, Alghadir A. Effect of isometric quadriceps exercise on muscle strength, pain, and function in patients with knee osteoarthritis: A randomized controlled study. Journal of Physical Therapy Science. 2014;**26**(5):745-748

[56] Widodo AF, Tien CW, Chen CW, Lai SC. Isotonic and isometric exercise interventions improve the hamstring muscles' strength and flexibility: A narrative review. In: Healthcare. Vol. 10, No. 5. Basel, Switzerland: MDPI; April 2022. p. 811

[57] Keles SB, Sekir U, Gur H, Akova B. Eccentric/concentric training of ankle evertor and dorsiflexors in recreational athletes: Muscle latency and strength. Scandinavian Journal of Medicine & Science in Sports. 2014;**24**(1):e29-e38

[58] Flore Z, Hambly K, De Coninck K, Welsch G. A rehabilitation algorithm after lateral ankle sprains in professional football (soccer): An approach based on clinical practice guidelines. International Journal of Sports Physical Therapy. 2024;**19**(7):910

[59] Kemler E, van de Port I, Backx F, van Dijk CN. A systematic review on the treatment of acute ankle sprain: Brace versus other functional treatment types. Sports Medicine. 2011;**41**:185-197

[60] Jay H, Corbett RO. An updated model of chronic ankle instability. Journal of Athletic Training (Allen Press). 2019;**54**(6):572-588

[61] Pfeifer CG, Grechenig S, Frankewycz B, Ernstberger A, Nerlich M, Krutsch W. Analysis of 213 currently

used rehabilitation protocols in foot and ankle fractures. Injury. 2015;**46**:S51-S57

[62] Black JDJ, Bhavikatti M, Al-Hadithy N, Hakmi A, Kitson J. Early weight-bearing in operatively fixed ankle fractures: A systematic review. The Foot. 2013;**23**(2-3):78-85

[63] Gould HP, Bano JM, Akman JL, Fillar AL. Postoperative rehabilitation following Achilles tendon repair: A systematic review. Sports Medicine and Arthroscopy Review. 2021;**29**(2):130-145

[64] Strom AC, Casillas MM. Achilles tendon rehabilitation. Foot and Ankle Clinics. 2009;**14**(4):773-782

[65] Alfredson H, Pietilä T, Jonsson P, Lorentzon R. Heavy-load eccentric calf muscle training for the treatment of chronic Achilles tendinosis. The American Journal of Sports Medicine. 1998;**26**(3):360-366

[66] Tarantino D, Palermi S, Sirico F, Corrado B. Achilles tendon rupture: Mechanisms of injury, principles of rehabilitation and return to play. Journal of Functional Morphology and Kinesiology. 2020;**5**(4):95

Chapter 2

Achilles Tendon Tears Treated with L.A.R.S. Augmentation

Luigi Corso, Giovanni Frezza and Chiara Cicuto

Abstract

The Achilles tendon ruptures management with synthetic augments remains controversial due to potential complications. Primary repair with Ligament Augmentation and Reconstruction System (LARS) offers a reliable technique for repair: it eliminates the need for graft harvesting, reduces the re-rupture rate, and complications related to immobilization. It is possible to associate the LARS technique with minimally invasive surgery, reducing problems related to wound management. LARS is an effective choice in acute trauma, even in young patients; combined with an early rehabilitation program, it improves functional outcomes.

Keywords: Achilles tendon rupture, L.A.R.S. and LARS, tendon reconstruction, biocompatibility, synthetic graft

1. Introduction

Achilles tendon partial or complete tears may be caused by a direct or indirect trauma or may occur without an acute trauma, as the result of a chronic degenerative process.

Usually, in a complete rupture, the patient feels severe pain, frequently described as a sensation of having been kicked in the tendon, with immediate functional impotence in plantar flexion unable to walk without support. In partial rupture, the clinical picture may be similar, but usually, the pain is less localized, and the ability to flex the plantar may remain. It is very important not to underestimate these lesions, which can rapidly evolve if not adequately treated.

First of all, it is necessary to have a clinical framing of tendon injuries, with the distinction between chronic and acute lesions.

Achilles tendon degeneration symptoms are not uncommon, and ruptures that occur without trauma are a sign of degeneration. This symptoms often manifest themselves much earlier than observed under surgery.

In everyday clinical and surgical practice, in the discussion of the reconstruction technique, a common factor emerges: the Achilles tendon is subjected to degenerative phenomena even in young patients, and its rupture, as well as its repair, must be studied and carried out taking into account the ruptured tissue quality.

Achilles tendon rupture is a clinical diagnosis. In the objective examination, it is necessary to perform a Thompson test and appreciate by palpation, a clear depression in tendon, interruption, or thinning of the size of the tendon fibers.

Tendon tissue should be studied with an echographic exam in case of doubt in partial lesion or to check residual tendon quality.

Tendon quality must be tested at the beginning of the surgical operation. All good-quality tissue will be utilized in the reconstruction and must guarantee performance during the physiotherapy rehabilitation program, as well as in the gradual return to sports activities and everyday life.

2. Choice of surgical technique

Different surgical techniques to repair the Achilles tendon are still being discussed, and even conservative methods are considered and often used.

In the decision-making process, it is mandatory to analyze different genesis of tendon injuries, the patient's immediate and remote medical history, age, quality of life before trauma and, mostly, different functional request [1]. Every choice must be designed on patient's needs, let us imagine this process like the creation of a tailor-made suit.

In **Table 1**, two authors, Myerson and Kuwada, classified Achilles tendon lesions and showed how the severity is essentially linked to the size of the tendon loss and retraction: at any increasing gap created by the injury, there corresponds an increasing complexity of surgical tendon repair [2, 3].

As mentioned above, determining the type of injury, acute or chronic, has to be the first step.

Ligament augmentation and reconstruction system L.A.R.S. (**Figure 1**) is well-known among knee surgery specialists owing to its consolidated use in anterior cruciate ligament reconstruction [4–7] but is also often used in chronic Achilles tendon injuries.

Undoubtedly, LARS reconstructions have proven fundamental importance to repair inveterate injuries, re-ruptures, or to revise previously operated tendons [8].

Grade	Gap	Surgery
Myerson		
I	Gap <2 cm	End-to-end anastomosis and posterior compartment fasciotomy
II	Gap 2–5 cm	V-Y plasty augmented with tendon transfer if needed
III	Gap >5 cm	Tendon transfer alone or in combination with V-Y plasty (advancement or turndown)
Kuwada		
I	Partial rupture	Nonoperative treatment
II	Complete rupture Gap <3 cm	End-to-end tenorrhaphy
III	Gap 3–6 cm	Biological graft +/− augmentation with artificial graft
IV	Gap >6 cm	Gastrocnemius recession, biological/artificial graft

Table 1.
Myerson classification and Kuwada classification of Achilles tendon rupture [2, 3].

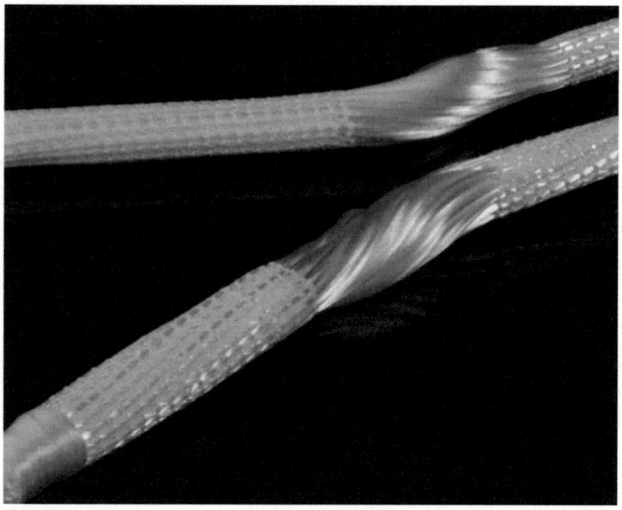

Figure 1.
L.A.R.S. ligament augmentation and reconstruction system.

Although the LARS technique used in chronic lesions is the most widely documented in the literature, some types of acute injuries may need LARS treatment as well. Acute rupture often involves a degenerated tendon, poor in fiber quality, associated with a degenerated peritenon, which makes it difficult to obtain a good direct reconstruction.

Acute trauma should also cause a severe tendon loss, which hesitates in an important tendon shortening if end-to-end sutures are used. In all these acute lesions it is difficult to obtain a valid end-to-end tenorrhaphy also with the use of V-Y plasty, tendon reinforcement (e.g., Chigot-Ganier technique) or reconstructions with flaps (e.g., Bosworth technique) [8–12].

Table 2 lists briefly different methods to perform reinforcement, advancement, plasty, local tendon transfer, or free tissue transfer (AUTOGRAFT – ALLOGRAFT—XEONOGRAFT). All these techniques help the functional tendon reconstruction in cases of lack of tissue [13, 14].

We also have to mention the development of percutaneous and minimally invasive suture techniques: Ma & Griffiths, Webb & Bannister, Carmont & Maffulli, Assal & Achillon, and the Tenolig prosthesis [10, 15, 16]. Percutaneous procedures have the advantage of respecting the skin layer, already affected by trauma, avoiding local skin and subcutaneous complications. This results in a lower risk of scar dehiscence and local infections. Furthermore, percutaneous and minimally invasive procedures have a greater respect for the site of rupture, which, similarly to fractures, is not directly exposed to the surgical insult. On the other hand, the lack of exposure of the rupture site does not allow for the evaluation of the state of the tendon stumps, their vitality, the quality of the peritenon, and its integrity. This may result in a failure of tenorrhaphy.

In the most recent years, Achilles tendon reconstruction has given new solutions to the problems that have been discussed so far [17]. Artificial ligaments seem to represent a suitable option to reinforce injured tendons as well as to obtain fast functional recovery.

Moreover, artificial ligaments should represent a sort of scaffold for biological regeneration. Follow-up through *in vivo* histological study shows within the structure of the implanted LARS, a new fibrovascular growth but also chronic inflammatory factors presence. The entity of its regeneration potential is still a matter of debate [18, 19].

Flaps reversed/advancement/reinforcement
• V–Y advancement flap (Abraham, Pankovich)
• Proximal reversed flap (Bosworth)
• Plantar gracilis tendon reinforcement (Chigot-Garnier)
Tendon transfer
• Peroneus brevis tendon (Teuffer, Turco, Spinella)
• Flexor longus hallucis tendon (Wapner)
Free tissue transfer (AUTOGRAFT, ALLOGRAFT, XENOGRAFT)
• Fascia lata (Bugg, Boyd)
• Gracilis tendon (Maffulli)
• Semitendinousus tendon (Sarzaeem)
• Extracellular Matrix Xenograft (e.g., xenogenic collagen matrix)
• Growth factor addiction: Platelet-rich plasma (PRP), lipoaspirated adipose tissue (e.g., Lipogems)
Percutaneous and Minimally invasive suture techniques
• Ma & Griffiths
• Webb & Bannister
• Carmont & Maffulli
• Assal & Achillon
• Tenolig prosthesis
• PARS Achilles jig system
Artificial ligaments
• Poli-tape
• LARS
• Dacron patch
• Marlex mesh
• Carbon-fiber implants

Table 2.
Achilles tendon salvage procedures.

3. Ligament advanced reinforcement system (L.A.R.S.)

The Ligament Augmentation and Reconstruction System or Ligament Advanced Reinforcement System (L.A.R.S.) is made of a nonabsorbable polyethylene terephthalate (PET), treated with a technology meant to reduce reactive phlogosis and keep a high resistance capacity under traction [4, 18, 20].

LARS ligaments can withstand forces between 2700 N and 5000 N.

Previous synthetic ligaments have faced a high incidence of synovitis and chronic inflammation due to wear and cyclic stress, which causes a release of pro-inflammatory microparticles [21].

LARS for Achilles tendon reconstruction consists of three sections:

- Muscular-tendon joint section (inverse warp knitted fibers in flat section)

- Intra-tendinous section (free longitudinal fibers in a circular section)
- Intra-osseous section (inverse warp knitted fibers in a circular section)

From the histologic point of view, free orientation of the longitudinal fibers and its porosity facilitate the adherence and ingrowth of osteoblasts, fibroblasts and tenocytes. These features promote better resistance to fatigue during flexion and extension. Newly formed collagen gradually overtake the synthetic ligament, improving biocompatibility [21].

LARS has historically been a surgical strategy in chronic injuries as re-ruptures, treatment of previously operated Achilles tendons, and inveterate injuries with stumps diastasis.

Examining acute injury, it is common to observe degenerated tissue, which is the real cause of the rupture. Tendon tissue deficit higher than 3 cm is commonly considered a risk factor for re-ruptures according to the classification of Kuwada (**Table 1**).

LARS ligament repair of acute Achilles tendon ruptures provides a reliable and effective technique for repair, with survivorship data to more than 10 years. It eliminates the need for graft harvesting, decreases postoperative complications, but most importantly, patients have improved functional outcomes. Also, patients with acute bilateral tendon ruptures treated with LARS benefit from shorter recovery time and rehabilitation time compared to patients treated with traditional surgery [22].

As we will learn in the next paragraph, this surgical technique involves an anchorage of the artificial ligament at the level of myotendinous junction. If this area appears to be injured and compromised, LARS is absolutely contraindicated.

4. L.A.R.S. Surgical technique

Prior to LARS implant and tendon repair, the Achilles tendon has to be examined through the usual access technique for injury assessment. We usually perform a postero-medial approach, with minimal medial deviation from the midline to preserve the sural nerve (**Figure 2**).

Although experienced orthopedic surgeons can easily learn the LARS technique, it is recommended to initially perform some implants with the open technique and later, to use LARS with minimally invasive technique. The minimally invasive technique requires three mini-incisions form proximal to distal: at the myotendinous junction, the Achilles tendon rupture site and its distal calcaneal insertion.

First of all, it is essential to identify and preserve the peritenon at the rupture site, then it is necessary to prepare the tendon stumps by removing the nonviable tissue (**Figure 3**).

After tendon injury evaluation, the middle part of the myotendinous junction must be identified. The key point to avoid failure is a good proximal LARS fixation.

A longitudinal incision of less than 1 cm is made in the median part of the myotendinous junction. Through a special curved tube, the artificial graft, appropriately oriented, is inserted inside the proximal tendon. In this way, the LARS is positioned in the central part of the tendon, completely covered by the proximal stump (**Figure 4**). We would like to underline that it is also really important for the LARS to maintain its central position, where free tendon fibers are present at the injury level.

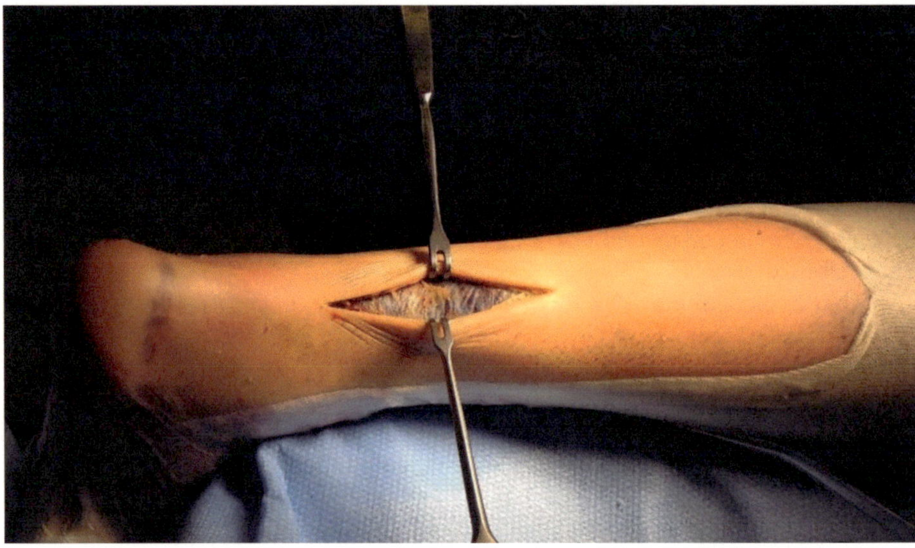

Figure 2.
Postero-medial approach: minimal medial deviation to respect sural nerve.

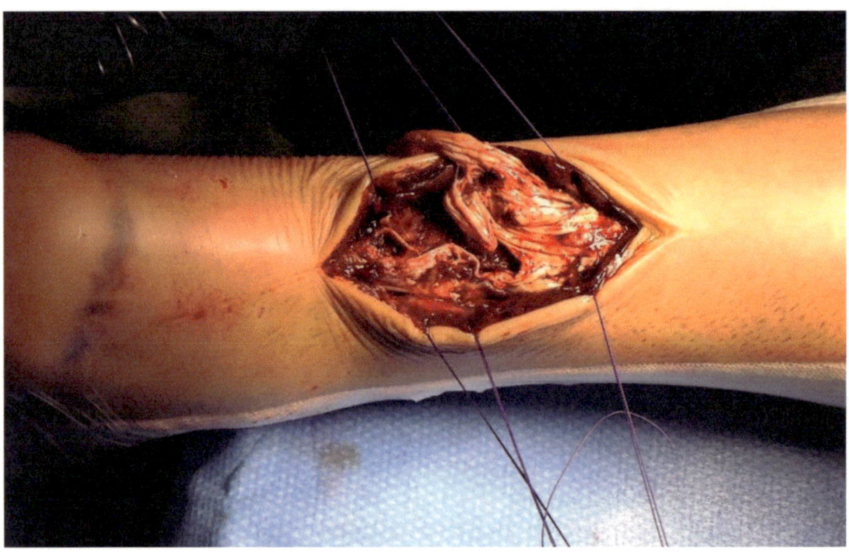

Figure 3.
Debridement and cleaning of tendon rupture site, the distal tendon stump is poorly represented.

The flat proximal LARS portion is sutured at the myotendinous level. We use absorbable sutures in polyglactin (continues Lembert sutures and Lock-stitch sutures). Secondly, the myotendinous tissue is sutured to cover the LARS (**Figure 5**).

It is of primary importance to cover the entire proximal LARS with myotendinous tissue to avoid microtraumas or friction of the LARS on the overlying layers. This allows the prevention secondary inflammation of the fascia, subcutaneous tissue and skin.

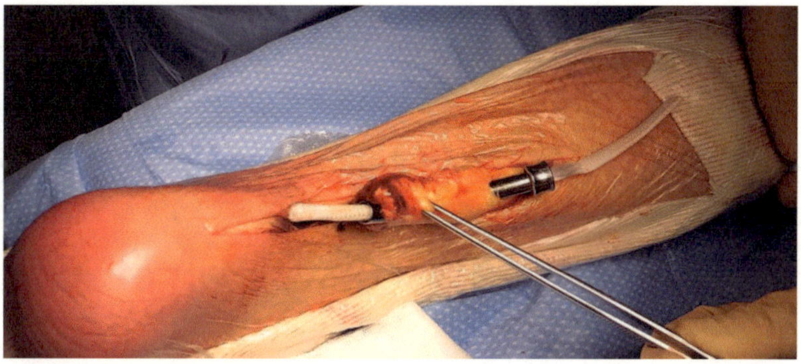

Figure 4.
Proximal insertion of the LARS at the myotendinous junction.

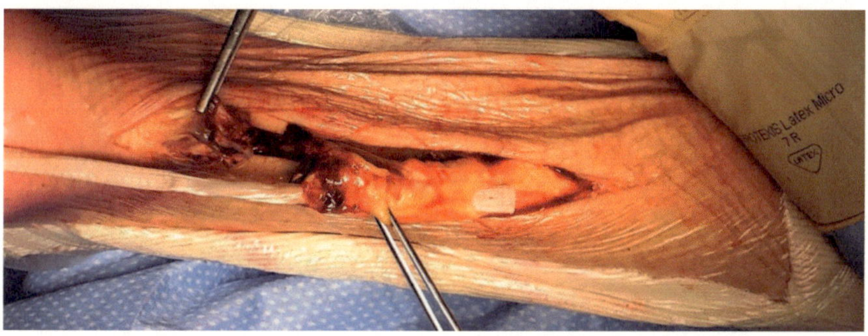

Figure 5.
Myotendinous junction covers proximal LARS insertion.

The next step is to prepare the distal end for LARS implantation.

We identify and prepare the postero-superior calcaneal tuberosity, respecting the periosteum, the distal stump, and the distal insertion of the Achilles tendon. Using a dedicated Kirschner wire with a proximal metal loop, we determine an angle of approximately 50°. This is the angulation that we want to give to the insertion of the LARS at the calcaneal level. The K-wire passing through the calcaneal bone perforates the heel plantarly (**Figure 6**).

We verify the correct positioning of the K-wire by intraoperative x-ray. Then, using this wire, the preparation of the half-tunnel is performed with an appropriate reamer (**Figure 7**).

The distal cylindrical LARS portion is prepared with two non-absorbable high resistance threads, which are passed inside the K-wire proximal hole, then the K-wire is extracted plantarly by means of a motorized drill. In this way, LARS is guided inside the distal tunnel. By pulling the threads that come out of the heel skin, it is possible to decide the correct tension to give to the LARS. It is suggested to position it and then fix it with the foot in slight equinus (max 20°). Intraoperatively, we perform the first tests with equinus/pronation stress, dorsal-plantar flexion of the foot, and comparison with the contralateral tendon to verify the correct rate of tendon tension and the good seal of the proximal LARS sutures.

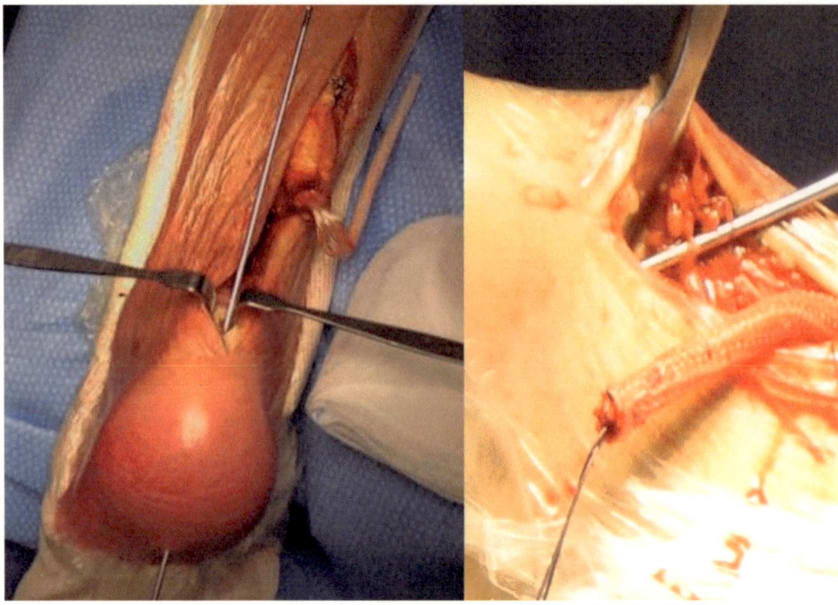

Figure 6.
K-wire insertion through calcaneal bone (posterior and medial observation point).

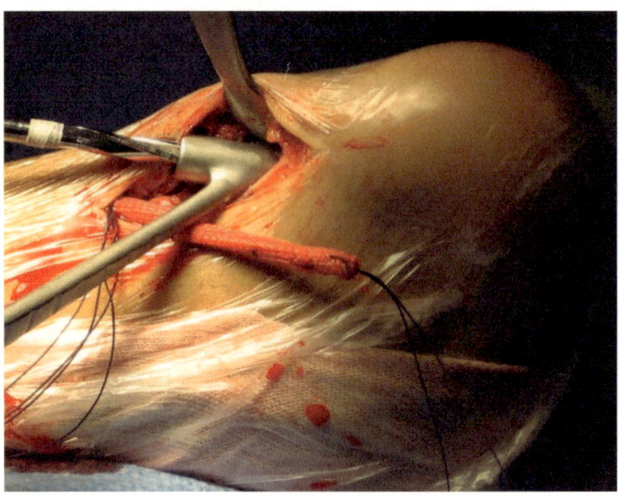

Figure 7.
Half-tunnel reaming.

Maintaining the chosen position of the tendon and foot, an interference screw distally locks the LARS implant. We verify the correct positioning of the screw by intraoperative x-ray (**Figure 8**).

In the end, the threads that emerge from the heel are cut close to the skin with light pressure, so that after cutting, the threads migrate under the subcutaneous tissue and do not create discomfort during load on the heel. Recently, to minimize this possibility, we replaced the high resistance non-re-absorbable threads with re-absorbable threads in polyglactin to prepare the distal LARS.

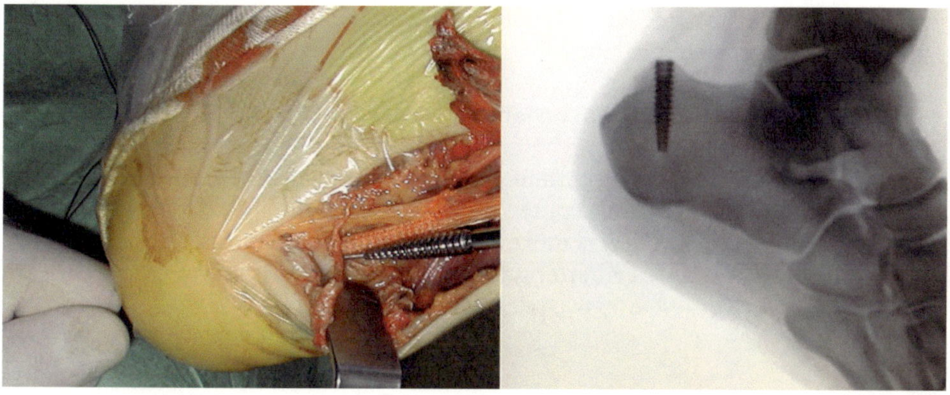

Figure 8.
Interference screw positioning and x-ray intraoperative control.

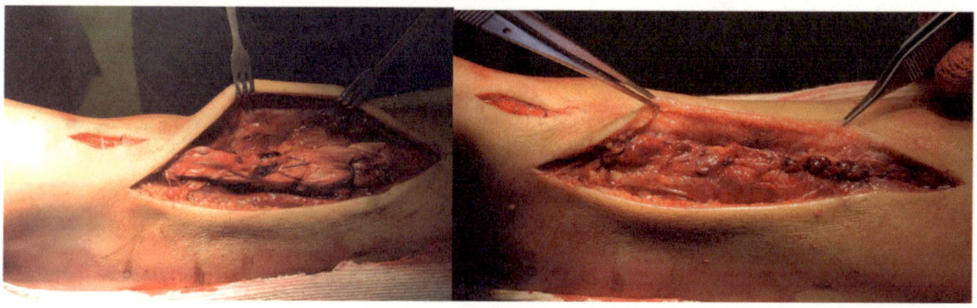

Figure 9.
Tendon stumps sutures (right) and peritenon suture (left). Distal median mini-incision for K-wire positioning is visible.

Last, but not least, at the site of the tendon lesion we perform, where possible, a Krachow suture or an end-to-end suture of the residual tendon fibers to cover the LARS and maximize the biological recovery capacity of the tendon. For this reason, it is also really important to carefully suture the peritenon, where is possible.

Finally, surgical access is carefully sutured (**Figure 9**).

5. Postoperative program

Postoperative treatment in our team has reached the best performance with the following indications:

- Weekly wound dressing in orthopedic clinic for 3 weeks (until sutures are removed)
- First and second week: 90° ankle walker boot (even during night) without load
- Third and fourth week: Start rehabilitation with removal of the Walker Boot for 20 minutes, 4 times a day for active mobilization without load; removal of the Walker boot during night

- Fifth week: Start of free load (depending on pain), if necessary for the patient, with the initial use of crutches

- From the sixth week: Gradual restart of sports activity

Technically, LARS allows the patient to walk from the first postoperative day [22], but we believe that a better result comes from the association of LARS and biological response. The second one requires more time, so our strategy promotes both repair approaches. We also obtained a better management of the surgical wound with weekly dressing performed only by specialized personnel.

6. Discussion

Rupture of the Achilles tendon is a considerable cause of morbidity, with an incidence of 18 per 100,000, and has been shown to be increasing [10].

In the literature, regardless of treatment, is reported that major functional deficits persist 2 years after acute Achilles tendon rupture and only 50–60% of elite sportsmen return to pre-injury levels following rupture [17, 18, 23].

Meta-analyses have shown that nonoperative management has an increased risk of re-rupture. Nonoperative risk of re-rupture 40% versus operative risk 5%. Surgical intervention has risks of complications related to the wound and iatrogenic nerve injury.

Minimally invasive surgery has been adopted to reduce these complications, and it seems to be particularly effective on superficial and deep wound infection rates. **Table 3** shows the major surgical complications [10, 24–30].

The authors' group treated with LARS 200 patients in 17 years (from 01/01/2008 to 01/03/2025). The age of patients who present this kind of lesion is increasing [25]. In their study group, the average age is 57 years range 31–79, with different comorbidities and functional requests. In this heterogeneity, the choice of treatment decided by the surgeon is fundamental. It is based not only on the biological age but also on the

Surgical complications reported in literature	**Percentage (%)**
Foreign body rejection	Rare, no percentage available
Wound recovery delay—dehiscence	6
Superficial wound infection	4
Deep wound infection	1.8
Low tolerance of the calcaneal screw (LARS system)	0.3
Calcaneal algodistrofia	0.2
Re-rupture	2
Nerve and vascular injuries	3.4
Chronic calcaneal and ankle pain	3.8
Achilles Tendon stiffness	7
Deep vein thrombosis	0.2

Table 3.
Surgical complications in Achilles tendon primary reconstruction.

functional requests of the patient and on the real repair potential without augmentations, which is often evident only in the operating room.

In their experience, treatment of Achilles tendon with LARS delivers good clinical results, with very low surgical complication rates in chronic and acute injuries. Calcaneal screw removal due to intolerance (0.5%), proximal re-rupture (1%), local superficial infection (3%), and wounds recovery delay (4%). In the LARS technique, re-ruptures usually are due to failure of the proximal suture LARS-myotendinous junction.

Other studies have reported that reconstruction with LARS decreases postoperative complications, but most importantly, patients have improved functional outcomes [22, 31].

All the outcomes were significantly correlated with patient global satisfaction.

The American Orthopedic Foot Ankle Society (AOFAS) scores were satisfactory in their patient group, with an average score of 85/100, but Achilles-tendon-specific problems, such as decreased jumping ability and muscle atrophy, have not been taken into consideration in the AOFAS score. This score seems not to be so reliable in athletes [32]. In young patients, acute Achilles tendon ruptures mainly occur in sports like soccer and basketball, which are popular sports in Italy. The goal of treatment is a return to play at the pre-injury level.

The authors interviewed the group of patients treated with LARS reconstruction who practiced sport at a precompetitive and competitive level (n = 12) and eight of them stated they returned to play at the same level as before surgery, in an average time of 7 months after injury. Rehabilitation plays a key role in this type of patients; the other four patients reduce sport activity to a non-competitive level [33]. Reconstruction with the LARS technique seems to have better results compared to most of the other techniques for this specific kind of patient. The recovery of functional capacity could be explained by that the augmented repair was stable enough to allow an accelerated functional rehabilitation protocol with early weight-bearing and range of motion.

All other patients in the study, with lower functional requests (n = 188), returned to work or to their level of activity before injury at an average of 20 weeks.

Low re-rupture rate is a prerequisite for any reliable surgical technique. In the authors' study re-rupture rate of the Achilles tendon with LARS augment was less than 2%. Although good clinical results have been reported with other techniques, long-lasting functional deficits such as reduced plantar flexion strength, increased tendon stiffness, and sural nerve deficit may occur. None of the complications just mentioned occurred in the authors' study.

Wound irritation and superficial wound infections are common complications after tendon reconstruction if LARS is anchored too superficially in the proximal part and does not entirely cover by myotendinous junction.

These data are comparable to the complication rate of most reviews about minimally invasive and percutaneous reconstruction techniques [10, 27].

There are few reports of the use of various synthetic materials to augment the repair of acute AT rupture, such as Dacron vascular graft, Polypropylene (PP) braid, and polyethylene mesh. The biomechanical advantages of synthetic graft augmentation have been demonstrated in laboratory studies, including decreasing gapping and increasing repair construct stiffness and ultimate failure load [23].

Based on the authors' experience, no difference was found in the timing of surgery in acute trauma. Patients operated after 5 days had the same outcomes as those who underwent immediate surgery within the first 48 hours of trauma. In timing decision, the evaluation of trauma-related skin swelling and tension is fundamental.

Finally, we can state that primary repair with Ligament Augmentation and Reconstruction System (LARS) provides a reliable technique, even in young patients with high functional demands. It eliminates the need for graft harvesting and reduces complications such as re-rupture and those related to immobilization. After acquiring good practice with LARS implants in open surgery (we suggest at least 10 interventions), it is possible to associate the LARS technique with minimally invasive surgery (3 mini-incisions, as previously described), thus also reducing complications related to wound management. The LARS technique, combined with an early rehabilitation program, improves functional outcomes.

Conflict of interest

The authors declare no conflict of interest.

Author details

Luigi Corso[1*], Giovanni Frezza[2] and Chiara Cicuto[3]

1 Santa Maria degli Angeli Hospital, Head of Orthopedic and Traumatology, Pordenone, Italy

2 Santa Maria della Misericordia Hospital, Udine, Italy

3 Maria degli Angeli Hospital, Pordenone, Italy

*Address all correspondence to: luigi.corso@asfo.sanita.fvg.it

References

[1] Atkinson TS, Easley M. The expert opinion: Complete ruptures of the Achilles tendon. Medscape Orthopedics. 2001;**5**(3)

[2] Kuwada GT. Critical analysis of tendo Achillis repair using Achilles tendon rupture classification system and repair. The Journal of Foot and Ankle Surgery. 1993;**32**(6):611-616

[3] Myerson MS. Achilles tendon Ruptures. Instructional Course Lectures. 1999;**48**:219-230

[4] Ebert J, Annear P. ACL reconstruction using autologous hamstrings augmented with the ligament augmentation and reconstruction system. Orthopaedic Journal of Sports Medicine. 2019;7(10):2325967119879079. DOI: 10.1177/2325967119879079

[5] Newman SDS, Atkinson HDE, Willis-Owen CA. Anterior cruciate ligament reconstruction with the ligament augmentation and reconstruction system: A systematic review. International Orthopaedics. 2013;**37**:321-326

[6] Chen S, Chen T, Wan F, Jiang J, Feller JA. Synthetic ligaments for ACL reconstruction. In: Controversies in the Technical Aspects of ACL Reconstruction: An Evidence-Based Medicine Approach. Berlin Heidelberg: Springer; 2017. pp. 333-341

[7] Gliatis J, Anagnostou K, Tsoumpos P, Billis E, Papandreou M, Plessas S. Complex knee injuries treated in acute phase: Long-term results using ligament augmentation and reconstruction system artificial ligament. World Journal of Orthopedics. 2018;**9**(3):24-34

[8] Ibrahim S. Surgical treatment of chronic Achilles tendon rupture. The Journal of Foot & Ankle Surgery. 2009;**48**(3):340-346. DOI: 10.1053/j.jfas.2009.02.007

[9] LARS ligament. Available from: https://www.coringroup.com/legacy/medical_professionals/products/lars_ligaments/overview/index.html.

[10] Carmont M, Rossi R, Scheffler S, Mei-Dan O, Beaufils P. Percutaneous & Mini Invasive Achilles tendon repair. Sports Medicine, Arthroscopy, Rehabilitation, Therapy & Technology: SMARTT. 2011;**3**(28). DOI: 10.1186/1758-2555-3-28

[11] Bosworth DM. Repair of defects in the tendon Achillis. Journal of Bone and Joint Surgery. 1956;**38**:111-114

[12] Chigot P, Garnier C, Cloutier M. Contribution à étude anatomo-patologique et on traitement chirurgical des ruptures sions-cutanèes du tendon d'Achille. Review Orthopedic. 1952;**38**:513

[13] Bussewitz BW. Repair of neglected Achilles rupture. Clinics in Podiatric Medicine and Surgery. 2017;**34**(2):263-274. DOI: 10.1016/j.cpm.2016.10.012

[14] Magnussen RA, Glisson RR, Moorman CT. Augmentation of Achilles tendon repair with extracellular matrix Xenograft a biomechanical analysis. The American Journal of Sports Medicine. 2011;**39**(7):1522-1527. DOI: 10.1177/0363546510397815

[15] PARS Achilles Jig System. Available from: https://www.gemes.it/pars-achilles-jig-system/.

[16] Magnan B, Samaila E, Merlini M, Bartolozzi P. Minimally invasive

repair of acute tear of Achilles tendon. Three different options. G.I.O.T. 2010;**36**:125-130

[17] Olsson N, Nilsson-Helander K, Karlsson J, Eriksson BI, Thomee R, Faxen E, et al. Major functional deficits persist 2 years after acute Achilles tendon rupture. Knee Surgery, Sports Traumatology, Arthroscopy. 2011;**19**:1385-1393

[18] Arya N, Sasun A, Burile G, et al. From trauma to recovery: A Comprehensive Management of Achilles Tendon Injury in a young female. Cureus. 2024;**16**(1):e52286. DOI: 10.7759/cureus.52286

[19] Di Benedetto P, Giardini P, Causero A. Histological analysis of ACL reconstruction failures due to synthetic-ACL (LARS) ruptures. Acta Biomed. 2020;**91**(4S):136-145. DOI: 10.23750/abm.v91i4-S.9702

[20] Corin Group. LARS TM ACL. Corin P; 2010. Available from: https://www.coringroup.com/assets/product-resources/LARS/Resources-Product-Literature-LARS-ACL-Your-Questions-Answered.pdf [Accessed: September 12, 2020]

[21] Mao Z, Fan B, Wang X, et al. A systematic review of tissue engineering scaffold in tendon bone healing in vivo. Frontiers in Bioengineering and Biotechnology. 2021;**9**:621483. DOI: 10.3389/fbioe.2021.621483

[22] Soo C, Mungovan S, Kwa A. Lars ligament repair of acute tendon Achilles rupture. Orthopaedic Proceedings. 2012;**94**(B-XLI):95-95

[23] Haroun HK, Elrahman AAA, Morsi A. Synthetic graft augmentation is safe and effective for the repair of acute achilles tendon rupture in patients with preexisting tendinopathy. Arthroscopy, Sports Medicine, and Rehabilitation. 2022;**14**(6):2079-2087. DOI: 10.1016/j.asmr.2022.10.001

[24] Bullock M, Pierson Z. Achilles Tendon rupture. Clinics in Podiatric Medicine and Surgery. 2024;**41**(3):535-549

[25] Nilsson-Helander K, Silbernagel KG, Thomee R, Faxen E, Olsson N, Eriksson BI, et al. Acute Achilles tendon rupture: A randomized controlled study comparing surgical and non surgical treatments using validated outcome measure. The American Journal of Sports Medicine. 2010;**38**:2186-9315

[26] Pean CA, William CA, Rubenstein J, Konda SR, Egol KA. Risk factors for complications after primary repair of Achilles tendon ruptures. Journal of Orthopaedics. 2018;**15**(1):226-229. DOI: 10.1016/j.jor.2018.01.017

[27] Attia AK, Mahmoud K, D'Hooghe P, Bariteau J, Labib SA, Myerson SM. Outcomes and complications of open versus minimally invasive repair of acute Achilles tendon ruptures: A systematic review and meta-analysis of randomized controlled trials. The American Journal of Sports Medicine. 2023;**51**(3):825-836. DOI: 10.1177/03635465211053619

[28] Fitzpatrick N, Balakrishnan T, Pillai A. Foreign body reaction following Achilles tendon reconstruction with the ligament advanced reconstructive system: Patient outcomes and clinical course. Cureus. 2023;**15**(11). DOI: 10.7759/cureus.48686

[29] Niazi N, Aljawadi A, Khan M, et al. Foreign body reaction with granuloma 10 years after Achilles tendon reconstruction with the Lars ligament. International Journal of Regenerative Medicine. 2022;**4**(2):2-3

[30] Maffulli N, Via AG, Oliva F. Chronic Achilles tendon rupture. The Open Orthopaedics Journal. 2017;**11**:660-669. DOI: 10.2174/1874325001711010660

[31] Feibel J, Bernacki B. A review of salvage procedures after failed Achilles tendon repair. Foot and Ankle Clinics. 2003;**8**(1):105-114

[32] Paget LDA, Sierevelt IN, Tol JL, Kerkhoffs GMMJ, Reurink G. The completely patient-reported version of the American Orthopaedic Foot and Ankle Society (AOFAS) score: A valid and reliable measurement for ankle osteoarthritis. Journal of ISAKOS. 2023;**8**(5):345-351

[33] Christensen M, Zellers JA, Kjær IL, Silbernagel KG, Rathleff MS. Resistance exercises in early functional rehabilitation for Achilles tendon ruptures are poorly described: A scoping review. Journal of Orthopaedic & Sports Physical Therapy. 2020;**50**(12):681-690

Chapter 3

Ankle Fractures in Diabetes Mellitus: A Narrative Review of Pathophysiology, Management, and Complications

Sedeek M. Mosaid, Ahmed Khalil, Khaled Elawady, Munier Hossain and Nijil Vasukutty

Abstract

The combination of neuropathy, vasculopathy, and impaired bone repair makes ankle fractures in people with diabetes mellitus a serious clinical concern. Complications, including infection, nonunion, Charcot neuroarthropathy, and even amputation, are more likely to occur in these individuals. This chapter analyses the biochemical and physiological impacts of diabetes on bone health and recovery, reviews specific assessment and evaluation methods for affected patients, and delineates both nonsurgical and surgical treatment alternatives. This study evaluates various surgical techniques, including standard, trans-syndesmotic, transarticular, hybrid fixation, and primary arthrodesis, within the framework of diabetic conditions. The significance of selecting a suitable fixation technique, evaluating vascular health, and utilising a multidisciplinary approach is highlighted. In addition, this chapter discusses complications such as Charcot arthropathy, fixation failure, and infection. The objective is to provide orthopaedic surgeons and clinicians with a practical, evidence-based guide for the effective management of diabetic ankle fractures.

Keywords: diabetic ankle fractures, diabetes mellitus, peripheral neuropathy, surgical management, pathophysiology, complications

1. Introduction

Ankle fractures are a common type of orthopaedic injury, and the incidence is increasing in the elderly population due to increased life expectancy [1].

Diabetic patients make up about 12% of all ankle fracture cases, and management of this group is of interest due to complications and cost to overall healthcare. Diabetes mellitus is a chronic metabolic disorder characterised by hyperglycaemia, either due to the pancreas's inability to produce enough insulin due to autoimmune causes (type 1) or the body's acquired resistance to insulin (type 2) [2].

Diabetes is associated with an increased risk of fractures and bone health; fragility fractures affect different age groups depending on the type of diabetes, disease duration and presence of other comorbidities. Many of these patients also have other comorbidities like peripheral vascular disease and diabetic neuropathy, which adds to the challenge after an ankle fracture [3].

Impaired wound healing and subsequent infection can complicate the decision to operate. However, conservative management carries the risk of loss of reduction, impaired fracture healing, and further complications. Both operative and nonoperative management in diabetic patients can increase the risk of Charcot neuroarthropathy and joint destruction, bone loss and deformity. Managing complications of diabetic ankle fractures not only puts an additional burden on healthcare resources but also affects the quality of life and well-being of the patient [4, 5].

Patients with diabetes mellitus, particularly those with diabetes-related comorbidities, might have serious consequences from foot and ankle fractures. Patients with diabetes mellitus had 7.4 times greater risk of amputation following ankle fracture surgery compared to a nondiabetic patients [6, 7].

2. Biochemical effects of diabetes on bone

Type 1 and type 2 diabetes have several common traits influencing bone health. This includes high blood glucose levels and the increased synthesis of compounds such as advanced glycation end products (AGEs), reactive oxygen species (ROS), and inflammatory mediators. These factors work together to increase osteoclast activity while reducing osteoblast production and bone growth, resulting in an increased risk of fractures and compromised fracture healing [4, 8]. Hyperglycemia, inflammation, advanced glycation end products (AGEs), and reactive oxygen species (ROS) are variables that several studies suggest affect the differentiation of osteoclasts and osteoblasts, which are essential for bone remodelling [4, 9].

Chronic hyperglycemia elevates blood viscosity, impairing red blood cells' oxygen transport capacity. It also influences nitric oxide, an antioxidant and neurotransmitter, and results in microvascular complications [4, 10].

Diabetes mellitus and associated hyperglycemia may lead to consequences including neuropathy, retinopathy, nephropathy, and cardiovascular impairment [4, 9].

3. Pathophysiology: Diabetic neuropathy

Peripheral neuropathy is a common and serious consequence in patients with diabetes, affecting up to 50% of those who may experience sensory impairments, including paraesthesia and loss of protective feeling, over their lives. This disorder is more common in patients over 60 years of age, who are at an increased risk for ankle fractures. Lack of protective sensation significantly raises the prevalence of undetectable damage, ulceration, and severe infection [11–13].

Further impairing motor and autonomic systems in diabetic neuropathy, which reduces balance, increases fall risk and raises fracture rates [4, 11].

Chronic hyperglycemia and dyslipidemia pathophysiologically generate oxidative stress *via* inflammatory pathways and excessive reactive oxygen species (ROS), resulting in direct neuronal damage and microvascular ischaemia. Reduced sodium-potassium pump function decreases nerve conduction velocity and neuronal excitability [4, 11].

The buildup of advanced glycation end products diminishes neurotrophic support, whereas vascular impairment intensifies progressive nerve damage [4, 11].

4. Diabetic vasculopathy

Diabetes affects the macro and microvascular systems, leading to decreased angiogenesis and peripheral arterial disease. Reduced oxygen supply, local tissue ischaemia and poor wound healing environment follow these changes in blood vessels. Advanced glycation end products (AGEs), impaired fibroblast activity, poor collagen synthesis, and increased vascular calcification explain delayed healing and a higher risk of postoperative complications. Preoperative vascular assessment is key in diabetic patients with ankle fractures to guide surgical planning and minimise complications [4, 10, 14].

5. Differences between complicated and uncomplicated diabetes

Addressing fractures and dislocations of the foot and ankle requires an awareness of the differences between individuals with uncomplicated and complicated diabetes. For this review, complicated diabetes is defined as "end organ damage, which includes patients with neuropathy, peripheral vascular disease, and/or chronic kidney disease [6, 15].

Peripheral neuropathy in diabetic people points to tissue and organ damage, therefore indicating extended suboptimal glycaemic management. Managing foot and ankle fractures in patients with complicated diabetes mellitus poses difficulties as surgical operations increase the risk of poor wound healing, delayed fracture repair, malunion, infection, and the requirement of revision surgery [4, 16].

6. Assessment and evaluation

6.1 History taking

The initial assessment and evaluation of foot and ankle fractures in patients with diabetes mellitus (DM) begins with a comprehensive history of the mechanism of injury and the time elapsed since the injury occurred. Of those with diabetes, 39% had osteoporosis, and 74% had bone density below osteopenia. A low-energy mechanism with a complex fracture pattern may indicate poor bone quality. The timing of injury and duration of diabetes are important factors [17, 18].

The absence of pain and the ability to walk on a fractured foot or ankle may indicate peripheral neuropathy that delays proper treatment and presentation. Additionally, Patients with less sensation may continue walking on the injured leg, worsening the fracture and causing further soft tissue injury [15, 17].

Given that they increase the risk of complications, the history should also include questions about comorbidities, as 89% of patients with diabetes have at least one comorbidity, and 15% have four or more. Other questions should include the history of ulcers, amputations, or infections, smoking, insulin or other medication use, and use of mobility aids before the accident [17, 19].

6.2 Physical examination

Comprehensive physical examinations should cover thorough evaluations of the dermatological, circulatory, neurological, and musculoskeletal systems. Carefully assessment for wounds can help rule out open fractures [17, 20]. It is vital to look for changes in skin colour, temperature fluctuations, or any bony prominences upon palpation to rule out the possibility of starting skin necrosis. Moreover, the presence of tense compartments or fracture blisters would imply that the extremity is not yet ready for surgical fixation [17].

Assessing peripheral neuropathy requires a comprehensive neurological examination of the foot and ankle. Patients are asked if they experience tingling, numbness, or a sensation of insects crawling on their skin. Autonomic dysfunction is suspected in individuals with dry, cracked, and hyperaemic skin. Motor dysfunction with intrinsic muscle atrophy can present as toe clawing. Loss of vibratory sense, pinprick sense, proprioception or absence of deep tendon reflexes at the ankle may indicate neuropathy, which can be hard to assess in cases of fracture [17, 21, 22].

A nerve conduction study is the gold standard for diagnosing peripheral neuropathy; however, a 5.07 (10-g) Semmes-Weinstein monofilament is the accepted method for testing loss of protective sensation. This simple test has a sensitivity of 91% and a specificity of 86%, respectively [23]. Testing at least four plantar locations improves these numbers: great toe, first metatarsal head, third metatarsal head and fifth metatarsal head [21].

The physical exam should include a vascular evaluation. This is significant as peripheral arterial disease (PAD) presents more than 40% of people with diabetes [17].

Visual clues pointing to peripheral artery disease(PAD) include dependent rubor, pallor with elevation of the extremities, dystrophic toenails, and hair loss [17].

The dorsal pedis, posterior tibial, and popliteal arteries should be palpated and then compared with the contralateral side. If pulses are still missing or weak following a reduction in the dislocation or improvement of the fracture alignment, Doppler ultrasound can help locate the vessels [15].

Palpable pedal pulses may not rule out PAD in individuals with diabetes and neuropathy; additionally, these patients may not show the usual PAD symptoms, including claudication [24].

While additional diagnostic testing should be done in individuals with abnormal vascular findings, it should not postpone the treatment of unstable fractures that need urgent reduction of fractures and dislocations [15, 17].

The ankle-brachial index (ABI) is often touted as a more sensitive and noninvasive assessment of a patient's vascular condition than other tests. It is considered normal when the value is between 0.91 and 1.3. An ABI greater than 1.3 denotes poor arterial compressibility; an ABI of 1.1 or greater may indicate arterial calcification in individuals with diabetes. Another method for evaluating tissue perfusion is transcutaneous oximetry (TcPO2) [15, 17, 25].

In patients with acute fractures, measuring the ankle-brachial index (ABI), toe-brachial index (TBI), and absolute toe pressure, as well as examining arterial waveforms, may not be possible or practicable; thus, further testing may be required [15, 25].

Patients with displaced foot and ankle fractures with dislocation are not unusual to have absent or reduced pulse. An immediate closed reduction should be performed, and the pulses should be reassessed; usually, this results in improved perfusion [15].

7. Radiologic and laboratory evaluations

Radiologic assessment should start with the standard anteroposterior (AP), lateral, and mortise views of the ankle joint. Additionally, X-rays of the foot may be conducted to check for any foot injuries [15, 17].

When an injury is suspected but not visible on X-rays, computed tomography (CT) can offer further insight. CT is also beneficial for planning surgery in cases of complex fracture patterns or injuries, particularly those involving intraarticular and periarticular damage [15, 17].

Magnetic resonance imaging (MRI) helps identify bone injuries that are not visible on plain films and in diagnosing injuries to ligaments, tendons, and cartilage. MRI can detect bone marrow oedema and stress injuries that might precede Charcot neuroarthropathy [15, 26].

In addition to the standard preoperative laboratory studies, every patient should have their glycaemic haemoglobin A1c (HbA1c) levels evaluated. A higher risk of complications and more extended hospital stays have been associated with levels over 6.5. Patients with HbA1c levels above eight have a 2.5 times higher risk of infections and poor surgical results. Although high HbA1c results should not halt surgery, they can help with postoperative diabetes control [17, 20].

As red blood cells have a shorter lifetime, HbA1c may not accurately reflect glycemic management for individuals undergoing frequent dialysis for chronic renal disease. In these situations, glycemic albumin or fructosamine levels may be used as alternative markers [27, 28].

Preoperative albumin levels can be evaluated. Low levels of serum albumin might indicate malnutrition, which can be a predictor of developing postoperative complications [17, 29].

A multidisciplinary diabetic team approach is advised, particularly in patients with complicated diabetes, as handling these medical problems goes beyond the knowledge of trauma and orthopaedic surgeons [27].

8. Fracture management

For ankle fractures, whether treated nonoperatively or operatively, the primary goals are to achieve a stable foot and ankle, restore function, and minimise complications [30].

Generally, uncomplicated diabetics who get an ankle fracture can be treated similarly to those without diabetes [30]. Before starting treatment, it is essential to have a thorough conversation with the patient about the management plan, including the potential need for additional nonoperative treatments to ensure sufficient healing and the possibility of nonweight-bearing and prolonged immobilisation. These additional treatments may include calcium, vitamin D, and protein supplements, as well as walking aids, wheelchairs, and devices such as a Charcot Restraint Orthotic Walker (CROW) boot. The management plan can be tailored to the patient's physiological condition and the injury pattern [17].

9. Nonoperative treatment

Nonoperative management can be controversial due to concerns about displacement. However, these patients can be managed successfully in specific indications.

Isolated Malleolar fractures without instability, confirmed by the fracture pattern and/or gravity stress radiographs, can be treated nonoperatively [27].

Treatment consists of closed contact casting and weight-bearing restriction until fracture healing is observed. After the casting period, patients are placed in a period of protected weight-bearing using a brace or boot for an additional 2–3 months [17, 27].

This management requires close observation and serial radiological assessment, especially in the early period, to monitor skin and soft tissue integrity and to detect subtle displacement. Patient compliance is key to this strategy. The treating surgeon should also be prepared to switch to another management plan if early complications arise that indicate nonoperative management is failing [17, 27].

There is limited research on the nonsurgical treatment of diabetic ankle fractures. Most existing studies involve a small number of patients and typically focus on nonsurgical methods as alternatives to surgical intervention. Complications noted in these studies include malunion due to the loss of initial reduction, nonunion, infections, and the formation of ulcers. Factors that increase the risk of complications include infrequent patient visits, early weight bearing, noncompliance, prolonged diabetes duration, neuropathy, insulin dependence, and a history of Charcot neuroarthropathy [5, 17, 27].

In a retrospective analysis spanning five years, Raheman et al. (2024) compared the outcomes of diabetic patients with ankle fractures treated conservatively versus surgically. Diabetic individuals reportedly had higher complication rates compared to nondiabetic ones. The incidence of complications under surgical and conservative treatment was almost the same. They concluded that nonoperative management might be suitable for some diabetic patients, especially those with multiple comorbidities [31].

10. Operative management

For closed, displaced ankle fractures, the initial step involves performing a closed reduction followed by splinting. If splinting fails to achieve and maintain bone stability or if there is a risk to the skin, a spanning external fixator may be used as an initial reduction measure. The first step in management should include elevating the injured limb on a frame or pillow to help reduce swelling. Monitoring injury-related swelling through clinical assessment is crucial for determining the appropriate timing for surgery when the soft tissues are ready [15, 32].

In cases of highly unstable fractures, reduction may be lost even with plaster backslabs, often due to swelling that does not improve with elevation or rest. When uncertain, it is essential to promptly assess the fracture position using suitable sequential imaging techniques in the backslab. An external fixator can be applied if the reduction is lost while allowing soft tissue swelling to subside before definitive surgical fixation is performed [15, 27].

Immediate open reduction and internal fixation (ORIF) is feasible if done before acute swelling begins. Otherwise, a waiting period of 7–10 days is generally necessary for postinjury swelling to decrease sufficiently for surgical intervention. This is indicated by reduced skin turgor and the appearance of skin wrinkles over the planned surgical incision sites [15, 27].

Displaced, unstable ankle fractures are optimally treated with ORIF, which involves careful handling of soft tissue, precise reduction of the articular surfaces, stable fixation of intraarticular fragments, and the use of suitable hardware to ensure the stability of the construct [27, 32].

11. Biological and mechanical aspects of fixation

In surgical treatments for diabetic foot and ankle fractures, fixation decisions must take into account two primary considerations: mechanical and biological. Local blood flow must be preserved, particularly in individuals with diabetes, where healing may be delayed [33].

Surgical techniques must be meticulously selected to preserve the soft tissue envelope surrounding the bone. More recent ideas, such as superconstructs, have been proposed to solve the problems with diabetic bone quality. These constructs provide additional stability by extending beyond the injured area.

Surgeons must choose between internal and external fixation. Every kind has benefits and drawbacks. Bone stability has been improved recently by developments in methods for applying external fixators—especially multiplanar and circular external fixators. Although external fixation maximises blood flow, it may not give as osseous stability as internal fixation. Alternatively, rigid stability is achieved by using screws and rigid compressive plates. It could, however, compromise the surrounding soft tissues and have negative consequences on the blood flow in the area [33].

Locking plates function as an "internal-external fixator," offering stability by maintaining a fixed angle between the screw and plate. The locking mechanism between the plate and screw head prevents movement and loosening, which can occur in osteoporotic bones. Current plate applications offer the biomechanical advantages of locking plates combined with the benefits of compression plate fixation [33].

The selection of fixation should be customised to every patient as it depends on various elements. Surgeons should have a strong awareness of the pathophysiology of the individual disease condition as well as of general fixation concepts. The surgeon should assess the pattern of the fracture, take into account the soft tissue envelope around it, and be aware of the possibility of Charcot neuroarthropathy development [33].

12. Surgical management procedures

There are five surgical techniques to manage diabetic ankle fractures: standard, trans-syndesmotic, circular external fixation, transarticular, and hybrid or a combination of these [17].

Standard fixation is suitable for patients with HbA1c < 7.0, BMI < 30, who can feel a 5.07 or smaller Semmes-Weinstein monofilament, have palpable pulses, nonosteoporotic bone, and no signs of autonomic dysfunction. This technique may involve small fragment fixation with a lag screw and plate for the fibula and cancellous screws for the medial malleolus [17, 32].

When installing hardware, a direct lateral incision with lateral plate application may increase lateral ankle volume, leaving insufficient tissue for closure. Even if closure is achieved, the combination of hardware under the skin and a splint or immobiliser above may cause incision necrosis and breakdown. An incision along the posterior border of the fibula or a traditional posterolateral approach is better, as it allows better skin mobility and hardware accommodation [32]. This approach also allows posterolateral fibula fixation, which cadaver studies have shown to be a stronger construct for supination and external rotation fractures compared to lateral locking plates [34]. Additionally, this incision also allows multi-layer closure over the hardware [32].

These patients may still require nonweight-bearing postoperatively for an extended period [32].

For patients who are not suitable for standard fixation techniques, three alternative methods are available. These approaches differ from traditional methods of ankle fixation, however still they are designed to preserve the anatomical mortise and reduce the likelihood of fixation failure before sufficient healing, which could result in a Charcot joint. Alongside extended immobilisation and nonweight-bearing, the surgical principles for these techniques involve using long, rigid locking plates with long bicortical or quadricortical screw placement, employing additional fixation, and considering bone grafting [17, 32].

The trans-syndesmotic fixation method stabilises the fibular fixation using the tibia. This technique involves restoring the fibula to its proper length, reducing the fracture, and attaching a 10-hole 3.5-mm or larger locking plate to the fibula. The surgeon then places as many quadricortical (crossing four cortices) locking screws as possible through the fibula into the tibia [17, 25].

Nwoko and colleagues recently noted challenges in reducing fibular fractures in diabetic ankle fractures due to glycation of the peroneal tendons and performed peroneal tendon lengthening as an additional procedure to assist in reducing the lateral malleolus [35].

The benefit of using a locking plate is its angular stability, which enhances its load-bearing capacity, making the locking plates four times stronger than load-sharing constructs. This means that for fixation failure to occur, all fixation points must fail, unlike the loosening of individual screws seen with traditional compression plating techniques. The fibula pro-tibial construct leverages the combined pullout strength of locking screws to create a biomechanically stronger construct. Using a fibula pro-tibial construct also ensures that the fixation is not as rigid as nonlocking tetracortical fixation and allows for some syndesmosis micro-movement. Therefore, removal before the patient begins weight-bearing is unnecessary [17, 36]. To complete the ankle fixation, long 4.0-mm bicortical screws can be used to stabilise the medial and posterior malleolar fractures. This construct enhances fixation stiffness without solely relying on the purchase of screws in the fibula. Although there is concern that this technique may alter the biomechanics of the syndesmosis, this has not been clinically demonstrated [20, 25].

The risk associated with these larger, more rigid fixation techniques is that bulky hardware may need to be removed if it becomes prominent or if wound dehiscence occurs [25].

Additionally, if medial cancellous screw fixation does not achieve stable fixation, these screws can be advanced obliquely into the tibial far cortex. A tension band wiring or plating technique may be used to enhance the medial fixation [25].

For unstable fractures or fracture dislocations, additional external and internal fixation methods may be used. The transarticular fixation can be done in two ways. Firstly, the patient is managed with standard reduction methods, and two or three large, smooth Steinmann pins are inserted antegrade or retrograde through the tibia, talus and calcaneus. Despite being an older method, it can help stabilise fixation when tibiotalar instability is a concern. This will cause some stiffness in the ankle and hindfoot, but the benefit is that it does not rely solely on standard fixation to maintain reduction [12, 17].

Transarticular fixation of subtalar and tibiotalar joints can be done independently or with traditional internal fixation or external fixation. Commonly, Smooth 1/8- or 5/32-inch axial Steinmann pins are inserted retrograde through the plantar surface of the calcaneus, engaging the distal tibial cortex to prevent upward movement. The pins are cut short under the skin, and a tamp is used to drive them deep enough to avoid protrusion on the plantar surface and subsequent ulceration. The pins are usually removed after 3–4 months. If there is an Achilles tendon contracture, a percutaneous triple-step tendon lengthening can be considered [25].

The other way is to use a retrograde tibial talar calcaneal intramedullary nail. While some calcification or fusion of the ankle or subtalar joints may occur, the difference between this method and arthrodesis is that neither the subtalar nor the ankle joint is exposed and prepared as in a formal arthrodesis [17].

Retrograde tibiotalocalcaneal (TTC) nailing, without careful joint preparation, may be considered in diabetic patients with pilon or ankle fractures as a limb salvage procedure. Schultz et al. (2025) analysed the outcomes of 25 diabetic patients who underwent this procedure, reporting an 84% limb salvage rate and 72% preservation of ambulation function [37].

The only two determinative factors regarding below-knee amputation (BKA) identified were the patient's HbA1c level and the Fracture-related Infection (FRI) [37].

These patients would gain from improved postoperative mobilisation and least invasive soft tissue dissection, preserving the periosteal blood supply. Patients with compromised wound healing or high infection rates will find these benefits very helpful. Therefore, the study found that TTC nailing without joint preparation provides a less disruptive approach to solid bone fixation, which may save certain susceptible patients from amputation despite concerns about potential complications [37].

The third method is a combined strategy. This combines the trans-syndesmotic method with two to three large, smooth Steinman pins inserted either antegrade or retrograde through the tibia, talus, and calcaneus. This gives excellent stability and is helpful for acute diabetic ankle fractures that cannot be fixed with standard fixation, especially in obese patients. Like other methods, the increased stiffness in the ankle does not appear to pose a clinical problem, as walking will gradually restore movement between the tibia and fibula. The Steinman pins in this combined approach can be left in for a minimum of 2–3 months before removal [17].

13. External fixators

External fixators generally can provide stability without the need for bulky internal hardware. An external fixator also eliminates the need for casting or splinting, allowing for inspection of the skin and wounds. Supplementary external fixation can remain in place for 6–12 weeks, provided the skin condition permits. Total contact casting is recommended once the external fixator is removed. Protected weight bearing is allowed only after radiographic evidence of fracture healing (usually at 12 weeks). This can be achieved with a total contact cast or a removable boot in compliant patients. External fixation also increases patient compliance with nonweight-bearing protocols [25].

The fixators can be circular or pin-and-bar external fixators. The decision to apply a pin-and-bar external fixation device versus a circular ring fixator should be considered carefully. The natural life of a pin-and-bar fixator in diabetic patients is 4–6 weeks. Beyond that, the pins may be loose, leading to loss of fixation and potential infection. Ilizarov-type external fixators are powerful devices that provide fracture stability in multiple planes while minimising soft tissue injury. They are used for more extended periods. They are more amenable to fixator maintenance, such as wire or pin augmentation, pin swapping, or even the late addition of internal fixation while keeping the external fixator in place. Additionally, olive wires, tensioning devices, and techniques can be used to aid in fracture reduction. If definitive treatment with external fixation is needed, it is advisable to use a ring-type external fixator at the beginning of treatment [25, 32, 38].

14. Ankle arthrodesis

Ankle arthrodesis, traditionally a salvage procedure, has become a primary procedure for some diabetic patients with acute ankle fractures. These patients often have multiple comorbidities such as peripheral neuropathy, vasculopathy, nephropathy or a history of Charcot arthropathy that makes conventional fixation methods unreliable [39, 40].

Primary arthrodesis, primarily achieved through tibiotalocalcaneal (TTC) fusion with hindfoot nails, provides immediate rigid stabilisation to prevent severe complications, such as deep infections or limb loss. However, it has a high complication rate [40].

A retrospective case series conducted by Grote et al. (2020) involving 13 high-risk diabetic patients who underwent arthrodesis. The study reported a complication rate of over 75% with infections (38.5%), wound problems (53.8%) and amputations (23.1%). Despite these figures, 89% of the patients healed, and patients had stable ankles that tolerated asymptomatic nonunion at the fusion site. Therefore, ankle arthrodesis can be considered a valuable option for diabetic patients with compromised soft tissue [40].

15. Complications

15.1 Infection

A comprehensive multidisciplinary team approach that includes orthopaedic surgeons, infectious disease specialists, endocrinologists, wound care experts, and sometimes plastic surgeons is required to manage diabetic ankle fracture complications. In real-life scenarios, multiple complications may arise simultaneously that require intervention, including osteomyelitis treatment, management of fixation failure, and both wound healing difficulties and nonunion management. In cases of infection, we first manage the infection before proceeding to definitive revision fixation using a staged approach [41].

Managing infections in patients is of a big concern, especially for those with diabetes and ankle fractures who are more prone to both superficial and deep surgical site infections [4].

Factors that increase the risk of infection include peripheral arterial disease, neuropathy, long-standing diabetes, poor glucose control (HbA1c over 8), Charcot joint, advanced age, obesity, a history of rheumatoid arthritis, previous ulcers, and open fractures. Neuropathy is a significant risk factor because it impairs patients' ability to detect infections, allowing even those not undergoing surgery to become infected [17, 42, 43].

Frequent checkups may not completely prevent this complication, but they can facilitate earlier intervention when infections are detected.

In a retrospective review by Wukich et al. of 1000 foot and ankle surgery cases, 19% were diabetic patients. The study found that post-op infections were more common in the diabetic group. Diabetic patients were five times more likely to have severe infections that required hospitalisation. Complicated diabetes increased the risk of post-op infection 10-fold compared to nondiabetics and 6-fold compared to those with uncomplicated diabetes. However, there was no significant increase in infection risk for those with uncomplicated diabetes compared to those without diabetes. Therefore, we need to identify diabetic complications early and ensure that those without complications adhere to their treatment plans [44].

Infections are often detected during cast changes. For superficial infections, managing the issue may involve creating a window in the cast for local daily wound care, oral antibiotics and weekly office visits. On the other hand, deep infections require irrigation and debridement, at least 6 weeks of IV antibiotics, and removal of loose implants. It is advisable to avoid taking a local swab of the area; instead, a deep culture or bone biopsy may be necessary to identify organisms if osteomyelitis is suspected. Once the infection is controlled, a local flap or free tissue transfer may be needed if the wound cannot be closed secondarily. If there is a significant loss of bone or articular surfaces after debridement, then ankle or double hindfoot arthrodesis may be needed to salvage the limb. Finally, if the limb cannot be salvaged, amputation may be necessary [17, 41].

15.2 Fixation failure

Fixation failure describes the early postoperative reduction loss occurring between 2 and 4 weeks without Charcot joint development. The combination of neuropathy in patients, along with their inability to avoid putting weight on the affected limb and inadequate initial fixation, can lead to this complication [17, 41].

The study by Shibuya et al. analysed variables related to nonunion and malunion, as well as delayed bone healing, in 165 diabetic patients who underwent surgical treatment for foot and ankle conditions. The research indicated that 25% of diabetic patients exhibited bone healing complications that were statistically related to surgical duration, peripheral neuropathy, and HbA1c levels above 7% [45].

Bone healing complications demonstrated the highest correlation with peripheral neuropathy among diabetic patients. Continuing conservative treatment for misaligned limbs frequently encounters malunion, nonunion, contracture formation, skin breakdown, and ulceration [45].

Combined surgical strategies, as described previously, can be used to address failed fixation, depending on the timing relative to the condition of the soft tissue envelope. When revision fixation cannot be performed, physicians might need to perform ankle or double hindfoot arthrodesis to preserve the limb [4, 17, 41].

16. Charcot arthropathy

Charcot arthropathy represents a neurodegenerative bone disease that usually appears in patients who suffer from advanced peripheral neuropathy caused by diabetes. Researchers continue to debate the pathophysiological mechanisms of this condition, with multiple theoretical frameworks presented in the scientific literature [46, 47]. The contemporary scientific consensus suggests that aetiopathogenesis involves a complex interplay between repetitive microtraumatic events, dysregulation of osseous metabolism, and sophisticated neurovascular alterations [46, 48].

Epidemiological data indicate that approximately 25–50% of affected individuals present with antecedent foot or ankle trauma, necessitating a comprehensive evaluation for Charcot arthropathy in all diabetic patients presenting with acute pedal and ankle injuries [46, 47].

The clinical management of this condition presents significant challenges, particularly when it develops after surgical intervention for ankle fractures, as it frequently receives erroneous classification as an infectious pathology in instances where a previously compliant patient who has undergone anatomical reduction of the mortise experiences fixation failure. Charcot joint disease should be included in the differential diagnosis. Acute exacerbations of Charcot arthropathy typically manifest with pronounced oedema, localised hyperthermia, and erythematous changes, which demonstrate considerable overlap with infectious processes. The diagnostic complexity is further compounded by elevations in inflammatory biomarkers, which demonstrate significant concordance with the patterns observed in acute infections. Differential diagnosis may be facilitated by the observation that erythematous manifestations in acute Charcot arthropathy typically diminish upon elevation of the affected extremity, despite otherwise similar clinical presentations [17, 46].

The therapeutic approach to these patients is frequently complicated by delayed presentation featuring malunion, nonunion, and contractile deformities of the extremities. When the affected extremity progresses to the subacute or chronic phase of pathology, reconstructive intervention could be considered [17].

17. Conclusion

Diabetic patients are more complex to manage than nondiabetic patients with ankle fractures. Neuropathy, vascular disease, and altered bone metabolism require a thorough preoperative assessment and a tailored treatment plan to obtain the best results. Mechanical stability while protecting soft tissue and vascular health is the key. Where internal fixation may not be possible or safe, superconstructs, hybrid fixation, or primary arthrodesis are valuable options, especially for complex diabetic patients. Success depends on the early identification of comorbidities, careful planning, and a team-based approach to postoperative care. Preventing infections and Charcot joint disease requires vigilance, patient education, and regular follow-up. A patient-centred and evidence-based approach will improve not only surgical outcomes but also the quality of life and limb preservation in this high-risk group.

DOI: http://dx.doi.org/10.5772/intechopen.1011938

Author details

Sedeek M. Mosaid[1*], Ahmed Khalil[2], Khaled Elawady[1], Munier Hossain[1] and Nijil Vasukutty[3]

1 Department of Trauma and Orthopaedics, United Lincolnshire Hospitals NHS Trust, Lincoln County Hospital, United Kingdom

2 Department of Surgery, United Lincolnshire Hospitals NHS Trust, Lincoln County Hospital, United Kingdom

3 Department of Trauma and Orthopaedics, United Lincolnshire Hospitals NHS Trust, Pilgrim Hospital, United Kingdom

*Address all correspondence to: sedeeko2000@hotmail.com

References

[1] Court-Brown CM, Duckworth AD, Clement ND, McQueen MM. Fractures in older adults. A view of the future? Injury. 2018;**49**(12):2161-2166

[2] Sundararaghavan V, Mazur MM, Evans B, Liu J, Ebraheim NA. Diabetes and bone health: Latest evidence and clinical implications. Therapeutic Advances in Musculoskeletal Disease [Internet]. 2017;**9**(3):67-74. Available from: https://www.ncbi.nlm.nih.gov/pmc/articles/PMC5349336/

[3] Lanzetti RM, Lupariello D, Venditto T, Guzzini M, Ponzo A, De Carli A, et al. The role of diabetes mellitus and BMI in the surgical treatment of ankle fractures. Diabetes/Metabolism Research and Reviews. 2017;**34**(2):e2954

[4] Amini B, Kadhm S, Trompeter A. The impact of diabetes mellitus on the management and outcome of ankle fractures. Injury [Internet]. 2025;**56**(4):112226. Available from: https://www.sciencedirect.com/science/article/pii/S0020138325000865

[5] Lovy AJ, Dowdell J, Keswani A, Koehler S, Kim J, Weinfeld S, et al. Nonoperative versus operative treatment of displaced ankle fractures in diabetics. Foot & Ankle International. 2016;**38**(3):255-260

[6] Liu JW, Ahn J, Raspovic KM, Liu GT, Nakonezny PA, Lavery LA, et al. Increased rates of readmission, reoperation, and mortality following open reduction and internal fixation of ankle fractures are associated with diabetes mellitus. The Journal of Foot and Ankle Surgery. 2019;**58**(3):470-474

[7] Pincus D, Veljkovic A, Zochowski T, Mahomed N, Ogilivie-Harris D, Wasserstein D. Rate of and risk factors for intermediate-term reoperation after ankle fracture fixation: A population-based cohort study. Journal of Orthopaedic Trauma. 2017;**31**(10):e315-e320

[8] Jiao H, Xiao E, Graves DT. Diabetes and its effect on bone and fracture healing. Current Osteoporosis Reports. 2015;**13**(5):327-335

[9] Catalfamo D, Britten T, Storch D, Calderon N, Sorenson H, Wallet S. Hyperglycemia induced and intrinsic alterations in type 2 diabetes-derived osteoclast function. Oral Diseases. 2012;**19**(3):303-312

[10] Wukich DK, Kline AJ. The management of ankle fractures in patients with diabetes. The Journal of Bone and Joint Surgery-American Volume. 2008;**90**(7):1570-1578

[11] Beeve AT, Brazill JM, Scheller EL. Peripheral neuropathy as a component of skeletal disease in diabetes. Current Osteoporosis Reports. 2019;**17**(5):256-269

[12] Jani MM, Ricci WM, Borrelli J, Barrett SE, Johnson JE. A protocol for treatment of unstable ankle fractures using transarticular fixation in patients with diabetes mellitus and loss of protective sensibility. Foot & Ankle International. 2003;**24**(11):838-844

[13] Hicks CW, Selvin E. Epidemiology of peripheral neuropathy and lower extremity disease in diabetes. Current Diabetes Reports [Internet]. 2019;**19**(10):1-8. Available from: https://www.ncbi.nlm.nih.gov/pmc/articles/PMC6755905/

[14] Marin C, Luyten FP, Van der Schueren B, Kerckhofs G, Vandamme K.

The impact of type 2 diabetes on bone fracture healing. Frontiers in Endocrinology. 2018;**9**:6

[15] Johnson M, Kandasamy S, Raspovic KM, Manchanda K, Liu GT, VanPelt MD, et al. Fractures and dislocations of the foot and ankle in people with diabetes: A literature review. Therapeutic. Advances in Endocrinology and Metabolism. 2023;**14**:204201882311637-204201882311637

[16] Wukich DK, Crim BE, Frykberg RG, Rosario BL. Neuropathy and poorly controlled diabetes increase the rate of surgical site infection after foot and ankle surgery. The Journal of Bone & Joint Surgery. 2014;**96**(10):832-839

[17] Herscovici DJ Jr, Scaduto JM. Management of acute diabetic fractures of the ankle. In: Herscovici DJ Jr, editor. The Surgical Management of the Diabetic Foot and Ankle. Cham: Springer; 2016. pp. 103-116

[18] Jones KB, Maiers-Yelden KA, Marsh JL, Zimmerman MB, Estin M, Saltzman CL. Ankle fractures in patients with diabetes mellitus. The Journal of Bone & Joint Surgery. 2005;**87-B**(4): 489-495

[19] O'Connell JM, Manson SM. Understanding the economic costs of diabetes and prediabetes and what we may learn about reducing the health and economic burden of these conditions. Diabetes Care [Internet]. 2019;**42**(9):1609-1611. Available from: https://www.ncbi.nlm.nih.gov/pmc/articles/PMC6702611/

[20] Chaudhary SB, Liporace FA, Gandhi A, Donley BG, Pinzur MS, Lin SS. Complications of ankle fracture in patients with diabetes. Journal of the American Academy of Orthopaedic Surgeons. 2008;**16**(3):159-170

[21] Herbst SA, Jones KB, Saltzman CL. Pattern of diabetic neuropathic arthropathy associated with the peripheral bone mineral density. The Journal of Bone and Joint Surgery British. 2004;**86-B**(3):378-383

[22] Armstrong DG, Lavery LA, Vela SA, Quebedeaux TL, Fleischli JG. Choosing a practical screening instrument to identify patients at risk for diabetic foot ulceration. Archives of Internal Medicine [Internet]. 1998;**158**(3):289. Available from: https://jamanetwork.com/journals/jamainternalmedicine/fullarticle/191320

[23] Smieja M, Hunt DL, Edelman D, Etchells E, Cornuz J, Simel DL. Clinical examination for the detection of protective sensation in the feet of diabetic patients. Journal of General Internal Medicine. 1999;**14**(7):418-424

[24] Wukich DK, Shen W, Raspovic KM, Suder NC, Baril DT, Avgerinos E. Noninvasive arterial testing in patients with diabetes. Foot & Ankle International. 2015;**36**(12):1391-1399

[25] Prisk VR, Wukich DK. Ankle fractures in diabetics. Foot and Ankle Clinics. 2006;**11**(4):849-863

[26] Chantelau E, Richter A. The acute diabetic Charcot foot managed on the basis of magnetic resonance imaging—A review of 71 cases. Swiss Medical Weekly. 2013;**143**:w13831

[27] Phyo N, Wee A. Managing acute ankle and hindfoot fracture in diabetic patients. Foot and Ankle Clinics. 2022;**27**(3):639-654

[28] Divani M, Georgianos PI, Didangelos T, Iliadis F, Makedou A, Hatzitolios AI, et al. Comparison of glycemic markers in chronic hemodialysis using continuous glucose monitoring.

American Journal of Nephrology. 2018;**47**(1):21-29

[29] Hoogwerf BJ, Sferra J, Donley BG. Diabetes mellitus--overview. Foot and Ankle Clinics [Internet]. 2006;**11**(4):703-715. Available from: https://www.ncbi.nlm.nih.gov/pubmed/17097511

[30] Gougoulias N, Oshba H, Dimitroulias A, Sakellariou A, Wee A. Ankle fractures in diabetic patients. EFORT Open Reviews [Internet]. 2020;**5**(8):457-463. Available from: https://pubmed.ncbi.nlm.nih.gov/32953131/

[31] Raheman F, Othieno-P'Otonya K, R eichert I, Ahluwalia R. The management of diabetic ankle fractures: Five year outcomes of extended fixation techniques. Foot & Ankle Orthopaedics. 2024;**9**(4)

[32] Manway JM, Blazek CD, Burns PR. Special considerations in the management of diabetic ankle fractures. Current Reviews in Musculoskeletal Medicine. 2018;**11**(3):445-455

[33] Bevilacqua NJ, Stapleton JJ. Advanced foot and ankle fixation techniques in patients with diabetes. Clinics in Podiatric Medicine and Surgery. 2011;**28**(4):661-671

[34] Minihane KP, Lee C, Ahn C, Zhang LQ, Merk BR. Comparison of lateral locking plate and antiglide plate for fixation of distal fibular fractures in osteoporotic bone: A biomechanical study. Journal of Orthopaedic Trauma. 2006;**20**(8):562-566

[35] Nwoko NC, Rodriguez-Collazo E, Goldflies ML. Peroneal tendon lengthening as an adjunct procedure to aid in the reduction of the lateral malleolus in diabetic ankle fractures: 2 case reports. The Journal of Foot and Ankle Surgery. 2019;**58**(6):1251-1256

[36] Okoro T, Teoh KH, Tanaka H. Fibula pro-tibia *vs* standard locking plate fixation in an ankle fracture saw bone model. World Journal of Orthopedics. 2021;**12**(8):548-554

[37] Schultz A, Poynter T, Wireman G, Sweeney M, Likine E, Ziegler C, et al. Outcomes in treatment of ankle and pilon fractures with retrograde tibiotalocalcaneal nailing without articular preparation in the setting of diabetes mellitus. Injury. 2025;**56**(3):112177

[38] Kapoor SS, Kataria H, Patra SK, Boruah T. Capsuloligamentotaxis and definitive fixation by an ankle-spanning Ilizarov fixator in high-energy pilon fractures. The Journal of Bone and Joint Surgery. 2010;**92-B**(8):1100-1106

[39] Ayoub MA. Ankle fractures in diabetic neuropathic arthropathy. The Journal of Bone and Joint Surgery British. 2008;**90-B**(7):906-914

[40] Grote CW, Tucker W, Stumpff K, Birt MC, Horton GA. Primary arthrodesis for diabetic ankle fractures. Foot & Ankle Orthopaedics. 2020;**5**(1):247301142090884

[41] Goldberg EM, Polachek WS, Hynes K. Ankle fractures in diabetic patients. JBJS Reviews. 2023;**11**(3)

[42] Pham H, Armstrong DG, Harvey C, Harkless LB, Giurini JM, Veves A. Screening techniques to identify people at high risk for diabetic foot ulceration: A prospective multicenter trial. Diabetes Care [Internet]. 2000;**23**(5):606-611. Available from: https://care.diabetesjournals.org/content/23/5/606?ijkey=1d97a26a58752ec45cf064d8bec548a63d222e35&keytype2=tf_ipsecsha

[43] Liu J, Ludwig T, Ebraheim NA. Effect of the blood HbA1c level on surgical

treatment outcomes of diabetics with ankle fractures. Orthopaedic Surgery. 2013;**5**(3):203-208

[44] Wukich DK, Lowery NJ, McMillen RL, Frykberg RG. Postoperative infection rates in foot and ankle surgery: A comparison of patients with and without diabetes mellitus. JBJS [Internet]. 2010;**92**(2):287-295

[45] Shibuya N, Humphers JM, Fluhman BL, Jupiter DC. Factors associated with nonunion, delayed union, and Malunion in foot and ankle surgery in diabetic patients. The Journal of Foot and Ankle Surgery. 2013;**52**(2):207-211

[46] Roepke WB, Haleem AM. Complications of foot and ankle fractures in diabetics. Foot and Ankle Clinics. Mar 2025;**30**(1):173-190. DOI: 10.1016/j.fcl.2024.04.004

[47] Trieb K. The charcot foot. The Bone & Joint Journal. 2016;**98-B**(9):1155-1159

[48] Rogers LC, Frykberg RG, Armstrong DG, Boulton AJM, Edmonds M, Van GH, et al. The charcot foot in diabetes. Diabetes Care [Internet]. 2011;**34**(9):2123-2129. Available from: https://www.ncbi.nlm.nih.gov/pubmed/21868781

Chapter 4

Matrix Metalloproteinases (MMPs) in Diabetic Foot Ulcers: Pathophysiology and Advances in Inhibitor Development

Satheesh Babu Natarajan, Gayathri Anbumani Alamelu, Saravanakumar Parameswaran, Suriyakala Perumal Chandran, Chadapully Kolumbu Ismail Sajeeth, S. M. Fazeela Mahaboob Begum and Anandarajagopal Kalusalingam

Abstract

Matrix metalloproteinases (MMPs) play a crucial role in extracellular matrix remodeling and wound healing. However, their dysregulation has been implicated in the pathogenesis of diabetic foot ulcers (DFUs), a severe complication of diabetes mellitus. Excessive MMP activity in DFUs leads to chronic inflammation, delayed wound healing, and tissue degradation by disrupting the balance between matrix deposition and degradation. Among MMPs, MMP-2 and MMP-9 are particularly elevated in chronic wounds, contributing to impaired angiogenesis and persistent infection. Understanding the role of MMPs in DFU pathophysiology has driven research into MMP inhibitors as potential therapeutic agents. Both natural and synthetic MMP inhibitors have been explored for their wound-healing properties. Natural inhibitors, including flavonoids, tannins, and polyphenols derived from medicinal plants, exhibit MMP-modulating effects through anti-inflammatory and antioxidant mechanisms. Synthetic inhibitors, such as hydroxamate-based compounds, have been developed to selectively target MMP activity, though their clinical application remains limited due to toxicity concerns. Recent advancements in nanotechnology and drug delivery systems have enabled the development of novel MMP inhibitors with improved specificity and reduced side effects. Current research focuses on optimizing these inhibitors to promote tissue regeneration while minimizing adverse effects. This review highlights the pathophysiological role of MMPs in DFUs and recent developments in MMP inhibitors of both natural and synthetic origins. A deeper understanding of these therapeutic strategies may pave the way for more effective treatments, improving clinical outcomes in diabetic patients suffering from chronic foot ulcers.

Keywords: matrix metalloproteinase enzyme, diabetic foot ulcers, nano-delivery, wound healing, growth factors

1. Introduction

Diabetic foot ulcers (DFUs) are a significant complication of diabetes mellitus, arising from a combination of peripheral neuropathy, peripheral arterial disease, and biomechanical abnormalities. Peripheral neuropathy leads to a loss of protective sensation, making individuals unaware of minor injuries or pressure points on their feet [1]. Concurrently, peripheral arterial disease impairs blood flow, reducing the delivery of oxygen and essential nutrients necessary for wound healing. Biomechanical changes, such as foot deformities and limited joint mobility, further contribute to abnormal pressure distribution during walking, increasing the risk of skin breakdown and ulcer formation as shown in **Figure 1** [2, 3]. The clinical significance of DFUs is profound. Approximately 34% of individuals with diabetes will develop a foot ulcer in their lifetime, and these ulcers precede 84% of all diabetes-related lower-leg amputations [4]. The presence of a DFU not only elevates the risk of infection, including cellulitis, osteomyelitis, and sepsis, but also significantly diminishes the patient's quality of life due to pain, restricted mobility, and the psychological burden associated with chronic wounds. Moreover, the five-year mortality rate following a diabetes-related amputation is alarmingly high, underscoring the severe implications of DFUs [5].

Effective management of DFUs necessitates a comprehensive approach. Off-loading techniques, such as total contact casting, are employed to redistribute pressure away from the ulcerated area, promoting healing [6]. Meticulous wound care, including debridement and appropriate dressings, is essential to prepare the wound bed for healing [7]. Infection control through the use of systemic antibiotics is critical when clinical signs of infection are present. Additionally, optimizing glycemic control and addressing comorbid conditions enhance the body's intrinsic healing capabilities [8]. Despite these interventions, the recurrence rate of DFUs remains high, with studies indicating that up to 65% of ulcers recur within 5 years, highlighting the necessity

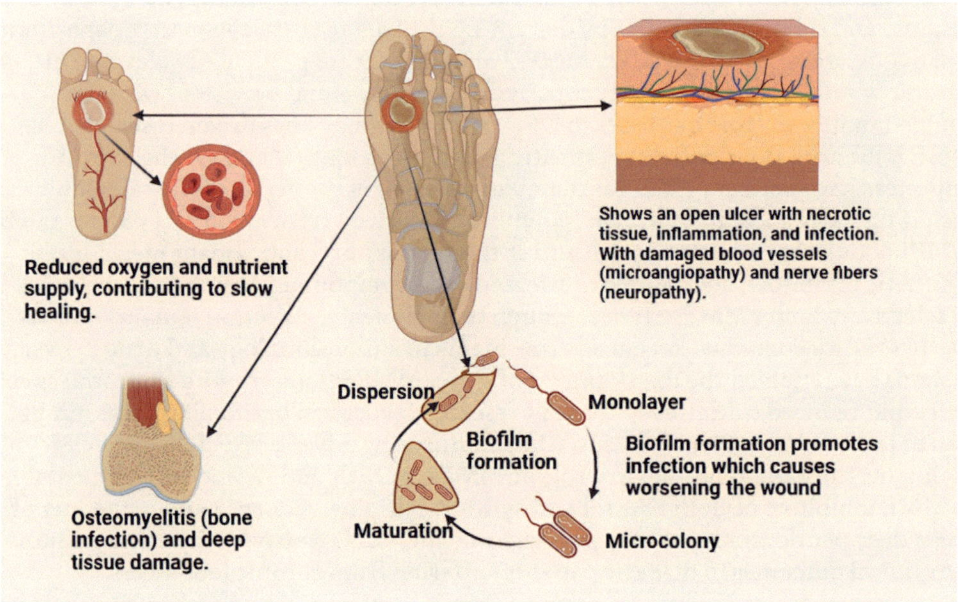

Figure 1.
Diabetic foot ulcer: Impaired healing and infection progression.

DOI: http://dx.doi.org/10.5772/intechopen.1010834

for ongoing preventive measures and patient education [9]. Chronic inflammation plays a pivotal role in the impaired wound healing observed in individuals with diabetes mellitus [10]. In a typical wound healing process, there are sequential phases: hemostasis, inflammation, proliferation, and remodeling. However, in diabetic patients, the inflammatory phase is often prolonged, leading to delayed progression to subsequent stages and resulting in chronic, nonhealing wounds [11].

One of the primary factors contributing to this impaired healing is the presence of advanced glycation end products (AGEs). Elevated blood glucose levels in diabetics lead to the formation of AGEs through nonenzymatic glycation of proteins and lipids [12]. These AGEs accumulate in various tissues, including the extracellular matrix (ECM), altering its properties and function [13]. Specifically, AGEs can increase the stiffness of collagen, disrupt normal cell-matrix interactions, and impede the migration of essential cells like fibroblasts and keratinocytes to the wound site. This disruption hinders the formation of new tissue and prolongs the inflammatory phase [14]. Moreover, AGEs interact with their receptors (RAGE) on the surface of various cells, including immune cells, leading to the activation of pro-inflammatory signaling pathways. This interaction results in the sustained release of pro-inflammatory cytokines such as tumor necrosis factor-alpha (TNF-α) and interleukins, which further perpetuate inflammation and tissue damage [15].

Another significant factor is the dysregulation of matrix metalloproteinases (MMPs) in diabetic wounds. MMPs are enzymes responsible for the degradation and remodeling of the ECM, a crucial step in wound healing [16]. In diabetic patients, there is an overexpression of MMPs, particularly MMP-2 and MMP-9, leading to excessive degradation of the ECM and growth factors necessary for tissue regeneration. This imbalance between MMPs and their natural inhibitors results in a hostile environment for cell proliferation and matrix deposition, further impairing wound closure [17]. Additionally, diabetic neuropathy contributes to impaired wound healing by reducing the sensation in extremities, leading to unrecognized injuries and persistent pressure points. This lack of sensation prevents timely protective actions, allowing minor wounds to progress to chronic ulcers [18]. Furthermore, diabetes is associated with impaired nitric oxide (NO) synthesis due to endothelial dysfunction. NO is vital for vasodilation and blood flow regulation; its deficiency leads to reduced blood supply to the wound area, depriving tissues of oxygen and essential nutrients necessary for healing [19].

Matrix metalloproteinases (MMPs) are a family of zinc-dependent endopeptidases that play a pivotal role in the remodeling of the extracellular matrix (ECM) during various physiological processes, including wound healing. They are capable of degrading a wide range of ECM components such as collagens, elastin, gelatin, and proteoglycans, thereby facilitating tissue repair and regeneration [20, 21]. The activity of MMPs is tightly regulated by tissue inhibitors of metalloproteinases (TIMPs), ensuring a balance between ECM degradation and formation. In the context of wound healing, MMPs contribute significantly to the different phases of the process [22]. During the inflammatory phase, MMPs such as MMP-9 are upregulated and assist in the migration of neutrophils across the basement membrane by degrading type IV and V collagens [23]. This degradation not only facilitates immune cell infiltration to combat infection but also helps in clearing the wound bed of damaged matrix components, setting the stage for subsequent tissue repair [24]. As healing progresses to the proliferative phase, MMPs continue to modulate the ECM environment. For instance, MMP-7, also known as matrilysin, degrades proteoglycans, fibronectin, and elastin, which is essential for epithelial cell migration and re-epithelialization of the wound surface [25].

The remodeling phase of wound healing involves the replacement of provisional ECM with a more organized and durable matrix [26]. MMPs such as MMP-1 (collagenase-1) and MMP-9 (gelatinase B) are instrumental in this phase, as they degrade interstitial collagens and gelatin, respectively, allowing for the reorganization of collagen fibers and restoration of normal tissue architecture. This controlled degradation is crucial for proper scar formation and the return of tissue functionality [27]. However, dysregulation of MMP activity can impair wound healing. Excessive MMP activity, often due to an imbalance between MMPs and TIMPs, can lead to chronic wounds characterized by persistent inflammation and ECM degradation [28]. Elevated levels of MMPs have been observed in nonhealing ulcers, where they degrade essential growth factors and receptors, further hindering the healing process. Therefore, maintaining the delicate balance between MMPs and their inhibitors is critical for effective wound repair [29].

Figure 1 illustrates the progression and complications of diabetic foot ulcers (DFUs). The ulcer results from reduced oxygen and nutrient supply, leading to slow healing. The presence of microangiopathy (damaged blood vessels) and neuropathy (damaged nerve fibers) further impairs tissue repair [30]. The ulcer develops necrotic tissue, inflammation, and infection, which can spread to deeper tissues, leading to osteomyelitis (bone infection) and deep tissue damage [31]. A significant factor worsening the condition is biofilm formation, where bacteria form protective layers that promote infection and delay healing. The biofilm progresses from a monolayer to microcolony, maturation, and dispersion, continuously aggravating the wound [32].

2. MMPs: Structure and function

Matrix metalloproteinases (MMPs) are a family of zinc-dependent endopeptidases that play a crucial role in the degradation and remodeling of the extracellular matrix (ECM) [20]. They are involved in various physiological processes, including embryonic development, tissue repair, and angiogenesis, as well as pathological conditions such as arthritis, cancer metastasis, and cardiovascular diseases [22]. MMPs are synthesized as inactive proenzymes and are activated through proteolytic cleavage. Their activity is tightly regulated by tissue inhibitors of metalloproteinases (TIMPs) to maintain tissue homeostasis. Alterations in MMP expression or activity can lead to pathological tissue remodeling, contributing to disease progression [33, 34]. The different types of MMPs and their biological function are shown in **Table 1**.

2.1 Extracellular matrix degradation

The ECM is a highly dynamic network composed of proteins such as collagen, elastin, fibronectin, and proteoglycans, which provide structural support to tissues and regulate various cellular activities, including proliferation, differentiation, and migration [73]. The process of ECM degradation and remodeling is critical in numerous biological processes such as tissue development, wound healing, fibrosis, and pathological events like cancer metastasis [74]. Mechanism involved in ECM degradation is given below.

Cysteine cathepsins are proteases that contribute to extracellular matrix (ECM) degradation, particularly in acidic environments like lysosomes [75]. Among them, cathepsin K degrades collagen and other ECM components,

MMP	Name	Primary substrates	Biological functions	References
MMP-1	Collagenase-1	Fibrillar collagens (types I, II, III), gelatin, aggrecan	Plays a key role in degrading interstitial collagens, which is crucial for tissue remodeling, wound healing, and fibrosis regulation. It is implicated in arthritis, tumor invasion, and fibrotic disorders.	[35, 36]
MMP-2	Gelatinase A	Gelatin, type IV collagen, elastin, fibronectin, laminin	Degrades basement membrane components, facilitating cell migration, angiogenesis, and tumor metastasis. Involved in cardiovascular diseases and fibrosis.	[37, 38]
MMP-3	Stromelysin-1	Proteoglycans, laminin, fibronectin, gelatin, non-fibrillar collagens	Plays a central role in tissue remodeling, wound healing, and inflammatory processes. Activates pro-MMPs and is involved in arthritis, atherosclerosis, and cancer progression.	[39, 40]
MMP-7	Matrilysin	Proteoglycans, fibronectin, elastin, casein, gelatin, entactin	Involved in epithelial repair, innate immunity, and cancer progression. Plays a role in regulating defensins in the intestinal mucosa and wound healing.	[41, 42]
MMP-8	Collagenase-2	Fibrillar collagens (types I, II, III), gelatin, aggrecan	Mainly associated with neutrophil-mediated inflammation and tissue remodeling. It plays a role in periodontal disease, rheumatoid arthritis, and wound healing.	[41, 43]
MMP-9	Gelatinase B	Gelatin, type IV and V collagens, elastin, fibronectin, laminin	Degrades extracellular matrix (ECM) components, facilitating leukocyte migration, angiogenesis, and blood–brain barrier disruption. Implicated in tumor invasion, neuroinflammation, and cardiovascular diseases.	[44, 45]
MMP-10	Stromelysin-2	Proteoglycans, fibronectin, gelatin, non-fibrillar collagens	Works in conjunction with MMP-3 in tissue remodeling and wound healing. Helps activate other MMPs and contributes to cartilage breakdown in arthritis.	[46, 47]
MMP-11	Stromelysin-3	Laminin, fibronectin, gelatin, aggrecan	Involved in tissue remodeling, adipose tissue homeostasis, and tumor progression by degrading ECM components. Plays a role in cancer cell invasion.	[48, 49]
MMP-12	Macrophage elastase	Elastin, fibronectin, laminin, type IV collagen	Major role in elastin degradation, which contributes to emphysema, atherosclerosis, and chronic inflammatory diseases such as COPD.	[50, 51]
MMP-13	Collagenase-3	Fibrillar collagens (types I, II, III), gelatin, aggrecan	Critical for cartilage remodeling and bone development. Overexpression is associated with osteoarthritis, rheumatoid arthritis, and bone metastasis.	[52, 53]

MMP	Name	Primary substrates	Biological functions	References
MMP-14	Membrane-type MMP-1	Progelatinase A, fibrillar collagens, gelatin, fibronectin	Plays a key role in pericellular proteolysis, cell migration, angiogenesis, and activation of MMP-2. Implicated in tumor metastasis and vascular remodeling.	[54, 55]
MMP-15	Membrane-type MMP-2	Progelatinase A, fibrillar collagens, gelatin, fibronectin	Contributes to ECM degradation, cell migration, and tissue invasion. Plays a role in embryonic development and tumor invasion.	[56, 57]
MMP-16	Membrane-type MMP-3	Progelatinase A, fibrillar collagens, gelatin, fibronectin	Involved in pericellular proteolysis and activation of MMP-2. Plays a role in tissue invasion, cancer progression, and angiogenesis.	[20, 58]
MMP-17	Membrane-type MMP-4	Fibrinogen, fibrin	Involved in blood clot remodeling, cell migration, and tissue invasion. Plays a role in immune responses and inflammation.	[59, 60]
MMP-19	RASI-1	Laminin, fibronectin, type IV collagen	Participates in wound healing, tissue remodeling, and immune regulation. Overexpression has been linked to inflammatory diseases.	[61, 62]
MMP-20	Enamelysin	Amelogenin, enamel proteins	Essential for enamel formation during tooth development. Plays a role in amelogenesis and dental tissue remodeling.	[63, 64]
MMP-21	X-MMP	Unknown	Involved in embryonic development, tissue remodeling, and morphogenesis. Overexpression has been linked to certain cancers.	[65, 66]
MMP-23	CA-MMP	Unknown	Plays a role in reproductive processes, immune regulation, and tissue remodeling. Involved in ovarian and testicular development.	[67, 68]
MMP-26	Matrilysin-2	Fibronectin, fibrinogen, type IV collagen	Contributes to tissue remodeling and wound healing. Overexpression has been linked to tumor progression and metastasis.	[69, 70]
MMP-28	Epilysin	Casein, fibronectin, type IV collagen	Plays a role in tissue homeostasis, wound healing, and epithelial cell turnover.	[71, 72]

Table 1.
Classification of MMPs and their function.

playing a crucial role in osteoclast-mediated bone resorption [76]. Cathepsin S is involved in proteoglycan breakdown and is linked to tissue destruction in inflammatory diseases such as rheumatoid arthritis, atherosclerosis, and cancer [77]. Heparanase, an enzyme that cleaves heparan sulfate chains of proteoglycans like perlecan and agrin, releases bound growth factors (FGF, VEGF, HGF), facilitating tissue remodeling, cell migration, tumor invasion, angiogenesis, and fibrosis. Elevated heparanase activity is implicated in cancer metastasis and inflammatory diseases [78].

Podosomes and invadopodia are actin-rich structures that facilitate ECM degradation and remodeling. Podosomes, found in macrophages, dendritic cells, and smooth muscle cells, localize MMPs at focal adhesion points to aid immune cell migration [79]. Invadopodia, present in invasive cancer cells, promote metastasis by secreting MMPs and degrading basement membranes, enabling tumor invasion [80]. Tissue Inhibitors of Metalloproteinases (TIMPs), including TIMP-1 to TIMP-4, regulate ECM turnover by inhibiting MMPs and maintaining tissue homeostasis [22]. Dysregulation of MMP-TIMP balance contributes to fibrosis, osteoarthritis, and cancer. Mechanical forces align ECM fibers, aiding wound healing by organizing collagen structure [81]. In cancer, ECM stiffening driven by tumor and stromal cells promotes tumor progression and therapy resistance, while in fibrosis, excessive tension leads to pathological ECM deposition and tissue scarring [82].

2.2 ECM remodeling and its role in biological processes

During embryogenesis and tissue development, ECM degradation and remodeling are essential for processes such as organ formation, vascularization, and tissue patterning. For example, the ECM in cartilage and bone is remodeled to allow for the growth of these tissues during development [83]. ECM remodeling plays a central role in wound healing. In the initial phase, ECM degradation is necessary to create space for new tissue growth. As healing progresses, the ECM is remodeled to restore tissue integrity and function [84]. This involves the deposition of new ECM components, such as fibronectin and collagen, which provide structural support for tissue regeneration [73]. In pathological conditions such as chronic inflammation, the ECM undergoes excessive deposition and remodeling, leading to fibrosis [85]. Fibrotic tissue is characterized by the accumulation of ECM components, particularly collagen, which impairs normal tissue function. Fibrosis is a hallmark of conditions such as pulmonary fibrosis, liver cirrhosis, and kidney fibrosis [86]. ECM remodeling is a crucial step in cancer metastasis. Tumor cells degrade the surrounding ECM to invade neighboring tissues and disseminate to distant organs. The ECM in the tumor microenvironment is often modified to facilitate tumor cell migration and resistance to chemotherapy [87].

2.3 Tissue inhibitors of metalloproteinases (TIMPs)

2.3.1 Regulation of MMP activity through tissue inhibitors of metalloproteinases (TIMPs)

MMP activity is mainly controlled by tissue inhibitors of metalloproteinases (TIMPs), endogenous proteins that inhibit MMPs. Humans have four TIMPs—TIMP-1, TIMP-2, TIMP-3, and TIMP-4—produced by cells like fibroblasts, endothelial cells, and smooth muscle cells [88]. These TIMPs balance MMP activity, preventing excessive ECM degradation. They bind to the catalytic domain of MMPs, blocking ECM breakdown [89]. The N-terminal domain of TIMPs binds MMPs, while the C-terminal domain varies, affecting binding specificity. For example, TIMP-1 binds strongly to MMP-9, and TIMP-2 prefers MMP-2 [90]. TIMP-1, for example, is known to promote cell survival and proliferation, particularly in the context of tumorigenesis and tissue repair. Additionally, TIMP-1 can modulate apoptosis by inhibiting caspase activity, providing anti-apoptotic effects [91].

2.3.2 The impact of cytokine signaling on MMP regulation

Cytokines are small signaling proteins that regulate immune responses and tissue homeostasis, significantly influencing MMP expression and ECM remodeling [92]. Pro-inflammatory cytokines like IL-1, TNF-α, and IL-6 upregulate MMPs during inflammation or injury by activating signaling pathways such as NF-κB [93]. Once activated, NF-κB translocates to the nucleus, inducing the transcription of MMP genes like MMP-1, MMP-3, and MMP-9, leading to ECM degradation and tissue remodeling. This regulation is crucial in processes such as wound healing, fibrosis, and inflammatory diseases [94]. Pro-inflammatory cytokines also regulate TIMP expression, influencing MMP activity balance. IL-1β induces TIMP-1 and TIMP-2 expression, while TNF-α increases TIMP-3 in a tissue-specific manner [22]. Conversely, anti-inflammatory cytokines like TGF-β and IL-10 inhibit MMP expression. TGF-β suppresses MMP production while promoting ECM synthesis, contributing to fibrosis and tissue repair [95].

2.3.3 Clinical implications and therapeutic targeting

The regulation of MMPs and TIMPs has significant clinical implications. Dysregulation of MMP and TIMP activity is implicated in a wide range of diseases, including cancer, cardiovascular disease, osteoarthritis, pulmonary diseases, and fibrosis [17]. For example, in cancer, inhibitors of MMPs (known as MMP inhibitors) have been developed as potential therapeutic agents to prevent metastasis and tumor growth. However, targeting MMPs has proven challenging, as MMPs have essential physiological roles, and their inhibition can have unintended side effects [96]. In diseases characterized by excessive fibrosis, such as pulmonary fibrosis or liver cirrhosis, strategies aimed at increasing the levels of TIMPs or inhibiting pro-inflammatory cytokine signaling pathways could help prevent ECM overaccumulation and tissue scarring [97]. Conversely, in diseases like osteoarthritis, where excessive ECM degradation occurs, promoting TIMP expression or inhibiting inflammatory cytokines may help preserve cartilage integrity [98].

3. Role of MMPs in diabetic foot ulcers (DFUs)

3.1 Matrix metalloproteinases (MMPs) and their role in ECM remodeling

Wound healing occurs through several overlapping phases such as hemostasis, inflammation, proliferation, and remodeling. During the proliferative phase, ECM remodeling plays a crucial role in the formation of granulation tissue, angiogenesis, and epithelialization [99]. MMPs facilitate the breakdown of the old ECM to allow for the deposition of new ECM components, such as collagen types I and III, fibronectin, and glycosaminoglycans [100]. In diabetic individuals, the wound healing process is significantly impaired, and this is partly due to the dysregulated activity of MMPs. Diabetes induces a hyperglycemic environment that leads to several pathological changes in immune function, inflammatory responses, and ECM remodeling [101]. Elevated glucose levels in diabetes promote an inflammatory state, marked by the overproduction of pro-inflammatory cytokines such as tumor necrosis factor-alpha (TNF-α) and interleukins (IL-1, IL-6). These cytokines, in turn, upregulate MMP expression [102]. Chronic inflammation in diabetic wounds leads to a prolonged presence of MMPs at the wound site, which disrupts the normal remodeling of ECM. In diabetic wounds, MMPs, particularly MMP-2 and MMP-9, are overexpressed, resulting in excessive ECM degradation [103].

Under normal conditions, TIMPs inhibit MMPs and maintain the balance between ECM degradation and deposition. In diabetic wounds, however, there is often a relative deficiency in TIMPs or an increase in their degradation, which exacerbates MMP activity [104]. This imbalance leads to uncontrolled ECM breakdown, preventing proper tissue regeneration and prolonging the inflammatory phase of wound healing. The dysregulation of TIMP expression in diabetes further exacerbates the problem [105]. Specifically, studies have found decreased levels of TIMP-1 in diabetic ulcers, which results in a reduced ability to inhibit the overexpression of MMPs and restrict excessive ECM turnover [103].

3.2 Hyperglycemia-induced oxidative stress

Hyperglycemia in diabetes leads to an increase in the production of reactive oxygen species (ROS) through several mechanisms. One primary pathway is the auto-oxidation of glucose, where glucose itself undergoes oxidation, generating ROS such as superoxide anion (O_2^-) [106]. Additionally, hyperglycemia increases the flux through polyol and hexosamine pathways, both of which contribute to ROS production. The polyol pathway, in particular, converts excess glucose to sorbitol, and this process generates NADH, which indirectly enhances ROS production [107]. In addition, hyperglycemia promotes the formation of advanced glycation end products (AGEs), which are products of nonenzymatic reactions between reducing sugars and proteins [108]. AGEs interact with receptors known as Receptor for AGEs (RAGE), activating signaling pathways that further promote oxidative stress, inflammation, and vascular damage [15]. The accumulation of ROS disrupts cellular functions and causes lipid peroxidation, DNA damage, and protein misfolding, which contribute to cell dysfunction. This oxidative burden impairs fibroblast and endothelial cell function, preventing effective tissue regeneration and prolonging the inflammatory phase of wound healing [109].

Elevated blood glucose exacerbates the upregulation of these MMPs through the generation of ROS, which activates signaling pathways like Nuclear Factor kappa-light-chain-enhancer of activated B cells (NF-kB) and Activator Protein 1 (AP-1), leading to increased transcription of MMP genes [110]. However, in diabetes, this balance is disrupted due to reduced TIMP expression or increased oxidative stress, leading to elevated MMP activity [111]. This results in excessive ECM breakdown, particularly collagen degradation, which weakens the wound site and impairs granulation tissue formation, ultimately delaying proper wound closure [26]. For instance, MMPs can cleave and inactivate platelet-derived growth factor (PDGF) and transforming growth factor-beta (TGF-β), both of which are pivotal in fibroblast proliferation, collagen synthesis, and wound contraction. This dysregulated ECM turnover contributes to delayed wound healing, poor tissue regeneration, and the chronicity of DFUs [112].

3.3 Involvement of MMP activity in diabetic wounds

In diabetic wounds, the activity of matrix metalloproteinases (MMPs) is significantly altered, contributing to impaired wound healing [103]. **Figure 2** illustrates the molecular mechanisms leading to impaired healing in diabetes. In normal wound

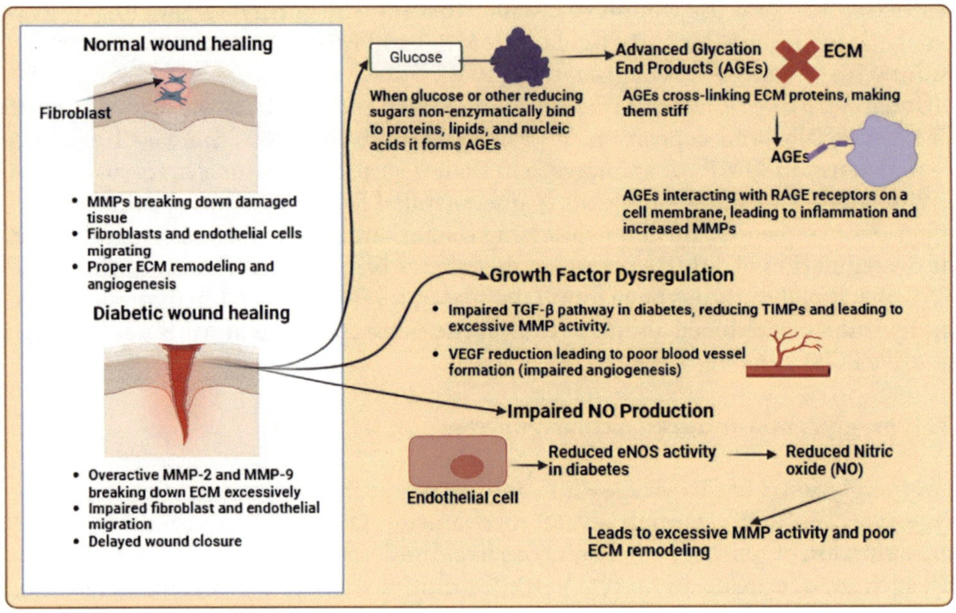

Figure 2.
Molecular mechanisms underlying impaired wound healing in diabetes.

healing, matrix metalloproteinases (MMPs) degrade damaged tissue, allowing fibroblasts and endothelial cells to migrate and facilitate extracellular matrix (ECM) remodeling and angiogenesis [113]. However, in diabetic wound healing, excessive MMP-2 and MMP-9 activity leads to excessive ECM breakdown, impairing fibroblast and endothelial cell migration, ultimately delaying wound closure [114]. The diagram highlights that glucose forms advanced glycation end products (AGEs) by nonenzymatically binding to proteins, lipids, and nucleic acids. AGEs cross-link ECM proteins, making them stiff, and interact with RAGE receptors, triggering inflammation and further increasing MMP activity [115]. Growth factor dysregulation in diabetes impairs the TGF-β pathway, reducing tissue inhibitors of metalloproteinases (TIMPs) and leading to excessive MMP activity, while VEGF reduction results in poor blood vessel formation and impaired angiogenesis [116]. Additionally, impaired nitric oxide (NO) production due to reduced endothelial nitric oxide synthase (eNOS) activity in diabetes exacerbates excessive MMP activity and poor ECM remodeling, further hindering wound healing [117].

4. Pathophysiological findings: MMPs as biomarkers in DFUs

Figure 3 illustrates the pathophysiology of diabetic foot ulcers (DFUs), a severe complication of diabetes mellitus. High glucose levels lead to neuropathy (nerve damage), causing a loss of sensation in the foot, and vasculopathy (blood vessel damage), reducing blood flow and oxygen supply. Additionally, diabetes impairs immune function, making it harder to fight infections and heal wounds [118]. The ulcer healing process is further disrupted by increased pro-inflammatory cytokine production, reduced angiogenesis, oxidative stress (hydroxyl radical formation), and damaged extracellular matrix (ECM), growth factors, and stroma cells. These impair

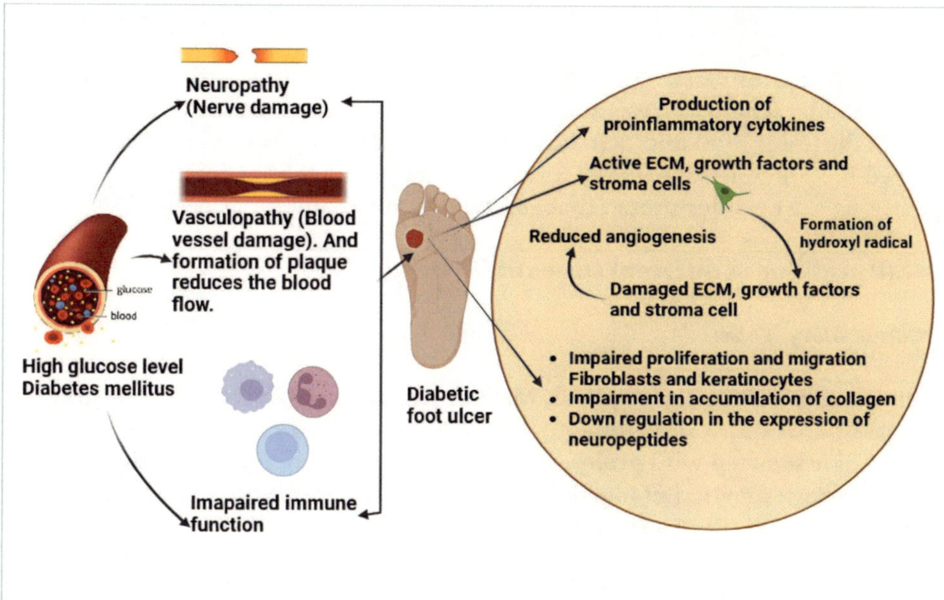

Figure 3.
Pathophysiology of diabetic foot ulcer.

fibroblast and keratinocyte migration, collagen accumulation, and neuropeptide expression, leading to chronic nonhealing ulcers [119, 120]. **Figure 4** illustrates that prolonged hyperglycemia leads to collagen cross-linking disorders, inflammation, impaired immune response, and disrupted angiogenesis, causing defective wound

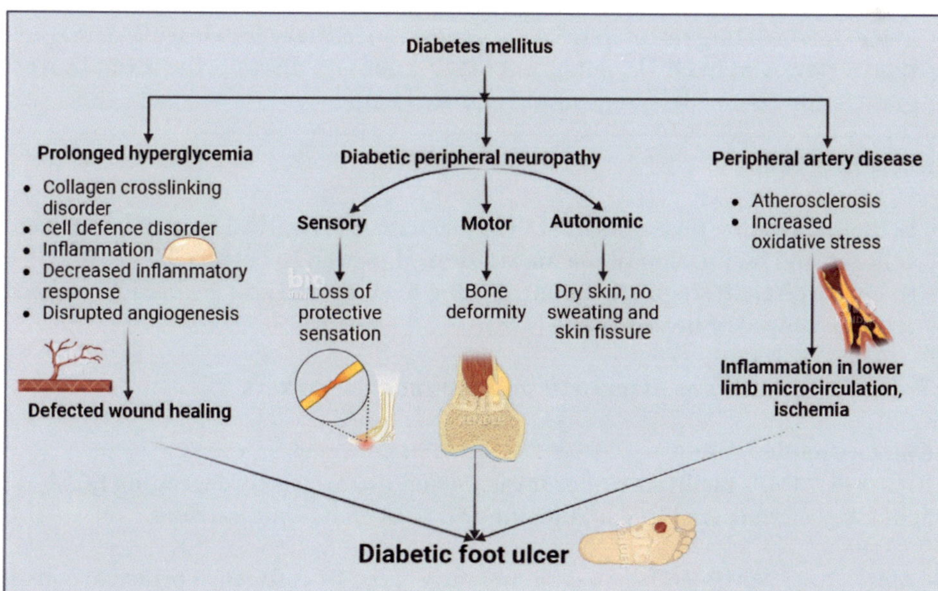

Figure 4.
Etiology of diabetic foot ulcer.

healing [121]. Diabetic peripheral neuropathy affects sensory, motor, and autonomic functions, resulting in loss of sensation, bone deformities, and dry skin with fissures, increasing the risk of ulcers [122]. Additionally, peripheral artery disease (PAD), characterized by atherosclerosis and oxidative stress, leads to ischemia and inflammation in the lower limb microcirculation, further delaying wound healing. These combined factors contribute to the formation and poor healing of diabetic foot ulcers, emphasizing the need for proper diabetes management and foot care [123].

4.1 MMP profiling in different stages of DFUs

Inflammatory phase:

- In the early inflammatory phase, MMP-8 (collagenase-2) and MMP-9 (gelatinase-B) are significantly upregulated. MMP-9, derived primarily from neutrophils, is associated with prolonged inflammation and delayed healing in DFUs. Studies have shown that high levels of MMP-9 correlate with increased wound size and poor healing outcomes [124].

- MMP-8, which degrades type I collagen, is also elevated in the inflammatory phase and contributes to tissue destruction if not regulated. The imbalance between MMP-8 and its inhibitor, TIMP-1, exacerbates ECM degradation [125].

Proliferative phase:

- During the proliferative phase, MMP-2 (gelatinase-A) and MMP-1 (collagenase-1) play a dual role. While MMP-2 is essential for angiogenesis and keratinocyte migration, its overexpression in DFUs leads to excessive degradation of basement membrane components, impairing re-epithelialization [126, 127].

- MMP-1, which targets interstitial collagens, is necessary for clearing damaged tissue. However, in DFUs, persistent MMP-1 activity disrupts the formation of granulation tissue, delaying wound closure [103].

Remodeling phase:

- In the remodeling phase, MMP-13 (collagenase-3) is critical for resolving excess collagen and facilitating tissue maturation. However, in chronic DFUs, MMP-13 levels are often dysregulated, contributing to abnormal scar formation and poor tensile strength of healed tissue [128].

4.2 Potential of MMPs as diagnostic and prognostic markers

Oncology applications.

In cancer, MMPs facilitate tumor invasion and metastasis by degrading ECM components, thereby enabling malignant cells to breach tissue barriers.

- *MMP-2 and MMP-9:* These gelatinases target type IV collagen, a principal constituent of basement membranes. Their heightened activity has been linked to increased metastatic potential in colorectal cancer, melanoma, breast, lung, ovarian, and prostate cancers [129]. Notably, MMP-2 mRNA levels in surrounding stromal tissue, rather than within the tumor itself, have been associated with metastasis, suggesting the tumor microenvironment's pivotal role in cancer progression [130].

- *MMP-28 (epilysin):* Overexpression of MMP-28 has been observed in various tumors, with associations to tumor diameter, invasion depth, and metastatic stage. Patients exhibiting high MMP-28 expression often face reduced survival rates, positioning it as a potential prognostic marker [131].

Cardiovascular Implications.

MMPs contribute to the pathophysiology of several cardiovascular conditions through ECM remodeling and modulation of inflammatory responses.

- *MMP-3:* This enzyme has been implicated in exacerbating traumatic brain injuries by disrupting the blood-brain barrier (BBB). Increased MMP-3 activity post-injury leads to degradation of tight junction proteins like claudin-5 and occludin, resulting in enhanced BBB permeability and subsequent neuronal damage [132].

- *MMP-9:* Elevated MMP-9 levels have been linked to the development of aortic aneurysms. Inhibition of MMP-9 activity, such as through doxycycline administration, has demonstrated a reduction in aneurysm progression, highlighting its potential as a therapeutic target and prognostic marker [133].

5. Therapeutic strategies targeting MMPs in diabetic foot

Various natural compounds such as EGCG, curcumin, and genistein have demonstrated MMP-inhibitory activity through diverse mechanisms (**Table 2**).

In addition to natural compounds, synthetic MMP inhibitors like batimastat, marimastat, and nanotechnology-based agents have been explored for DFU treatment (**Table 3**).

Natural MMPs inhibitor	Source	Mechanism of action	References
Epigallocatechin-3-gallate (EGCG)	Green tea (*Camellia sinensis*)	EGCG, a major green tea polyphenol, inhibits MMP-2, MMP-9, and MMP-14 through multiple mechanisms. It binds to the catalytic zinc ion of MMPs, blocking their activity, and suppresses MMP expression by inhibiting NF-κB and AP-1 signaling. Additionally, EGCG reduces oxidative stress by scavenging free radicals and enhancing antioxidant enzymes. It also upregulates TIMPs.	[134, 135]
Curcumin	Turmeric (*Curcuma longa*)	Curcumin, derived from turmeric, inhibits MMP-2, MMP-9, and MMP-14 by suppressing NF-κB, MAPK, and PI3K/Akt pathways essential for MMP transcription. It directly binds to the zinc-binding domain of MMPs, blocking their activity. Additionally, curcumin reduces ROS production and downregulates pro-inflammatory cytokines like TNF-α and IL-1β.	[136, 137]

Natural MMPs inhibitor	Source	Mechanism of action	References
Genistein	Soybeans (*Glycine max*)	Genistein, an isoflavone in soybeans, inhibits MMP-2 and MMP-9 by blocking ERK1/2 and PI3K/Akt pathways and acting as a tyrosine kinase inhibitor. It suppresses NF-κB and AP-1, enhances TIMP expression, and reduces oxidative stress.	[138, 139]
Resveratrol	Grapes (*Vitis vinifera*)	Resveratrol, a grape-derived polyphenol, inhibits MMP-2, MMP-9, and MMP-13 by suppressing NF-κB and AP-1 pathways. It upregulates TIMPs, reduces oxidative stress by enhancing antioxidant enzymes, and downregulates pro-inflammatory cytokines like TNF-α and IL-6.	[140]
Quercetin	Apples, onions, and berries	Quercetin, a flavonoid in apples and onions, inhibits MMP-2 and MMP-9 by suppressing MAPK and NF-κB pathways. It chelates the zinc ion in MMPs, directly inhibiting their activity, reduces oxidative stress by enhancing antioxidant enzymes, and downregulates pro-inflammatory cytokines.	[141, 142]
Catechins	Green tea (*Camellia sinensis*)	Catechins inhibit MMP-1, MMP-2, and MMP-9 by binding to their active sites and blocking proteolytic activity.	[143]
Sulforaphane	Broccoli (*Brassica oleracea*)	Sulforaphane inhibits MMP-2, MMP-9, and MMP-14 by suppressing NF-κB and MAPK pathways.	[144]
Ellagic Acid	Pomegranate (*Punica granatum*)	Ellagic acid inhibits MMP-2 and MMP-9 by suppressing NF-κB and MAPK pathways.	[145]
Berberine	*Berberis* species	Berberine inhibits MMP-2 and MMP-9 by suppressing AP-1 and NF-κB pathways. It upregulates TIMP-1 and TIMP-2, counteracting MMP activity, and reduces oxidative stress by enhancing antioxidant enzymes.	[146]
Luteolin	Celery, parsley, and chamomile	Luteolin inhibits MMP-2 and MMP-9 by blocking PI3K/Akt and MAPK pathways and suppressing NF-κB activation. Its antioxidant properties further reduce oxidative stress, limiting MMP expression.	[147]
Caffeic acid phenethyl ester (CAPE)	Propolis (beehive product)	CAPE inhibits MMP-2 and MMP-9 by suppressing NF-κB and MAPK pathways and directly blocking MMP activity. Its anti-inflammatory and antioxidant properties further enhance its MMP-inhibitory effects.	[148]
Silymarin	Milk thistle (*Silybum marianum*)	Silymarin inhibits MMP-2 and MMP-9 by suppressing NF-κB and AP-1 pathways. It reduces oxidative stress and inflammation, further limiting MMP expression.	[149]
Carnosol	Rosemary (*Rosmarinus officinalis*)	Carnosol inhibits MMP-9 by suppressing NF-κB and AP-1 pathways and upregulating TIMP-1. Its antioxidant properties further enhance its MMP-inhibitory effects.	[150]
Apigenin	Parsley, chamomile, and celery	Apigenin inhibits MMP-2 and MMP-9 by suppressing PI3K/Akt and MAPK pathways and reducing NF-κB signaling. Its antioxidant properties further enhance its MMP-inhibitory effects.	[151]

Natural MMPs inhibitor	Source	Mechanism of action	References
Kaempferol	Tea, broccoli, and grapes	Kaempferol inhibits MMP-2 and MMP-9 by suppressing NF-κB and MAPK pathways. It reduces oxidative stress and inflammation.	[152]
Marine-derived compounds			
Sulfated polysaccharide	Red algae (*Gelidium crinale*)	A sulfated polysaccharide inhibits MMP-2 and MMP-9 by suppressing NF-κB and PI3K/Akt pathways. It prevents IκBα degradation, reducing NF-κB activation and MMP transcription.	[153]
Astaxanthin	Marine microalgae (e.g., *Haematococcus pluvialis*)	Astaxanthin, a marine microalgae carotenoid, inhibits MMPs by scavenging ROS, which activates AP-1 and MAPK pathways.	[154]
Eckol	Brown algae (e.g., *Ecklonia cava*)	Eckol, a brown algae phlorotannin, inhibits MMP-1 and MMP-9 by blocking ERK and p38 phosphorylation in the MAPK pathway. It also reduces TNF-α and IL-1β levels, limiting MMP expression *via* NF-κB and AP-1.	[155]
Microbial-derived compounds			
Salinosporamide A	Marine bacterium (*Salinispora tropica*)	Salinosporamide A inhibits MMP-9 by blocking proteasome activity, preventing IκBα degradation and NF-κB activation. It also suppresses the MAPK pathway, reducing MMP-9 expression and activity.	[156]
Aspulvinone	Marine-derived	Aspulvinone MMP-9 by suppressing MAPK signaling and reducing ERK, JNK, and p38 phosphorylation.	[157]

Table 2.
Natural origin MMP inhibitors.

MMPs inhibitor	Structure	MOA	Reference
Small molecule inhibitor			
Batimastat	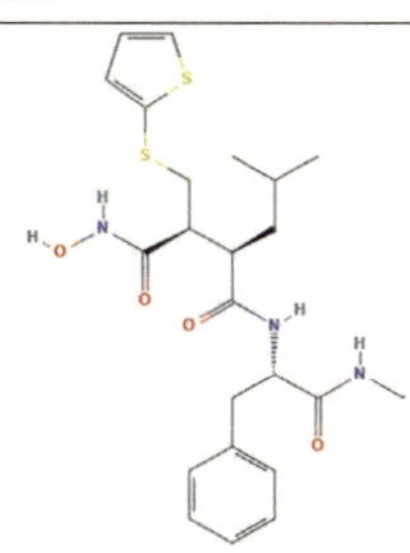	Batimastat is a broad-spectrum MMP inhibitor that chelates the zinc ion at the active site of MMPs, preventing substrate binding and catalytic activity. It specifically targets MMP-2, MMP-9, and MMP-14, which are involved in tumor invasion and angiogenesis.	[158]
Marimastat	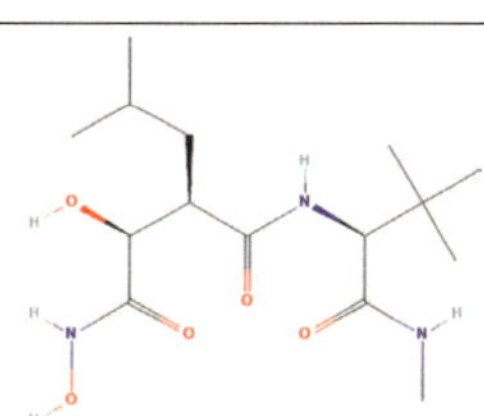	Marimastat is a synthetic hydroxamate-based inhibitor that binds to the zinc-binding domain of MMPs, inhibiting their proteolytic activity.	[159]

MMPs inhibitor	Structure	MOA	Reference
Prinomastat	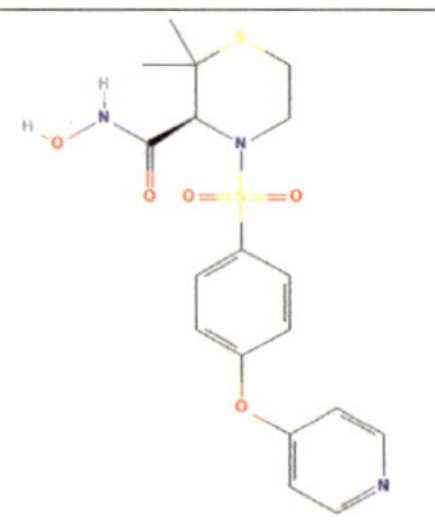	Prinomastat selectively inhibits MMP-2 and MMP-9 by mimicking the collagen substrate and binding to the active site. It also disrupts the interaction between MMPs and their natural inhibitors (TIMPs).	[160]
Tetracyclines as MMP inhibitors			
Doxycycline	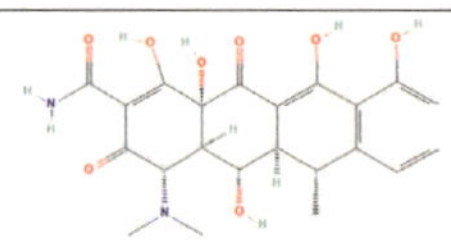	Doxycycline inhibits MMPs by chelating zinc and calcium ions at the catalytic site, reducing MMP-2, MMP-8, and MMP-9 activities.	[161]
Minocycline	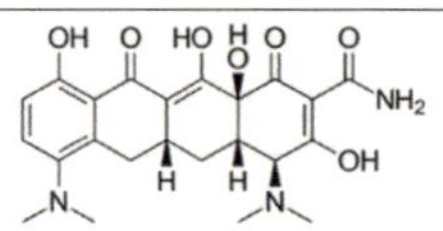	Minocycline inhibits MMP-9 by blocking its activation pathway, which involves the ERK1/2 and JNK signaling pathways. It also reduces oxidative stress, which indirectly suppresses MMP expression.	[162]
Nanotechnology-based MMP inhibitors			
Gold nanoparticles	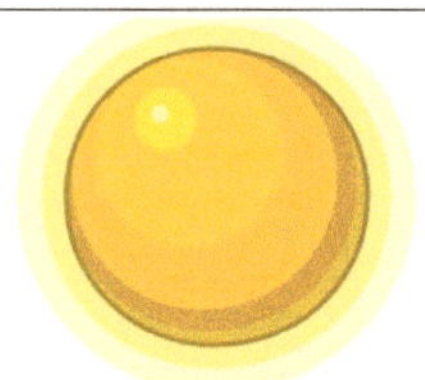	AuNPs functionalized with MMP-specific peptides (e.g., CTT peptide) selectively bind to MMP-2 and MMP-9, blocking their activity. The nanoparticles also enhance drug delivery to tumor sites.	[163]
Liposomal-encapsulated inhibitors	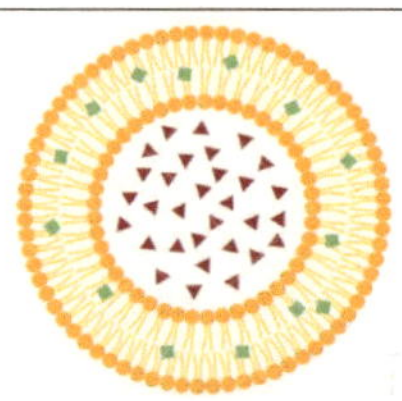	Liposomes encapsulating MMP inhibitors provide targeted delivery to tumor tissues. The liposomes release the inhibitor in response to the acidic tumor microenvironment, ensuring localized inhibition of MMP-2 and MMP-9.	[164]
Polymeric nanoparticles	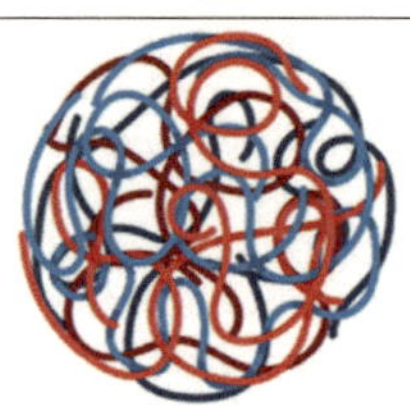	Polymeric nanoparticles (e.g., PLGA-based) loaded with MMP inhibitors degrade slowly, providing sustained release of the inhibitor. They also reduce systemic toxicity and enhance bioavailability.	[165]
Dendrimers	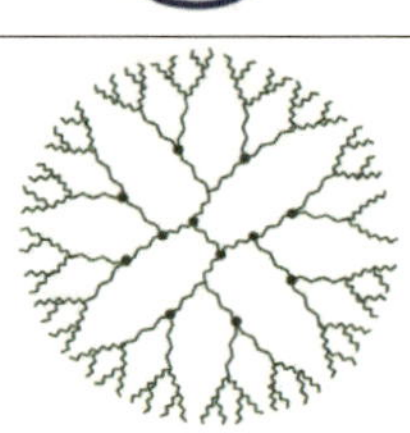	Dendrimers conjugated with MMP inhibitors target MMP-overexpressing cells. The dendrimers' multivalent surface allows for high-affinity binding to MMPs, enhancing inhibitory efficacy.	[166]

Table 3.
Synthetic MMP inhibitors.

6. Recent advances and future perspectives

6.1 Novel drug delivery approaches

Figure 4 illustrates the various novel drug delivery approaches for diabetic foot ulcers (DFUs). It categorizes different systems such as nanoparticle-based delivery, hydrogels, microneedle patches, liposomal delivery, electrospun nanofibers, topical gels and creams, and biological scaffolds. Each category highlights specific formulations, such as polymeric nanoparticles (PLGA, chitosan), hyaluronic acid-based hydrogels, biodegradable microneedles, lipid-based vesicles, ECM-mimicking scaffolds, and nanostructured lipid carriers [167–170]. The benefits of these advanced delivery systems include controlled release, enhanced wound penetration, sustained drug release, improved retention, and structural support, making them promising strategies for effective DFU treatment [171].

6.2 Gene therapy targeting and RNA-based therapeutics targeting MMPs in DFUs

Gene therapy offers a potential solution to modulate MMP expression and activity in DFUs. The approach involves delivering genetic material to cells to either upregulate or downregulate specific MMPs [172], depending on the therapeutic goal. Key strategies include:

Gene silencing:

Using small interfering RNA (siRNA) or short hairpin RNA (shRNA) to target and degrade MMP mRNA, thereby reducing MMP expression. For example, studies have shown that siRNA-mediated knockdown of MMP-9 can reduce excessive ECM degradation and promote wound healing in diabetic models [173].

Gene overexpression:

In some cases, overexpression of tissue inhibitors of metalloproteinases (TIMPs), which are natural inhibitors of MMPs, can restore the balance between MMPs and TIMPs. Gene therapy approaches using plasmid DNA or viral vectors to deliver TIMP genes have shown promise in preclinical studies [174, 175].

siRNA-based approaches:

siRNA targeting MMP-9 has been shown to reduce its expression in diabetic wound models, leading to improved wound healing outcomes [176]. Delivery systems such as lipid nanoparticles, hydrogels, or microneedles are being developed to enhance the stability and targeted delivery of siRNA to wound sites [171].

miRNA-based approaches:

miRNAs are small noncoding RNAs that regulate gene expression post-transcriptionally. Certain miRNAs, such as miR-21 and miR-29, have been implicated in the regulation of MMP expression [177]. For example, miR-29 has been shown to downregulate MMP-9, and its delivery *via* nanoparticles has demonstrated enhanced wound healing in diabetic models [103].

Antisense oligonucleotides (ASOs):

ASOs can bind to MMP mRNA and prevent its translation, effectively reducing MMP levels. Preclinical studies have shown that ASOs targeting MMP-2 and MMP-9 can improve wound healing by reducing ECM degradation and inflammation [178].

6.3 Clinical trials and emerging trends in DFU management

6.3.1 Clinical trials in DFU management

Clinical trials for diabetic foot ulcer (DFU) management focus on enhancing wound healing, preventing infections, and reducing amputations. Key areas of investigation include advanced wound care products, such as bioactive dressings containing growth factors (e.g., recombinant human epidermal growth factor), antimicrobial agents (e.g., silver, iodine), and collagen-based matrices, which aim to accelerate wound closure and reduce bacterial load [179]. Stem cell therapy, particularly using mesenchymal stem cells (MSCs) and platelet-rich plasma (PRP), is being explored for its regenerative potential in promoting angiogenesis and tissue repair [180]. Hyperbaric oxygen therapy (HBOT) is under clinical assessment for its ability to enhance oxygen delivery to hypoxic tissues, improving healing in refractory DFUs [181]. Gene therapy trials are investigating gene-based interventions, such as viral vector-mediated delivery of growth factor genes (e.g., VEGF), to modulate inflammation and promote tissue regeneration [182]. Given the rising concern of antibiotic resistance, researchers are testing alternatives like bacteriophages, antimicrobial peptides, and biofilm-disrupting agents for infected DFUs [183]. Additionally, wearable technologies that monitor wound parameters in real time (e.g., temperature, moisture, pH) are being evaluated to enable personalized treatment adjustments, potentially optimizing DFU management [184].

6.3.2 Emerging trends in DFU management

Emerging trends in diabetic foot ulcer (DFU) management emphasize personalized, multidisciplinary, and technology-driven approaches. Bioengineered skin substitutes, such as Apligraf and Dermagraft, provide scaffolds for tissue regeneration and growth factor delivery [185]. Research on microbiome modulation is exploring probiotics and microbiome-targeted therapies to restore microbial balance and enhance healing [186]. Artificial intelligence (AI) and machine learning are being applied to wound image analysis, outcome prediction, and treatment recommendations, improving diagnostic accuracy and reducing clinician workload [187].

6.4 Challenges in translating MMP inhibitors to clinical use in DFUs

Complex role of MMPs in wound healing:

MMPs are a family of zinc-dependent endopeptidases that play a dual role in wound healing. While they are essential for extracellular matrix (ECM) remodeling and tissue repair, their overexpression in chronic wounds, such as DFUs, leads to excessive degradation of ECM components, growth factors, and cytokines, impairing healing [126]. The challenge lies in selectively inhibiting pathological MMP activity without disrupting their beneficial roles in wound repair. Nonselective MMP inhibitors have shown adverse effects in clinical trials, such as impaired wound closure and musculoskeletal toxicity [188].

Lack of selectivity in MMP inhibitors:

Many early-generation MMP inhibitors (e.g., batimastat and marimastat) were broad-spectrum and targeted multiple MMPs, leading to off-target effects and toxicity [189]. For example, inhibition of MMP-1 (collagenase-1) has been associated with musculoskeletal syndrome, a significant side effect observed in clinical trials [190].

Heterogeneity of DFUs:

DFUs are highly heterogeneous in terms of etiology, microbial load, and inflammatory profile. This variability complicates the design of clinical trials and the identification of patient subgroups that may benefit most from MMP inhibition [191]. The presence of biofilms and persistent infections in DFUs further complicates the therapeutic efficacy of MMP inhibitors, as biofilms can alter the local MMP expression and activity [192].

Pharmacokinetic and delivery challenges:

MMP inhibitors often have poor bioavailability and stability, limiting their effectiveness when administered systemically [188]. Local delivery methods, such as topical formulations or biomaterial-based delivery systems, are being explored but face challenges in achieving sustained and controlled release at the wound site [193]. **Figure 5** illustrates the structured overview of strategies for developing selective matrix metalloproteinase (MMP) inhibitors for diabetic foot ulcers (DFUs). It highlights six key approaches: (1) Advances in structural biology and computational modeling for designing selective MMP inhibitors [194]; (2) Combination therapies involving antibiotics, growth factors, or stem cells to enhance healing [195]; (3) Biomaterial-based delivery systems using hydrogels, nanoparticles, and scaffolds for controlled release and improved bioavailability [196]; (4) personalized medicine approaches that tailor treatments based on patient-specific MMP expression and biomarkers [197]; (5) robust clinical trials focusing on larger sample sizes, standardized measures, and optimal therapy duration [198]; and (6) exploration of natural MMP inhibitors such as polyphenols and flavonoids, which may offer fewer side effects than synthetic inhibitors (**Figure 6**) [199].

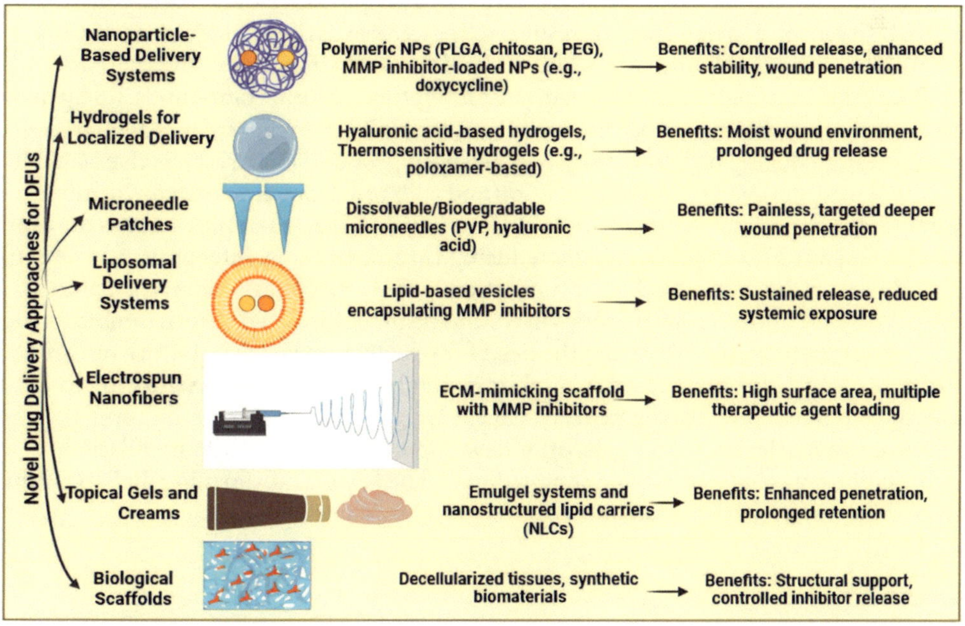

Figure 5.
Novel drug delivery approaches for DFUs.

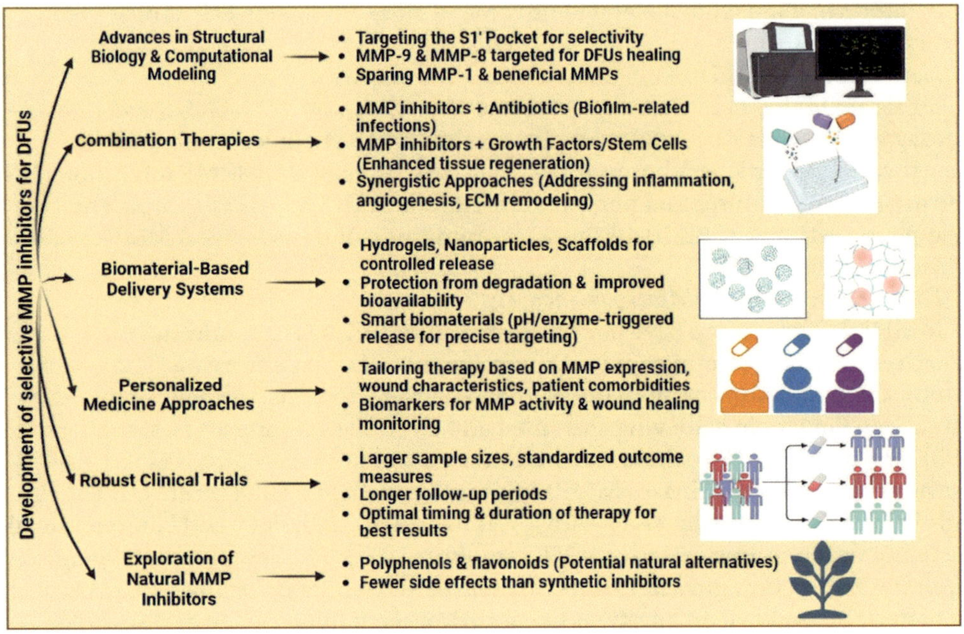

Figure 6.
Future directions for MMP inhibitors in DFUs.

7. Conclusion

Research on MMP-targeted therapies for diabetic wound healing underscores the critical role of matrix metalloproteinases (MMPs) in the impaired healing process seen in diabetic patients. Diabetic wounds often exhibit a dysregulated balance between MMPs and their tissue inhibitors (TIMPs), resulting in excessive extracellular matrix (ECM) degradation, chronic inflammation, and delayed tissue repair. Studies suggest that MMP-targeted therapies, including synthetic inhibitors, natural compounds, and gene-based approaches, show promise in preclinical models by restoring balance, enhancing angiogenesis, reducing inflammation, and promoting wound closure. Selective MMP-9 inhibition has improved re-epithelialization and collagen deposition in diabetic models, highlighting the potential of isoform-specific targeting. These therapies address the root causes of impaired healing, potentially reducing chronic wounds, infections, and amputations. However, challenges in clinical translation include specificity concerns, off-target effects, and the complex role of MMPs in wound healing. Broad-spectrum inhibitors have shown adverse effects, emphasizing the need for selective approaches. Future research should focus on developing targeted inhibitors, combination therapies with growth factors or stem cells, and robust clinical trials. Advances in biomaterials and drug delivery, such as nanoparticles and hydrogels, offer new opportunities for MMP modulation. Interdisciplinary collaboration and innovation will be key to transforming diabetic wound care and improving patient outcomes.

Abbreviations

DFU	diabetic foot ulcer
MMP	matrix metalloproteinase

ECM	extracellular matrix
RAGE	receptor for advanced glycation end products
TIMP	tissue inhibitor of metalloproteinase
NO	nitric oxide
TNF-α	tumor necrosis factor-alpha
AGE	advanced glycation end product
FGF	fibroblast growth factor
VEGF	vascular endothelial growth factor
HGF	hepatocyte growth factor
IL	interleukin
NF-κB	nuclear factor kappa-light-chain-enhancer of activated B cells
TGF-β	transforming growth factor-beta
ROS	reactive oxygen species
AP-1	activator protein 1
PDGF	platelet-derived growth factor
eNOS	endothelial nitric oxide synthase
PAD	peripheral artery disease
BBB	blood-brain barrier
EGCG	epigallocatechin-3-gallate
MAPK	mitogen-activated protein kinase
PI3K/Akt	phosphoinositide 3-kinase/protein kinase B
IL-1β	interleukin-1 beta
IL-6	interleukin-6
ERK	extracellular signal-regulated kinase
JNK	c-Jun N-terminal kinase
CAPE	caffeic acid phenethyl ester
PLGA	poly(lactic-co-glycolic acid)
AuNP	gold nanoparticle
SiRNA	small interfering RNA
ShRNA	short hairpin RNA
PRP	platelet-rich plasma
HBOT	hyperbaric oxygen therapy
MSC	mesenchymal stem cell
ASO	antisense oligonucleotide
RNA	ribonucleic acid
DNA	deoxyribonucleic acid
AI	artificial intelligence

Author details

Satheesh Babu Natarajan[1*], Gayathri Anbumani Alamelu[1], Saravanakumar Parameswaran[1], Suriyakala Perumal Chandran[2], Chadapully Kolumbu Ismail Sajeeth[3], S. M. Fazeela Mahaboob Begum[4] and Anandarajagopal Kalusalingam[5]

1 School of Pharmacy, Lincoln University College, Selangor, Malaysia

2 Faculty of Medicine, Lincoln University College, Selangor, Malaysia

3 Prime College of Pharmacy, Palakkad, India

4 School of Life Sciences, B S Abdur Rahman Crescent Institute of Science and Technology, Chennai, India

5 School of Pharmacy, KPJ Healthcare University, Nilai, Malaysia

*Address all correspondence to: satheeshbabumpharm@gmail.com

References

[1] Wang X, Yuan CX, Xu B, Yu Z. Diabetic foot ulcers: Classification, risk factors and management. World Journal of Diabetes. 2022;**13**(12):1049

[2] van Schie CH, Boulton AJ. Biomechanics of the diabetic foot: The road to foot ulceration. The Diabetic Foot. 2006;(10):185-200

[3] Schie CH, Boulton AJ. Biomechanics of the diabetic foot. The Diabetic Foot. 2006;(10):185-200. DOI: 10.1007/978-1-59745-075-1_10

[4] Botros M, Kuhnke J, Embil J, Goettl K, Morin C, Parsons L, et al. Prevention and management of diabetic foot ulcers. In: Canadian Association of Wound Care. Toronto: Wounds Canada; 2019

[5] Mairghani M. Diabetic foot ulcers (DFU) in Bahrain; An epidemiological profile of the prevalence, clinical care, economic cost and impact on quality of life [doctoral dissertation]. Dublin, Ireland: Royal College of Surgeons in Ireland; 2014

[6] Lazzarini PA, Jarl G. Knee-high devices are gold in closing the foot ulcer gap: A review of offloading treatments to heal diabetic foot ulcers. Medicina. 2021;**57**(9):941

[7] Attarde DV, Nawani N. Empowering wound care strategies: Best practices for effective wound healing. New Delhi, India: Springer Nature; 2021

[8] Harris AM, Hicks LA, Qaseem A, High Value Care Task Force of the American College of Physicians and for the Centers for Disease Control and Prevention. Appropriate antibiotic use for acute respiratory tract infection in adults: Advice for high-value care from the American College of Physicians and the Centers for Disease Control and Prevention. Annals of Internal Medicine. 2016;**164**(6):425-434

[9] Moore Z, Avsar P, Wilson P, Mairghani M, O'Connor T, Nugent L, et al. Diabetic foot ulcers: Treatment overview and cost considerations. Journal of Wound Care. 2021;**30**(10):786-791

[10] Pradhan L, Nabzdyk C, Andersen ND, LoGerfo FW, Veves A. Inflammation and neuropeptides: The connection in diabetic wound healing. Expert Reviews in Molecular Medicine. 2009;**11**:e2

[11] Landén NX, Li D, Ståhle M. Transition from inflammation to proliferation: A critical step during wound healing. Cellular and Molecular Life Sciences. 2016;**73**:3861-3885

[12] Van Putte L, De Schrijver S, Moortgat P. The effects of advanced glycation end products (AGEs) on dermal wound healing and scar formation: A systematic review. Scars, Burns & Healing. 2016;**2**:2059513116676828

[13] Bansode SB, Gacche RN. Glycation-induced modification of tissue-specific ECM proteins: A pathophysiological mechanism in degenerative diseases. Biochimica et Biophysica Acta (BBA)-General Subjects. 2019;**1863**(11):129411

[14] Blair MJ, Jones JD, Woessner AE, Quinn KP. Skin structure–function relationships and the wound healing response to intrinsic aging. Advances in Wound Care. 2020;**9**(3):127-143

[15] Xie J, Méndez JD, Méndez-Valenzuela V, Aguilar-Hernández MM. Cellular signalling of the receptor for advanced glycation end products

(RAGE). Cellular Signalling. 2013;**25**(11):2185-2197

[16] Jabłońska-Trypuć A, Matejczyk M, Rosochacki S. Matrix metalloproteinases (MMPs), the main extracellular matrix (ECM) enzymes in collagen degradation, as a target for anticancer drugs. Journal of Enzyme Inhibition and Medicinal Chemistry. 2016;**31**(Suppl. 1):177-183

[17] Wolosowicz M, Prokopiuk S, Kaminski TW. The complex role of matrix Metalloproteinase-2 (MMP-2) in health and disease. International Journal of Molecular Sciences. 2024;**25**(24):13691

[18] Bonham PA. Assessment and management of patients with venous, arterial, and diabetic/neuropathic lower extremity wounds. AACN Advanced Critical Care. 2003;**14**(4):442-456

[19] Triggle CR, Ding H. A review of endothelial dysfunction in diabetes: A focus on the contribution of a dysfunctional eNOS. Journal of the American Society of Hypertension. 2010;**4**(3):102-115

[20] Sekhon BS. Matrix metalloproteinases–an overview. Research and Reports in Biology. 2010;(1):1-20

[21] Ravanti L, Kähäri VM. Matrix metalloproteinases in wound repair. International Journal of Molecular Medicine. 2000;**6**(4):391-798

[22] Cabral-Pacheco GA, Garza-Veloz I, Castruita-De la Rosa C, Ramirez-Acuña JM, Perez-Romero BA, Guerrero-Rodriguez JF, et al. The roles of matrix metalloproteinases and their inhibitors in human diseases. International Journal of Molecular Sciences. 2020;**21**(24):9739

[23] Nissinen L, Kähäri VM. Matrix metalloproteinases in inflammation. Biochimica et Biophysica Acta (BBA)-General Subjects. 2014;**1840**(8):2571-2580

[24] Eming SA, Krieg T, Davidson JM. Inflammation in wound repair: Molecular and cellular mechanisms. Journal of Investigative Dermatology. 2007;**127**(3):514-525

[25] Martins VL, Caley M, O'Toole EA. Matrix metalloproteinases and epidermal wound repair. Cell and Tissue Research. 2013;**351**:255-268

[26] Xue M, Jackson CJ. Extracellular matrix reorganization during wound healing and its impact on abnormal scarring. Advances in Wound Care. 2015;**4**(3):119-136

[27] Thomas JT, Joseph B, Waltimo T. Matrix Metalloproteinases (MMPs). Advances in Gingival Diseases and Conditions. 2024:37

[28] Yanhan R, Guosheng G, Min Y, Driver VR. Role of matrix metalloproteinases in chronic wound healing: Diagnostic and therapeutic implications. Chinese Medical Journal. 2014;**127**(8):1572-1581

[29] Uccioli L, Izzo V, Meloni M, Vainieri E, Ruotolo V, Giurato L. Non-healing foot ulcers in diabetic patients: General and local interfering conditions and management options with advanced wound dressings. Journal of Wound Care. 2015;**24**(Sup. 4b):35-42

[30] Powell HC, Rosoff J, Myers RR. Microangiopathy in human diabetic neuropathy. Acta Neuropathologica. 1985;**68**:295-305

[31] Leone A, Vitiello C, Gullì C, Sikora AK, Macagnino S, Colosimo C. Bone and soft tissue infections in patients

with diabetic foot. La Radiologia Medica. 2020;**125**:177-187

[32] Afonso AC, Oliveira D, Saavedra MJ, Borges A, Simões M. Biofilms in diabetic foot ulcers: Impact, risk factors and control strategies. International Journal of Molecular Sciences. 2021;**22**(15):8278

[33] Murphy G, Stanton H, Cowell S, Butler G, Knäuper V, Atkinson S, et al. Mechanisms for pro matrix metalloproteinase activation. APMIS. 1999;**107**(1-6):38-44

[34] Philips N, Samuel M, Arena R, Chen YJ, Conte J, Natarajan P, et al. Direct inhibition of elastase and matrix metalloproteinases and stimulation of biosynthesis of fibrillar collagens, elastin, and fibrillins by xanthohumol (vol 61, pg 125, 2010). Journal of Cosmetic Science. 2010;**61**(6):485

[35] Pardo A, Selman M. MMP-1: The elder of the family. The International Journal of Biochemistry & Cell Biology. 2005;**37**(2):283-288

[36] Keskin ES, Keskin ER, Öztürk MB, Çakan D. The effect of MMP-1 on wound healing and scar formation. Aesthetic Plastic Surgery. 2021;**45**:2973-2979

[37] Lafuma C, El Nabout RA, Crechet F, Hovnanian A, Martin M. Expression of 72-kDa gelatinase (MMP-2), collagenase (MMP-1), and tissue metalloproteinase inhibitor (TIMP) in primary pig skin fibroblast cultures derived from radiation-induced skin fibrosis. Journal of Investigative Dermatology. 1994;**102**(6):945-950

[38] Bauvois B. New facets of matrix metalloproteinases MMP-2 and MMP-9 as cell surface transducers: Outside-in signaling and relationship to tumor progression. Biochimica et Biophysica Acta (BBA)-Reviews on Cancer. 2012;**1825**(1):29-36

[39] Kim IS, Yang WS, Kim CH. Physiological properties, functions, and trends in the matrix metalloproteinase inhibitors in inflammation-mediated human diseases. Current Medicinal Chemistry. 2023;**30**(18):2075-2112

[40] Zheng L, Amano K, Iohara K, Ito M, Imabayashi K, Into T, et al. Matrix metalloproteinase-3 accelerates wound healing following dental pulp injury. The American Journal of Pathology. 2009;**175**(5):1905-1914

[41] Laronha H, Caldeira J. Structure and function of human matrix metalloproteinases. Cells. 2020;**9**(5):1076

[42] Hayden DM, Forsyth C, Keshavarzian A. The role of matrix metalloproteinases in intestinal epithelial wound healing during normal and inflammatory states. Journal of Surgical Research. 2011;**168**(2):315-324

[43] Dejonckheere E, Vandenbroucke RE, Libert C. Matrix metalloproteinase8 has a central role in inflammatory disorders and cancer progression. Cytokine & Growth Factor Reviews. 2011;**22**(2):73-81

[44] Van den Steen PE, Dubois B, Nelissen I, Rudd PM, Dwek RA, Opdenakker G. Biochemistry and molecular biology of gelatinase B or matrix metalloproteinase-9 (MMP-9). Critical Reviews in Biochemistry and Molecular Biology. 2002;**37**(6):375-536

[45] Turner RJ, Sharp FR. Implications of MMP9 for blood brain barrier disruption and hemorrhagic transformation following ischemic stroke. Frontiers in Cellular Neuroscience. 2016;**10**:180751

[46] Salmela MT, Pender SL, Karjalainen-Lindsberg ML, Puolakkainen P,

Macdonald TT, Saarialho-Kere U. Collagenase-1 (MMP-1), matrilysin-1 (MMP-7), and stromelysin-2 (MMP-10) are expressed by migrating enterocytes during intestinal wound healing. Scandinavian Journal of Gastroenterology. 2004;**39**(11):1095-1104

[47] Rohani MG, McMahan RS, Razumova MV, Hertz AL, Cieslewicz M, Pun SH, et al. MMP-10 regulates collagenolytic activity of alternatively activated resident macrophages. Journal of Investigative Dermatology. 2015;**135**(10):2377-2384

[48] Vaalamo M. Matrix metalloproteinases and their inhibitors in normal and aberrant wound repair: Expression patterns of Collagenases-1 and-3, Stromelysins-1 and-2, matrilysin, metalloelastase and TIMPs-1,-2,-3 and-4 in healing cutaneous wounds and in chrome ulcers of the skin and the intestine [doctoral dissertation]. Helsinki, Finland: University of Helsinki; 1999

[49] Lijnen HR, Van Hoef B, Vanlinthout I, Verstreken M, Rio MC, Collen D. Accelerated neointima formation after vascular injury in mice with stromelysin-3 (MMP-11) gene inactivation. Arteriosclerosis, Thrombosis, and Vascular Biology. 1999;**19**(12):2863-2870

[50] Bauters D, Van Hul M, Lijnen HR. Macrophage elastase (MMP-12) in expanding murine adipose tissue. Biochimica et Biophysica Acta (BBA)-General Subjects. 2013;**1830**(4):2954-2959

[51] Molet S, Belleguic C, Lena H, Germain N, Bertrand CP, Shapiro SD, et al. Increase in macrophage elastase (MMP-12) in lungs from patients with chronic obstructive pulmonary disease. Inflammation Research. 2005;**54**:31-36

[52] Vaalamo M, Mattila L, Johansson N, Kariniemi AL, Karjalainen-Lindsberg ML, Kähäri VM, et al. Distinct populations of stromal cells express collagenase-3 (MMP-13) and collagenase-1 (MMP-1) in chronic ulcers but not in normally healing wounds. Journal of Investigative Dermatology. 1997;**109**(1):96-101

[53] Toriseva MJ, Ala-aho R, Karvinen J, Baker AH, Marjomäki VS, Heino J, et al. Collagenase-3 (MMP-13) enhances remodeling of three-dimensional collagen and promotes survival of human skin fibroblasts. Journal of Investigative Dermatology. 2007;**127**(1):49-59

[54] Hongqing QY, Maeda M, Fu-Shin XY, Azar DT. Differential expression of MT1-MMP (MMP-14) and collagenase III (MMP-13) genes in normal and wounded rat corneas. Investigative Ophthalmology & Visual Science. 2000;**41**(10):2894-2899

[55] Chang JH, Huang YH, Cunningham CM, Han KY, Chang M, Seiki M, et al. Matrix metalloproteinase 14 modulates signal transduction and angiogenesis in the cornea. Survey of Ophthalmology. 2016;**61**(4):478-497

[56] Armstrong DG, Jude EB. The role of matrix metalloproteinases in wound healing. Journal of the American Podiatric Medical Association. 2002;**92**(1):12-18

[57] Strong AL, Semon JA, Strong TA, Santoke TT, Zhang S, McFerrin HE, et al. Obesity-associated dysregulation of calpastatin and MMP-15 in adipose-derived stromal cells results in their enhanced invasion. Stem Cells. 2012;**30**(12):2774-2783

[58] Wang H, Qi C, Wan D. MicroRNA-377-3p targeting MMP-16 inhibits ovarian cancer cell growth, invasion,

and interstitial transition. Annals of Translational Medicine. 2021;**9**(2):124

[59] Lijnen HR, Collen D. Role of the plasminogen and MMP systems in wound healing. In: Plasminogen: Structure, Activation, and Regulation. Boston, MA: Springer US; 2003. pp. 189-200

[60] Clements KM, Flannelly JK, Tart J, Brockbank SM, Wardale J, Freeth J, et al. Matrix metalloproteinase 17 is necessary for cartilage aggrecan degradation in an inflammatory environment. Annals of the Rheumatic Diseases. 2011;**70**(4):683-689

[61] Sedlacek R. RASI-1, MMP-19. In: Handbook of Proteolytic Enzymes. San Diego, CA, USA: Academic Press; 2004. pp. 559-561

[62] Beck IM, Rückert R, Brandt K, Mueller MS, Sadowski T, Brauer R, et al. MMP19 is essential for T cell development and T cell-mediated cutaneous immune responses. PLoS One. 2008;**3**(6):e2343

[63] Llano E, Pendás AM, Knäuper V, Sorsa T, Salo T, Salido E, et al. Identification and structural and functional characterization of human enamelysin (MMP-20). Biochemistry. 1997;**36**(49):15101-15108

[64] Cuéllar-Rivas E, Pustovrh-Ramos MC. The role of enamelysin (MMP-20) in tooth development. Systematic review. Revista Facultad de Odontología Universidad de Antioquia. 2015;**27**(1):154-176

[65] Marchenko GN, Marchenko ND, Strongin AY. The structure and regulation of the human and mouse matrix metalloproteinase-21 gene and protein. Biochemical Journal. 2003;**372**(2):503-515

[66] Wu T, Li Y, Lu J, Qiao Q, Bao G, Wang N, et al. Increased MMP-21 expression is associated with poor overall survival of patients with gastric cancer. Medical Oncology. 2013;**30**:1-6

[67] Galea CA, Nguyen HM, George Chandy K, Smith BJ, Norton RS. Domain structure and function of matrix metalloprotease 23 (MMP23): Role in potassium channel trafficking. Cellular and Molecular Life Sciences. 2014;**71**:1191-1210

[68] Moogk D, da Silva IP, Ma MW, Friedman EB, de Miera EV, Darvishian F, et al. Melanoma expression of matrix metalloproteinase-23 is associated with blunted tumor immunity and poor responses to immunotherapy. Journal of Translational Medicine. 2014;**12**:1

[69] Pirilä E, Korpi JT, Korkiamäki T, Jahkola T, Gutierrez-Fernandez A, Lopez-Otin C, et al. Collagenase-2 (MMP-8) and matrilysin-2 (MMP-26) expression in human wounds of different etiologies. Wound Repair and Regeneration. 2007;**15**(1):47-57

[70] Yamamoto H, Vinitketkumnuen A, Adachi Y, Taniguchi H, Hirata T, Miyamoto N, et al. Association of matrilysin-2 (MMP-26) expression with tumor progression and activation of MMP-9 in esophageal squamous cell carcinoma. Carcinogenesis. 2004;**25**(12):2353-2360

[71] Illman SA, Lohi J, Keski-Oja J. Epilysin (MMP-28)–structure, expression and potential functions. Experimental Dermatology. 2008;**17**(11):897-907

[72] Saarialho-Kere U, Kerkelä E, Suomela S, Jahkola T, Keski-Oja J, Lohi J. Epilysin (MMP-28) expression is associated with cell proliferation during

epithelial repair. Journal of Investigative Dermatology. 2002;**119**(1):14-21

[73] Halper J, Kjaer M. Basic components of connective tissues and extracellular matrix: Elastin, fibrillin, fibulins, fibrinogen, fibronectin, laminin, tenascins and thrombospondins. Progress in Heritable Soft Connective Tissue Diseases. 2014:31-47

[74] Afshar K, Sanaei MJ, Ravari MS, Pourbagheri-Sigaroodi A, Bashash D. An overview of extracellular matrix and its remodeling in the development of cancer and metastasis with a glance at therapeutic approaches. Cell Biochemistry and Function. 2023;**41**(8):930-952

[75] Fonović M, Turk B. Cysteine cathepsins and extracellular matrix degradation. Biochimica et Biophysica Acta (BBA)-General Subjects. 2014;**1840**(8):2560-2570

[76] Löfvall H, Newbould H, Karsdal MA, Dziegiel MH, Richter J, Henriksen K, et al. Osteoclasts degrade bone and cartilage knee joint compartments through different resorption processes. Arthritis Research & Therapy. 2018;**20**:1-3

[77] Yasuda Y, Kaleta J, Brömme D. The role of cathepsins in osteoporosis and arthritis: Rationale for the design of new therapeutics. Advanced Drug Delivery Reviews. 2005;**57**(7):973-993

[78] Mayfosh AJ, Nguyen TK, Hulett MD. The heparanase regulatory network in health and disease. International Journal of Molecular Sciences. 2021;**22**(20):11096

[79] Linder S, Cervero P, Eddy R, Condeelis J. Mechanisms and roles of podosomes and invadopodia. Nature Reviews Molecular Cell Biology. 2023;**24**(2):86-106

[80] Jacob A, Prekeris R. The regulation of MMP targeting to invadopodia during cancer metastasis. Frontiers in Cell and Developmental Biology. 2015;**3**:4

[81] Lin J, Shi Y, Men Y, Wang X, Ye J, Zhang C. Mechanical roles in formation of oriented collagen fibers. Tissue Engineering Part B: Reviews. 2020;**26**(2):116-128

[82] Wei J, Yao J, Yan M, Xie Y, Liu P, Mao Y, et al. The role of matrix stiffness in cancer stromal cell fate and targeting therapeutic strategies. Acta Biomaterialia. 2022;**150**:34-47

[83] Paiva KB, Granjeiro JM. Bone tissue remodeling and development: Focus on matrix metalloproteinase functions. Archives of Biochemistry and Biophysics. 2014;**561**:74-87

[84] Lu P, Takai K, Weaver VM, Werb Z. Extracellular matrix degradation and remodeling in development and disease. Cold Spring Harbor Perspectives in Biology. 2011;**3**(12):a005058

[85] Herrera J, Henke CA, Bitterman PB. Extracellular matrix as a driver of progressive fibrosis. The Journal of Clinical Investigation. 2018;**128**(1):45-53

[86] Zhao M, Wang L, Wang M, Zhou S, Lu Y, Cui H, et al. Targeting fibrosis: Mechanisms and clinical trials. Signal Transduction and Targeted Therapy. 2022;**7**(1):206

[87] Henke E, Nandigama R, Ergün S. Extracellular matrix in the tumor microenvironment and its impact on cancer therapy. Frontiers in Molecular Biosciences. 2020;**6**:160

[88] Vaalamo M, Leivo T, Saarialho-Kere U. Differential expression of tissue inhibitors of metalloproteinases (TIMP-1,-2,-3, and-4) in normal and aberrant

wound healing. Human Pathology. 1999;**30**(7):795-802

[89] Arpino V, Brock M, Gill SE. The role of TIMPs in regulation of extracellular matrix proteolysis. Matrix Biology. 2015;**44**:247-254

[90] Moore CS, Crocker SJ. An alternate perspective on the roles of TIMPs and MMPs in pathology. The American Journal of Pathology. 2012;**180**(1):12-16

[91] Justo BL, Jasiulionis MG. Characteristics of TIMP1, CD63, and β1-integrin and the functional impact of their interaction in cancer. International Journal of Molecular Sciences. 2021;**22**(17):9319

[92] Vaday GG, Lider O. Extracellular matrix moieties, cytokines, and enzymes: Dynamic effects on immune cell behavior and inflammation. Journal of Leukocyte Biology. 2000;**67**(2):149-159

[93] Wang T, He C. Pro-inflammatory cytokines: The link between obesity and osteoarthritis. Cytokine & Growth Factor Reviews. 2018;**44**:38-50

[94] Chen Q, Jin M, Yang F, Zhu J, Xiao Q, Zhang L. Matrix metalloproteinases: Inflammatory regulators of cell behaviors in vascular formation and remodeling. Mediators of Inflammation. 2013;**2013**(1):928315

[95] Schiller M, Javelaud D, Mauviel A. TGF-β-induced SMAD signaling and gene regulation: Consequences for extracellular matrix remodeling and wound healing. Journal of Dermatological Science. 2004;**35**(2):83-92

[96] Hidalgo M, Eckhardt SG. Development of matrix metalloproteinase inhibitors in cancer therapy. Journal of the National Cancer Institute. 2001;**93**(3):178-193

[97] Roeb E. Matrix metalloproteinases and liver fibrosis (translational aspects). Matrix Biology. 2018;**68**:463-473

[98] Clutterbuck AL, Asplin KE, Harris P, Allaway D, Mobasheri A. Targeting matrix metalloproteinases in inflammatory conditions. Current Drug Targets. 2009;**10**(12):1245-1254

[99] Gonzalez AC, Costa TF, Andrade ZD, Medrado AR. Wound healing-A literature review. Anais Brasileiros de Dermatologia. 2016;**91**(5):614-620

[100] Stamenkovic I. Extracellular matrix remodelling: The role of matrix metalloproteinases. The Journal of Pathology: A Journal of the Pathological Society of Great Britain and Ireland. 2003;**200**(4):448-464

[101] Shahen VA, Gerbaix M, Koeppenkastrop S, Lim SF, McFarlane KE, Nguyen AN, et al. Multifactorial effects of hyperglycaemia, hyperinsulinemia and inflammation on bone remodelling in type 2 diabetes mellitus. Cytokine & Growth Factor Reviews. 2020;**55**:109-118

[102] Maqsood M, Sharif S, Naz S, Farasat T, Manzoor F, Cheema M, et al. Expression of pro-inflammatory cytokines (IL-6 & IL-18) exacerbate the risk of diabetic nephropathy in the Pakistani population. Molecular Biology Reports. 2023;**50**(4):3249-3257

[103] Chen J, Qin S, Liu S, Zhong K, Jing Y, Wu X, et al. Targeting matrix metalloproteases in diabetic wound healing. Frontiers in Immunology. 2023;**14**:1089001

[104] McCarty SM, Percival SL. Proteases and delayed wound healing. Advances in Wound Care. 2013;**2**(8):438-447

[105] Basu S, Shukla V. Complications of wound healing. Measurements in Wound Healing: Science and Practice. 2012:109-144

[106] Kassab A, Piwowar A. Cell oxidant stress delivery and cell dysfunction onset in type 2 diabetes. Biochimie. 2012;**94**(9):1837-1848

[107] Garg SS, Gupta J. Polyol pathway and redox balance in diabetes. Pharmacological Research. 2022;**182**:106326

[108] Khalid M, Petroianu G, Adem A. Advanced glycation end products and diabetes mellitus: Mechanisms and perspectives. Biomolecules. 2022;**12**(4):542

[109] Juan CA, Pérez de la Lastra JM, Plou FJ, Pérez-Lebeña E. The chemistry of reactive oxygen species (ROS) revisited: Outlining their role in biological macromolecules (DNA, lipids and proteins) and induced pathologies. International Journal of Molecular Sciences. 2021;**22**(9):4642

[110] Kumar Rajendran N, George BP, Chandran R, Tynga IM, Houreld N, Abrahamse H. The influence of light on reactive oxygen species and NF-κB in disease progression. Antioxidants. 2019;**8**(12):640

[111] Kadoglou NP, Vrabas IS, Sailer N, Kapelouzou A, Fotiadis G, Noussios G, et al. Exercise ameliorates serum MMP-9 and TIMP-2 levels in patients with type 2 diabetes. Diabetes & Metabolism. 2010;**36**(2):144-151

[112] Pakyari M, Farrokhi A, Maharlooei MK, Ghahary A. Critical role of transforming growth factor beta in different phases of wound healing. Advances in Wound Care. 2013;**2**(5):215-224

[113] Rohani MG, Parks WC. Matrix remodeling by MMPs during wound repair. Matrix Biology. 2015;**44**:113-121

[114] Caley MP, Martins VL, O'Toole EA. Metalloproteinases and wound healing. Advances in Wound Care. 2015;**4**(4):225-234

[115] Zgutka K, Tkacz M, Tomasiak P, Tarnowski M. A role for advanced glycation end products in molecular ageing. International Journal of Molecular Sciences. 2023;**24**(12):9881

[116] Raeeszadeh-Sarmazdeh M, Do LD, Hritz BG. Metalloproteinases and their inhibitors: Potential for the development of new therapeutics. Cells. 2020;**9**(5):1313

[117] Ahmed R, Augustine R, Chaudhry M, Akhtar UA, Zahid AA, Tariq M, et al. Nitric oxide-releasing biomaterials for promoting wound healing in impaired diabetic wounds: State of the art and recent trends. Biomedicine & Pharmacotherapy. 2022;**149**:112707

[118] Jais S. Various types of wounds that diabetic patients can develop: A narrative review. Clinical Pathology. 2023;(16):2632010X231205366

[119] Swarnakar S, Ganguly K, Paul S. Regulating functions of angiogenesis in prevention and therapy of gastric ulcers. In: Angiogenesis: Insights from a Systematic Overview. 2013. pp. 159-171

[120] Feng J, Wang J, Wang Y, Huang X, Shao T, Deng X, et al. Oxidative stress and lipid peroxidation: Prospective associations between ferroptosis and delayed wound healing in diabetic ulcers. Frontiers in Cell and Developmental Biology. 2022;**10**:898657

[121] Baltzis D, Eleftheriadou I, Veves A. Pathogenesis and treatment of impaired

wound healing in diabetes mellitus: New insights. Advances in Therapy. 2014;**31**:817-836

[122] Haider R. Foot problems in patients with diabetes. Clinical Trials and Clinical Research. 2023;**2**(4):1-14. DOI: 10.31579/2834- 5126/029

[123] Hinchliffe RJ, Brownrigg JR, Apelqvist J, Boyko EJ, Fitridge R, Mills JL, et al. IWGDF guidance on the diagnosis, prognosis and management of peripheral artery disease in patients with foot ulcers in diabetes. Diabetes/Metabolism Research and Reviews. 2016;**32**:37-44

[124] Lazaro JL, Izzo V, Meaume S, Davies AH, Lobmann R, Uccioli L. Elevated levels of matrix metalloproteinases and chronic wound healing: An updated review of clinical evidence. Journal of Wound Care. 2016;**25**(5):277-287

[125] Luchian I, Goriuc A, Sandu D, Covasa M. The role of matrix metalloproteinases (MMP-8, MMP-9, MMP-13) in periodontal and peri-implant pathological processes. International Journal of Molecular Sciences. 2022;**23**(3):1806

[126] Fu K, Zheng X, Chen Y, Wu L, Yang Z, Chen X, et al. Role of matrix metalloproteinases in diabetic foot ulcers: Potential therapeutic targets. Frontiers in Pharmacology. 2022;**13**:1050630

[127] Wu S, Zhou Z, Li Y, Jiang J. Advancements in diabetic foot ulcer research: Focus on mesenchymal stem cells and their exosomes. Heliyon. 2024;**10**(17):e37031

[128] Toriseva M. The Regulation and Function of Collagenase-3 (MMP-13) in Cutaneous Wound Healing and Squamous Cell Carcinoma. Turku, Finland: University of Turku; 2012

[129] Augoff K, Hryniewicz-Jankowska A, Tabola R, Stach K. MMP9: A tough target for targeted therapy for cancer. Cancers. 2022;**14**(7):1847

[130] Neophytou CM, Panagi M, Stylianopoulos T, Papageorgis P. The role of tumor microenvironment in cancer metastasis: Molecular mechanisms and therapeutic opportunities. Cancers. 2021;**13**(9):2053

[131] Jian P, Yanfang T, Zhuan Z, Jian W, Xueming Z, Jian N. MMP28 (epilysin) as a novel promoter of invasion and metastasis in gastric cancer. BMC Cancer. 2011;**11**:1-8

[132] Sulhan S, Lyon KA, Shapiro LA, Huang JH. Neuroinflammation and blood–brain barrier disruption following traumatic brain injury: Pathophysiology and potential therapeutic targets. Journal of Neuroscience Research. 2020;**98**(1):19-28

[133] McMillan WD, Pearce WH. Increased plasma levels of metalloproteinase-9 are associated with abdominal aortic aneurysms. Journal of Vascular Surgery. 1999;**29**(1):122-129

[134] Singh BN, Shankar S, Srivastava RK. Green tea catechin, epigallocatechin-3-gallate (EGCG): Mechanisms, perspectives and clinical applications. Biochemical Pharmacology. 2011;**82**(12):1807-1821

[135] Ahmed S, Wang N, Lalonde M, Goldberg VM, Haqqi TM. Green tea polyphenol epigallocatechin-3-gallate (EGCG) differentially inhibits interleukin-1β-induced expression of matrix metalloproteinase-1 and-13 in human chondrocytes. The Journal

of Pharmacology and Experimental Therapeutics. 2004;**308**(2):767-773

[136] Yodkeeree S, Chaiwangyen W, Garbisa S, Limtrakul P. Curcumin, demethoxycurcumin and bisdemethoxycurcumin differentially inhibit cancer cell invasion through the down-regulation of MMPs and uPA. The Journal of Nutritional Biochemistry. 2009;**20**(2):87-95

[137] Kumar D, Kumar M, Saravanan C, Singh SK. Curcumin: a potential candidate for matrix metalloproteinase inhibitors. Expert Opinion on Therapeutic Targets. 2012;**16**(10):959-972

[138] Lima A, Oliveira J, Saúde F, Mota J, Ferreira RB. Proteins in soy might have a higher role in cancer prevention than previously expected: Soybean protein fractions are more effective MMP-9 inhibitors than non-protein fractions, even in cooked seeds. Nutrients. 2017;**9**(3):201

[139] Gupta A, Jain P, Nagori K, Adnan M. Treatment strategies for psoriasis using flavonoids from traditional Chinese medicine. Pharmacological Research-Modern Chinese Medicine. 2024;(4):100463

[140] Gonçalves AC, Rodrigues S, Rodrigues R, Silva LR. Potential Role of Dietary Phenolic Compounds in the Prevention and Treatment of Rheumatoid Arthritis: Current Reports. Pharmaceuticals. 6 May 2024;**17**(5):590

[141] Zaborowski MK, Długosz A, Błaszak B, Szulc J, Leis K. The role of quercetin as a plant-derived bioactive agent in preventive medicine and treatment in skin disorders. Molecules. 2024;**29**(13):3206

[142] Li Y, Yao J, Han C, Yang J, Chaudhry MT, Wang S, et al. Quercetin, inflammation and immunity. Nutrients. 2016;**8**(3):167

[143] Kim-Park WK, Allam ES, Palasuk J, Kowolik M, Park KK, Windsor LJ. Green tea catechin inhibits the activity and neutrophil release of matrix Metalloproteinase-9. Journal of Traditional and Complementary Medicine. 2016;**6**(4):343-346

[144] Rose P, Huang Q, Ong CN, Whiteman M. Broccoli and watercress suppress matrix metalloproteinase-9 activity and invasiveness of human MDA-MB-231 breast cancer cells. Toxicology and Applied Pharmacology. 2005;**209**(2):105-113

[145] Liu H, Zeng Z, Wang S, Li T, Mastriani E, Li QH, et al. Main components of pomegranate, ellagic acid and luteolin, inhibit metastasis of ovarian cancer by down-regulating MMP2 and MMP9. Cancer Biology & Therapy. 2017;**18**(12):990-999

[146] Liu SJ, Yin CX, Ding MC, Xia SY, Shen QM, Wu JD. Berberine suppresses in vitro migration of human aortic smooth muscle cells through the inhibitions of MMP-2/9, u-PA, AP-1, and NF-κB. BMB Reports. 2014;**47**(7):388

[147] Rocchetti MT, Bellanti F, Zadorozhna M, Fiocco D, Mangieri D. Multi-faceted role of luteolin in cancer metastasis: EMT, angiogenesis, ECM degradation and apoptosis. International Journal of Molecular Sciences. 2023;**24**(10):8824

[148] Sun W, Xie W, Huang D, Cui Y, Yue J, He Q, et al. Caffeic acid phenethyl ester attenuates osteoarthritis progression by activating NRF2/HO-1 and inhibiting the NF-κB signaling pathway. International Journal of Molecular Medicine. 2022;**50**(5):134

[149] Zare Z, Dizaj TN, Lohrasbi A, Sheikhalishahi ZS, Asadi A, Zakeri M, et al. Silibinin inhibits TGF-β-induced MMP-2 and MMP-9 through Smad Signaling pathway in colorectal cancer HT-29 cells. Basic & Clinical Cancer Research. 2020;**12**(2):81-90

[150] Alsamri H, El Hasasna H, Al Dhaheri Y, Eid AH, Attoub S, Iratni R. Carnosol, a natural polyphenol, inhibits migration, metastasis, and tumor growth of breast cancer via a ROS-dependent proteasome degradation of STAT3. Frontiers in Oncology. 2019;**9**:743

[151] Javed Z, Sadia H, Iqbal MJ, Shamas S, Malik K, Ahmed R, et al. Apigenin role as cell-signaling pathways modulator: Implications in cancer prevention and treatment. Cancer Cell International. 2021;**21**:1-1

[152] Chen HJ, Lin CM, Lee CY, Shih NC, Peng SF, Tsuzuki M, et al. Kaempferol suppresses cell metastasis via inhibition of the ERK-p38-JNK and AP-1 signaling pathways in U-2 OS human osteosarcoma cells. Oncology Reports. 2013;**30**(2):925-932

[153] Zheng H, Pei Y, He YL, Liu Y, Chen M, Hong P, et al. A Sulfated polysaccharide from red algae (Gelidium crinale) to suppress cells metastasis and MMP-9 expression of HT1080 cells. Food. 2022;**11**(15):2360

[154] Chou HY, Lee C, Pan JL, Wen ZH, Huang SH, Lan CW, et al. Enriched astaxanthin extract from Haematococcus pluvialis augments growth factor secretions to increase cell proliferation and induces MMP1 degradation to enhance collagen production in human dermal fibroblasts. International Journal of Molecular Sciences. 2016;**17**(6):955

[155] Besednova NN, Andryukov BG, Zaporozhets TS, Kuznetsova TA, Kryzhanovsky SP, Ermakova SP, et al. Molecular targets of brown algae phlorotannins for the therapy of inflammatory processes of various origins. Marine Drugs. 2022;**20**(4):243

[156] Ahn KS, Sethi G, Chao TH, Neuteboom ST, Chaturvedi MM, Palladino MA, et al. Salinosporamide a (NPI-0052) potentiates apoptosis, suppresses osteoclastogenesis, and inhibits invasion through down-modulation of NF-κB–regulated gene products. Blood, The Journal of the American Society of Hematology. 2007;**110**(7):2286-2295

[157] Qiu Y, Chen S, Yu M, Shi J, Liu J, Li X, et al. Natural products from marine-derived fungi with anti-inflammatory activity. Marine Drugs. 2024;**22**(10):433

[158] Brown PD, Giavazzi R. Matrix metalloproteinase inhibition: A review of anti-tumour activity. Annals of Oncology. 1995;**6**(10):967-974

[159] Rasmussen HS, PP MC. Matrix metalloproteinase inhibition as a novel anticancer strategy: A review with special focus on batimastat and marimastat. Pharmacology & Therapeutics. 1997;**75**(1):69-75

[160] Garcia CR, Bartsch DU, Rivero ME, Hagedorn M, McDermott CD, Bergeron-Lynn G, et al. Efficacy of Prinomastat®(AG3340), a matrix metalloprotease inhibitor, in treatment of retinal neovascularization. Current Eye Research. 2002;**24**(1):33-38

[161] Smith GN Jr, Mickler EA, Hasty KA, Brandt KD. Specificity of inhibition of matrix metalloproteinase activity by doxycycline: Relationship to structure of the enzyme. Arthritis & Rheumatism: Official Journal of the American College of Rheumatology. 1999;**42**(6):1140-1146

[162] Afshari AR, Mollazadeh H, Sahebkar A. Minocycline in treating glioblastoma multiforme: Far beyond a conventional antibiotic. Journal of Oncology. 2020;**2020**(1):8659802

[163] Sun R, Wang Y, Sun Q, Su Y, Zhang J, Liu D, et al. MMP-2 responsive gold Nanorods loaded with HSP-70 siRNA for enhanced photothermal tumor therapy. Molecular Pharmaceutics. 2024;**21**(11):5455-5468

[164] Lyu Y, Xiao Q, Yin L, Yang L, He W. Potent delivery of an MMP inhibitor to the tumor microenvironment with thermosensitive liposomes for the suppression of metastasis and angiogenesis. Signal Transduction and Targeted Therapy. 2019;**4**(1):26

[165] Li H, Yu SS, Miteva M, Nelson CE, Werfel T, Giorgio TD, et al. Matrix metalloproteinase responsive, proximity-activated polymeric nanoparticles for siRNA delivery. Advanced Functional Materials. 2013;**23**(24):3040-3052

[166] Haiba NS, Khalil HH, Bergas A, Abu-Serie MM, Khattab SN, Teleb M. First-in-class star-shaped triazine dendrimers endowed with MMP-9 inhibition and VEGF suppression capacity: Design, synthesis, and anticancer evaluation. ACS Omega. 2022;**7**(24):21131-21144

[167] Singh R, Lillard JW Jr. Nanoparticle-based targeted drug delivery. Experimental and Molecular Pathology. 2009;**86**(3):215-223

[168] Soppimath KS, Aminabhavi TM, Dave AM, Kumbar SG, Rudzinski WE. Stimulus-responsive "smart" hydrogels as novel drug delivery systems. Drug Development and Industrial Pharmacy. 2002;**28**(8):957-974

[169] Nazary Abrbekoh F, Salimi L, Saghati S, Amini H, Fathi Karkan S, Moharamzadeh K, et al. Application of microneedle patches for drug delivery; doorstep to novel therapies. Journal of Tissue Engineering. 2022;**13**:20417314221085390

[170] Li WJ, Mauck RL, Tuan RS. Electrospun nanofibrous scaffolds: Production, characterization, and applications for tissue engineering and drug delivery. Journal of Biomedical Nanotechnology. 2005;**1**(3):259-275

[171] Liu M, Wei X, Zheng Z, Li Y, Li M, Lin J, et al. Recent advances in nano-drug delivery systems for the treatment of diabetic wound healing. International Journal of Nanomedicine. 2023;(18):1537-1560

[172] Shaabani E, Sharifiaghdam M, Faridi-Majidi R, De Smedt SC, Braeckmans K, Fraire JC. Gene therapy to enhance angiogenesis in chronic wounds. Molecular Therapy-Nucleic Acids. 2022;**29**:871-899

[173] Waghode P, Quadir SS, Choudhary D, Sharma S, Joshi G. Small interfering RNA (siRNA) as a potential gene silencing strategy for diabetes and associated complications: Challenges and future perspectives. Journal of Diabetes & Metabolic Disorders. 2024;**23**(1):365-383

[174] Jean M, Alameh M, Buschmann MD, Merzouki A. Effective and safe gene-based delivery of GLP-1 using chitosan/plasmid-DNA therapeutic nanocomplexes in an animal model of type 2 diabetes. Gene Therapy. 2011;**18**(8):807-816

[175] Wong MS, Hawthorne WJ, Manolios N. Gene therapy in diabetes. Self/Nonself. 2010;**1**(3):165-175

[176] Li N, Luo HC, Yang C, Deng JJ, Ren M, Xie XY, et al. Cationic

star-shaped polymer as an siRNA carrier for reducing MMP-9 expression in skin fibroblast cells and promoting wound healing in diabetic rats. International Journal of Nanomedicine. 2014;(9):3377-3387

[177] Rubiś P, Totoń-Żurańska J, Wiśniowska-Śmiałek S, Holcman K, Kołton-Wróż M, Wołkow P, et al. Relations between circulating microRNAs (miR-21, miR-26, miR-29, miR-30 and miR-133a), extracellular matrix fibrosis and serum markers of fibrosis in dilated cardiomyopathy. International Journal of Cardiology. 2017;**231**:201-206

[178] Hong HJ, Jin SE, Park JS, Ahn WS, Kim CK. Accelerated wound healing by smad3 antisense oligonucleotides-impregnated chitosan/alginate polyelectrolyte complex. Biomaterials. 2008;**29**(36):4831-4837

[179] Deng X, Gould M, Ali MA. A review of current advancements for wound healing: Biomaterial applications and medical devices. Journal of Biomedical Materials Research Part B: Applied Biomaterials. 2022;**110**(11):2542-2573

[180] Anitua E, Troya M, Tierno R, Zalduendo M, Alkhraisat MH. The effectiveness of platelet-rich plasma as a carrier of stem cells in tissue regeneration: A systematic review of pre-clinical research. Cells, Tissues, Organs. 2021;**210**(5-6):339-350

[181] Goldman RJ. Hyperbaric oxygen therapy for wound healing and limb salvage: A systematic review. PM&R. 2009;**1**(5):471-489

[182] Eming SA, Krieg T, Davidson JM. Retracted: Gene therapy and wound healing. Clinics in Dermatology. 2007;**25**(1):79-92

[183] Larson D, Neelon J, Karna SR, Nuutila K. Local treatment of wound infections: A review of clinical trials from 2013 to 2024. Advances in Wound Care. 2025;**14**(1):14-32

[184] Lu SH, Samandari M, Li C, Li H, Song D, Zhang Y, et al. Multimodal sensing and therapeutic systems for wound healing and management: A review. Sensors and Actuators Reports. 2022;**4**:100075

[185] Mansbridge J. Skin substitutes to enhance wound healing. Expert Opinion on Investigational Drugs. 1998;**7**(5):803-809

[186] Al-Smadi K, Leite-Silva VR, Filho NA, Lopes PS, Mohammed Y. Innovative approaches for maintaining and enhancing skin health and managing skin diseases through microbiome-targeted strategies. Antibiotics. 2023;**12**(12):1698

[187] Dabas M, Schwartz D, Beeckman D, Gefen A. Application of artificial intelligence methodologies to chronic wound care and management: A scoping review. Advances in Wound Care. 2023;**12**(4):205-240

[188] Vandenbroucke RE, Libert C. Is there new hope for therapeutic matrix metalloproteinase inhibition? Nature Reviews Drug Discovery. 2014;**13**(12):904-927

[189] Roy R, Yang J, Moses MA. Matrix metalloproteinases as novel biomarker s and potential therapeutic targets in human cancer. Journal of Clinical Oncology. 2009;**27**(31):5287-5297

[190] Renkiewicz R, Qiu L, Lesch C, Sun X, Devalaraja R, Cody T, et al. Broad-spectrum matrix metalloproteinase inhibitor marimastat–induced musculoskeletal side effects in

rats. Arthritis & Rheumatism: Official Journal of the American College of Rheumatology. 2003;**48**(6):1742-1749

[191] Sadeghpour Heravi F, Zakrzewski M, Vickery K, G. Armstrong D, Hu H. Bacterial diversity of diabetic foot ulcers: Current status and future prospectives. Journal of Clinical Medicine. 2019;**8**(11):1935

[192] Srivastava P, Sondak T, Sivashanmugam K, Kim KS. A review of immunomodulatory reprogramming by probiotics in combating chronic and acute diabetic foot ulcers (DFUs). Pharmaceutics. 2022;**14**(11):2436

[193] Kaur G, Narayanan G, Garg D, Sachdev A, Matai I. Biomaterials-based regenerative strategies for skin tissue wound healing. ACS Applied Bio Materials. 2022;**5**(5):2069-2106

[194] Rao BG. Recent developments in the design of specific matrix metalloproteinase inhibitors aided by structural and computational studies. Current Pharmaceutical Design. 2005;**11**(3):295-322

[195] Jackson WM, Nesti LJ, Tuan RS. Mesenchymal stem cell therapy for attenuation of scar formation during wound healing. Stem Cell Research & Therapy. 2012;**3**:1-9

[196] Trucillo P. Biomaterials for drug delivery and human applications. Materials. 2024;**17**(2):456

[197] Kumar A, Mazumder A, Bansal P, Tyagi PK, Kaur A. Integrating Precision Medicine in Diabetes Mellitus: Enhancing Wound Healing and Shaping Future Therapies, Recent Advances in Inflammation & Allergy Drug Discovery. 2024;**18**:e27722708335238. DOI: 10.2174/0127722708335238240920035556

[198] Bolton LL. Quality randomized clinical trials of topical diabetic foot ulcer healing agents. Advances in Wound Care. 2016;**5**(3):137-147

[199] Kumar S, Bharali A, Sarma H, Kushari S, Gam S, Hazarika I, et al. Traditional complementary and alternative medicine (TCAM) for diabetic foot ulcer management: A systematic review. Journal of Ayurveda and Integrative Medicine. 2023;**14**(4):100745

Chapter 5

Perspective Chapter: Minimally Invasive Treatment for Post-Traumatic Neuropathic Pain

Giorgio Pietramaggiori, Federico Ricci, Franco Bassetto and Saja Scherer

Abstract

Addressing post-traumatic lower limb neuropathic pain is challenging. Several invasive and non-invasive approaches have been described with mixed results including wide neurolysis, neurectomy, and neuroma resection. Recently, minimally invasive techniques as adipose fat transfer showed good effectiveness and low complication rate. Adipose fat transfer is surgical technique in which the patient's own fat is harvested and injected to regenerate another area. The aim of this chapter is to examine the different techniques used to treat neuropathic pain after trauma and scar entrapment, focusing on our experience on minimally invasive techniques such as adipose fat transfer for scar regeneration and pain relief.

Keywords: neuropathic pain, regenerative surgery, adipose fat transfer, post-traumatic pain, nerve surgery, selective denervation, chronic pain

1. Introduction

Post-traumatic neuropathic pain (PTNP) refers to a specific type of chronic pain that arises because of an injury to the nervous system, typically following physical trauma [1, 2]. It is characterized by pain that results from nerve damage, which may involve the mostly the peripheral nerves and the spinal cord. The pain is often described as burning, tingling, stabbing, or shooting and is usually accompanied by sensory disturbances such as hyperalgesia (increased sensitivity to pain) or allodynia (pain from stimuli that do not normally provoke pain, like light touch) [3]. Unlike acute pain, which typically resolves as the body heals, PTNP can persist long after the initial injury has been treated. These symptoms not only cause physical discomfort but also significantly affect mental and emotional well-being, leading to issues such as anxiety, depression, and social withdrawal [4].

Post-traumatic neuropathic pain is a significant clinical issue, affecting many individuals worldwide. The exact prevalence varies depending on the population being studied, but it is estimated that approximately 10–30% of individuals with

IntechOpen

traumatic injuries will develop some form of neuropathic pain [5]. This can vary with the type of injury, with those suffering spinal cord injuries, amputations, or severe burns being at particular risk.

The impact of PTNP is multifaceted and profound. The chronic nature of the pain can lead to decreased mobility, muscle atrophy, and loss of functionality in the affected area, leading to physical disability [5, 6]. Chronic pain is a well-known risk factor for developing mental health conditions such as depression, anxiety, and post-traumatic stress disorder (PTSD). Patients with PTNP may experience feelings of helplessness, frustration, and despair due to the drug resistant nature of their pain [7]. This can impact the social and occupational aspect too. These patients often face difficulty in maintaining work and social relationships. As a consequence the financial burden is dramatic [5]. Chronic pain leads to substantial direct and indirect costs, including frequent medical visits, physical therapy, medications and loss of work ability.

Post-traumatic neuropathic pain can result from a variety of traumatic events, including:

- *Physical trauma:* This is the most common cause, including motor vehicle accidents, industrial accidents, combat injuries, falls, or sporting injuries. These events often lead to direct injury to the nerves, such as lacerations, crush injuries, or stretch injuries.

- *Surgical interventions:* In some cases, PTNP may develop after surgical procedures, particularly when nerves are inadvertently damaged during surgery or as a consequence of the post-operation scarring process.

- *Amputation:* One of the more specific forms of PTNP is phantom limb pain, which occurs after an amputation. In this condition, patients feel pain in a limb that no longer exists, often due to the brain's response to the loss of sensory input.

- *Spinal cord injury:* Injuries to the spinal cord can lead to widespread changes in both the central and peripheral nervous systems, causing neuropathic pain below the level of injury.

- *Burns:* Severe burns, particularly third-degree burns, can damage sensory nerves and lead to chronic pain that is neuropathic in nature.

- *Other traumatic events:* Even less common injuries, such as gunshot wounds, chemical exposures, or electrical burn, can lead to PTNP, depending on the nerves that are affected.

Understanding the mechanisms behind PTNP requires a basic grasp of how the nervous system processes pain.

The development of post-traumatic neuropathic pain involves complex neurophysiological processes. When nerves are damaged, whether through direct injury or inflammation, they may begin to send abnormal pain signals to the cortex. This abnormal signaling can cause persistent pain sensations, even when there is no ongoing injury [8].

DOI: http://dx.doi.org/10.5772/intechopen.1009949

Some of the key processes in the pathophysiology of PTNP include:

- Peripheral sensitization
- Central sensitization
- Ectopic activity
- Neuroinflammation

Damaged peripheral nerves become more sensitive, responding to stimuli that would normally not be painful. This damage can cause the nerve fibers to send abnormal signals to the cortex, even in the absence of a painful stimulus. Over time, these abnormal signals can lead to changes in the central nervous system, a process known as central sensitization. This makes the nervous system more sensitive to pain, creating a vicious cycle that perpetuates discomfort. This amplifies the pain sensation. In this context, injured nerves can fire spontaneously, leading to pain sensation not related to stimuli. The pain signals can be perpetuated by chronic inflammation of nerves [9].

Traditional treatments for PTNP often focus on managing symptoms rather than addressing the underlying causes. Medications such as antidepressants, anticonvulsants, and opioids are commonly prescribed as first-line therapeutics, but have limited efficacy and come with significant side effects. Physical therapy and psychological support are essential components of a holistic treatment plan, but may not provide sufficient relief for all patients. These challenges have driven the development of minimally invasive techniques that target the sources of pain more directly while reducing the risks associated with traditional surgical procedures.

Minimally invasive treatments, such as nerve blocks, adipose fat transfer (AFT), and selective denervation, represent a paradigm shift in how PTNP is managed. These approaches leverage advances in medical technology and regenerative medicine to offer precise and effective solutions. They aim to not only alleviate pain, but also improve nerve function and promote tissue healing, providing patients with a better quality of life [10, 11].

This chapter provides an in-depth exploration of the minimally invasive options available for PTNP, with a focus on their mechanisms, applications, and outcomes. By understanding these innovative treatments, patients and healthcare providers can make informed decisions about managing this debilitating condition.

2. Pathophysiology

The pathophysiology of post-traumatic neuropathic pain (PTNP) is multifaceted, involving a range of molecular, cellular, and neural adaptations that occur following injury. These changes occur both in the peripheral nerves and the central nervous system (CNS) and contribute to the abnormal and chronic pain that characterizes neuropathic pain syndromes. The hallmark of PTNP is that pain persists long after the tissue injury has healed, driven by maladaptive changes in the nervous system itself.

2.1 Peripheral sensitization

Peripheral sensitization refers to the increased responsiveness of sensory neurons to stimuli in the area surrounding the injury. This phenomenon occurs as the result of molecular changes within the injured nerves and the local environment in the tissues surrounding the nerve.

- Release of inflammatory mediators: After a traumatic injury, inflammatory mediators such as prostaglandins, bradykinin, substance P, interleukins, calcitonin gene-related peptide, and histamine are released by damaged tissues and immune cells. These molecules directly activate pain receptors (nociceptors) located on sensory nerve endings. They also enhance the excitability of these neurons, making them more responsive to stimuli.

- Activation of toll-like receptors: Damage to the peripheral nerve or surrounding tissues can activate the Toll-like receptors (TLRs) on the surface of immune cells. These receptors play a crucial role in recognizing danger signals from the injured tissue and triggering the release of pro-inflammatory cytokines and other mediators. This, contributes to sustained inflammation and pain hypersensitivity at the site of injury.

- Ion channel modulation: Following nerve injury, ion channels in the nerve membranes, particularly voltage-gated sodium channels (Nav), are altered. For instance, Nav1.7 and Nav1.8 sodium channels are upregulated in injured nerves, contributing to increased excitability of nociceptors. This reduction in the threshold for firing means that normally non-painful stimuli, such as touch or slight pressure, may be perceived as painful (allodynia).

- Neurotrophic factors and growth factors: In response to nerve injury, nerve growth factor (NGF) and brain-derived neurotrophic factor (BDNF) are upregulated. These growth factors promote the survival and sensitization of neurons and contribute to the persistence of pain signaling. NGF, in particular, increases the expression of certain ion channels and receptors that enhance the pain signal transmission.

- Ectopic nerve activity: The damaged peripheral nerve can begin firing spontaneously or at irregular rates. This ectopic activity occurs due to changes in the excitability of the nerve after injury. Injured axons may form neuromas, which are clusters of abnormal nerve growths that can generate spontaneous pain signals, even in the absence of external stimuli [1, 12].

2.2 Central sensitization

Central sensitization refers to the amplification of pain signals within the CNS, particularly within the dorsal horn of the spinal cord, where peripheral sensory neurons transmit their signals to second-order neurons. This process involves changes in the spinal cord and brain that increase the sensitivity of pain pathways and cause the nervous system to become more reactive to noxious and non-noxious stimuli alike.

- Glutamatergic transmission and NMDA (N-methyl-D-aspartate) receptor activation: One of the central mechanisms in sensitization is the increased release of the excitatory neurotransmitter glutamate in the dorsal horn of the spinal cord.

Glutamate binds to NMDA receptors on spinal neurons, leading to an increase in calcium influx. This influx of calcium enhances the transmission of pain signals and leads to synaptic plasticity, making pain pathways more efficient and persistent [9].

- Wind-up phenomenon: Wind-up is a process that occurs when repeated stimulation of sensory neurons in the spinal cord leads to a progressive increase in pain perception. This is caused by a long-term potentiation (LTP) of synapses in the dorsal horn, resulting in an exaggerated response to pain stimuli. This mechanism is thought to be responsible for the heightened sensitivity to pain, even in the absence of an ongoing injury [9, 13].

- Increased sensory processing: The somatosensory cortex and thalamus, which are key brain regions responsible for pain perception, may also undergo neuroplastic changes as a result of chronic pain. These changes lead to an increased sensitivity to pain (hyperalgesia) and the phenomenon of allodynia (pain from non-painful stimuli). This occurs because these brain regions "re-map" pain perception in response to chronic pain, leading to an amplification of sensory input [9, 13].

- Reduced inhibitory control: Under normal conditions, inhibitory neurons in the spinal cord (such as those utilizing GABA or glycine) help to dampen excessive pain signaling. However, in PTNP, these inhibitory pathways can become dysfunctional. A reduction in inhibitory signaling from the descending pain control pathways (which include serotonergic and noradrenergic systems) allows pain signals to be transmitted without adequate regulation, thus amplifying the pain experience [9, 13].

- Microglial activation: Microglia, the resident immune cells of the CNS, become activated following nerve injury and play a significant role in central sensitization. These cells release pro-inflammatory cytokines (e.g., TNF-alpha, IL-1β, IL-6) that increase the excitability of spinal cord neurons and contribute to the persistent pain state. Microglial activation is particularly important in chronic pain states, as they contribute to the sustained central amplification of pain signals [9].

2.3 Neuroinflammation

Neuroinflammation is a critical factor in the maintenance and progression of PTNP. The activation of immune cells and the release of inflammatory mediators both in the periphery and within the CNS can perpetuate pain.

- Peripheral neuroinflammation: Following traumatic nerve injury, there is often an influx of immune cells, such as macrophages, which release pro-inflammatory cytokines (e.g., TNF-alpha, IL-6) and chemokines. These mediators sensitize the peripheral nociceptors and increase pain transmission by enhancing nerve excitability. Chronic inflammation can also lead to tissue remodeling, further contributing to pain [3, 9].

- CNS neuroinflammation: After a peripheral injury, neuroinflammation spreads to the spinal cord and brain, where it activates microglia and astrocytes. These glial cells release additional pro-inflammatory cytokines and chemokines that sensitize pain-processing neurons in the spinal cord. This spinal neuroinflammation is a key driver of central sensitization and contributes to the persistence of pain even when the original injury has healed [3, 9].

- Astrocyte activation: Astrocytes, another type of glial cell in the spinal cord and brain, become activated after injury. In the case of PTNP, activated astrocytes release signaling molecules such as glutamate, ATP, and pro-inflammatory cytokines, which contribute to the hyperactivity of pain-processing neurons and the amplification of pain signals. Astrocytes play a pivotal role in mediating the cross-talk between neurons and glial cells, which amplifies and sustains pain [3, 9].

2.4 Ectopic activity and abnormal nerve firing

Ectopic activity refers to the abnormal firing of neurons following injury. This occurs both in peripheral nerves and in the spinal cord, and it is a major contributor to the experience of neuropathic pain.

- Peripheral ectopic activity: In response to nerve injury, peripheral axons can form neuromas—clumps of disorganized nerve fibers. These neuromas are prone to spontaneous firing and can generate abnormal pain signals that are transmitted to the spinal cord. This is one of the key mechanisms by which pain becomes persistent and independent of the original injury [14].

- Spinal cord ectopic activity: In the dorsal horn of the spinal cord, damaged sensory neurons can transmit abnormal signals to second-order neurons, even in the absence of external stimuli. This ectopic firing leads to an ongoing pain experience, including spontaneous pain and allodynia [14].

2.5 Descending modulation dysfunction

The descending pain modulation system involves pathways from the brainstem to the spinal cord that help to regulate pain. In PTNP, these pathways are often impaired.

- Dysfunction of descending inhibition: The brain has an innate ability to modulate pain through inhibitory pathways, which releases neurotransmitters such as serotonin and norepinephrine. These pathways normally reduce the transmission of pain signals from the spinal cord to the brain. However, in PTNP, there is often impaired descending inhibition, leading to reduced control over pain signals and contributing to the persistence of pain.

- Increased facilitation: In contrast, facilitatory pathways—such as those involving the neurotransmitter glutamate—may become upregulated after injury. This leads to an increase in pain signal transmission, further enhancing pain perception [12].

The pathophysiology of post-traumatic neuropathic pain (PTNP) is rooted in complex molecular and cellular processes involving peripheral sensitization, central sensitization, neuroinflammation, abnormal nerve activity, and dysfunction in descending pain control systems. Together, these factors create a persistent, maladaptive pain state that can be difficult to treat. Understanding the mechanisms at the molecular, cellular, and system levels is critical for developing targeted therapies that address the underlying causes of PTNP, rather than merely masking its symptoms.

This detailed understanding provides the foundation for effective interventions aimed at breaking the cycle of pain amplification and improving the patient outcomes.

3. Diagnosis

Diagnosing post-traumatic neuropathic pain (PTNP) requires a comprehensive approach, combining clinical assessment, detailed patient history, and diagnostic tests. PTNP is a complex condition where nerve damage following an injury leads to chronic, persistent pain, and diagnosing it accurately is crucial for determining the most appropriate treatment plan. The goal of diagnosis is to confirm that the pain is neuropathic in nature and that it arises from damage to the peripheral or central nervous system, rather than from other pain sources such as nociceptive pain or inflammatory pain [1, 10, 11].

3.1 Patient history

A thorough patient history is a critical first step in diagnosing PTNP. The clinician should focus on several key aspects:

Nature of the trauma: The history should include a detailed description of the traumatic event, including the type of injury (e.g., blunt force trauma, fracture, laceration, burn, surgical procedure, amputation) and the body areas affected. Certain types of injuries are more likely to lead to neuropathic pain, such as spinal cord injuries, nerve lacerations, or severe burns.

Pain characteristics and intensity: Describing the quality of the pain is central to diagnosing neuropathic pain. Patients typically describe PTNP as burning, shooting, stabbing, electric shock-like, or tingling. The clinician should inquire about the pain's intensity, location, and specific triggers, as well as any changes in pain sensation over time. The presence of spontaneous pain (pain without external stimuli) and paroxysmal pain (pain that comes in sudden bursts) are important indicators of neuropathic pain.

Onset and duration of pain: The clinician should establish when the pain started in relation to the trauma. PTNP typically persists for weeks or months after the initial injury, with some patients experiencing pain long after the tissue has healed. The onset of pain is often delayed, and it may not appear immediately after the injury.

Sensory disturbances: A history of sensory changes, such as numbness, tingling (paresthesia), or hyperalgesia (increased pain sensitivity), should be noted. Additionally, allodynia (pain in response to non-painful stimuli, such as light touch or brushing clothing) is a hallmark symptom of neuropathic pain and should be specifically queried.

Comorbidities and risk factors: The clinician should assess the patient's medical history to identify risk factors for neuropathic pain. This includes conditions such as diabetes mellitus, vascular disease, previous surgeries that may have affected nerves and infections (e.g., shingles). Psychological conditions, such as depression or anxiety, are also common in patients with chronic pain and may exacerbate the perception of pain.

3.2 Clinical examination

A comprehensive clinical examination helps identify the location, severity, and nature of neuropathic pain, and it is essential for determining whether the pain is due to nerve injury.

Sensory testing: Sensory function is assessed through a variety of tests that evaluate the presence of neuropathy or nerve damage [15]:

Light touch: A cotton wisp or monofilament can be used to test the skin's sensitivity to light touch. Decreased or absent sensation may suggest nerve damage.

Pinprick sensation: This test involves pricking the skin with a sterile pin to assess the patient's ability to feel sharp stimuli. An abnormal response, such as hypersensitivity or the inability to feel the stimulus, may indicate neuropathy.

Temperature sensation: Using cold or warm objects, the clinician can test the ability to distinguish between hot and cold sensations.

Vibration sense: Vibration is tested by applying a tuning fork over bony prominences to assess the function of the large nerve fibers responsible for proprioception and vibration sense.

Motor function: Motor function should be tested to assess whether the nerve damage has affected the motor components of the nerve. This includes checking for muscle weakness, atrophy, or abnormal reflexes. Nerve damage can result in weakness, paralysis, or diminished reflexes in the affected areas.

Deep tendon reflexes (DTRs): Reflexes are checked for abnormalities such as hyperreflexia (increased reflex responses) or hyporeflexia (diminished or absent reflexes), which can be signs of nerve dysfunction.

Hyperalgesia and allodynia testing: The presence of hyperalgesia (exaggerated pain in response to normally painful stimuli) and allodynia (pain caused by non-painful stimuli) is a hallmark of neuropathic pain. The clinician should use light touch, pressure, and thermal stimuli to assess the presence of these phenomena. For example, gently brushing the skin with a cotton swab or applying light pressure to the skin can reveal whether the patient experiences pain from non-noxious stimuli.

3.3 Diagnostic imaging

While imaging studies are not typically used to diagnose neuropathic pain, they can be helpful in ruling out other potential causes of pain or assessing the extent of nerve damage [16]:

Ultrasound and dynamic ultrasound: Static and dynamic ultrasound may identify focal caliber changes, or adherences to scar tissue along the course of the studied nerve.

Magnetic resonance imaging (MRI): MRI is often used to visualize soft tissue damage, including the spinal cord, nerve roots, and peripheral nerves. MRI can identify structural damage, such as spinal cord compression, herniated discs, or nerve impingement, which might contribute to PTNP. Functional MRI (fMRI) can be used in research settings to study brain activity related to pain perception [10].

Computed tomography (CT) Scan: CT scans are useful for assessing bone fractures or structural abnormalities that may be affecting nerve function. For example, after a traumatic injury or surgery, a CT scan can identify bone spurs or fractures that may be compressing peripheral or spinal nerves [10].

X-rays: Standard X-rays may be used to rule out fractures or dislocations that could be causing nerve compression or injury.

3.4 Electrophysiological studies (nerve conduction studies and electromyography - EMG)

Electrodiagnostic tests are important for assessing the integrity and function of peripheral nerves. These tests may help distinguish between neuropathic and musculoskeletal pain sources [17].

Nerve conduction studies (NCS): NCS measure the speed at which electrical signals travel along a nerve. Slower conduction speeds or decreased amplitudes of nerve signals can indicate nerve damage or dysfunction. This test can help localize the site of injury and assess the degree of nerve involvement in PTNP.

Electromyography (EMG): EMG measures the electrical activity of muscles at rest and during contraction. It can identify neuropathy, radiculopathy, or other conditions affecting the motor nerves. Abnormal spontaneous activity or low-amplitude motor unit potentials suggest nerve damage.

Quantitative sensory testing (QST): QST is a more specialized test used to evaluate sensory nerve function. It involves applying controlled stimuli (such as pressure, vibration, or temperature) to different skin areas and measuring the patient's sensory response. This can help determine whether there is any abnormal sensory processing or central sensitization [17].

3.5 Pain scales and questionnaires

Standardized pain assessment tools are used to evaluate the intensity, quality, and impact of pain on daily life. These tools help to quantify pain and provide a systematic approach to diagnosis and management.

Visual analog scale (VAS): VAS is a simple method for assessing pain intensity. The patient rates their pain on a scale from 0 (no pain) to 10 (worst pain imaginable). In our opinion, the ease of application makes this scale the most useful (**Figure 1**).

PTNP arises often early or immediately after the injury and is most of times unremitting.

Neuropathic pain scale (NPS): The NPS is specifically designed to assess the sensory and emotional characteristics of neuropathic pain, including pain quality (burning, shooting), and the presence of sensory disturbances (e.g., allodynia or hyperalgesia).

Douleur neuropathique 4 (DN4): The DN4 questionnaire is a widely used screening tool for diagnosing neuropathic pain. It includes questions about pain quality and specific sensory disturbances, such as the presence of burning sensations, shooting pains, and skin hypersensitivity.

McGill pain questionnaire: This tool assesses both the sensory and affective dimensions of pain. It helps to capture the complexity of neuropathic pain, which is often more than just physical discomfort and involves emotional and cognitive components [18, 19].

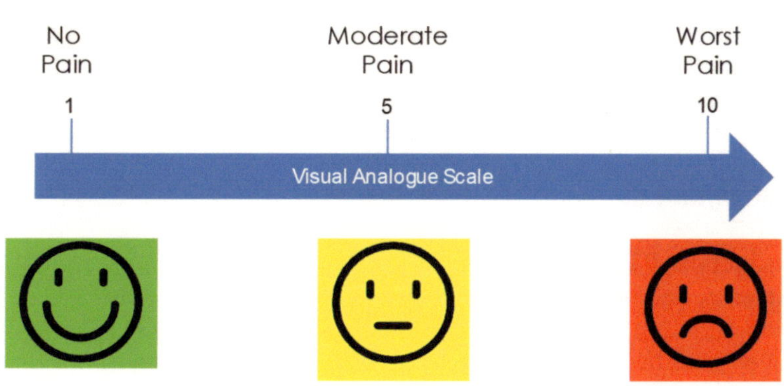

Figure 1.
Visual analogue scale (VAS) for pain assessment.

3.6 Differential diagnosis

One of the most challenging aspects of diagnosing PTNP is distinguishing it from other types of pain. Differential diagnoses should rule out:

Nociceptive pain: This is the pain resulting from injury to tissues, such as bone, muscle, or skin. Nociceptive pain typically responds well to analgesics and anti-inflammatory drugs, unlike neuropathic pain, which may require other therapeutic approaches.

Visceral pain: Pain arising from internal organs can sometimes mimic neuropathic pain. Conditions such as gastrointestinal or cardiovascular problems should be ruled out if symptoms overlap.

Psychogenic pain: Although psychogenic factors (e.g., stress, anxiety) can exacerbate pain, they are not the primary cause of PTNP. However, clinicians should consider whether a psychological component contributes to the pain experience.

Diagnosing post-traumatic neuropathic pain requires careful and comprehensive evaluation using a combination of detailed patient history, clinical examination, diagnostic imaging, electrophysiological testing, and pain scales. The goal is to differentiate PTNP from other types of pain, confirm the presence of nerve damage, and identify the most appropriate treatment approach. Early and accurate diagnosis is crucial for effectively managing PTNP and improving the patient's quality of life.

4. Treatment

The treatment of post-traumatic neuropathic pain (PTNP) involves a range of therapeutic options that span from pharmacological interventions to more invasive surgical procedures. Pharmacological treatments, such as antidepressants and anticonvulsants, are often the first line of defense, targeting the underlying mechanisms of nerve pain. If these medications are insufficient, interventional techniques such as nerve blocks, spinal cord stimulation, and radiofrequency ablation may be considered. In cases where pain persists despite other approaches, surgical options, including nerve decompression, neurolysis, adipose fat transfer, or selective denervation, offer a more definitive solution. A multimodal, personalized treatment strategy is typically employed to manage PTNP effectively, with a focus on improving quality of life and reducing pain [10, 11].

4.1 Physical therapy

Physical therapy (PT) is a crucial part of managing lower limb neuropathic pain (LLNP), especially for chronic pain that does not respond to pharmacological treatments alone. PT focuses on improving function, reducing pain, and enhancing quality of life through non-invasive techniques, including exercises and various modalities [20].

4.1.1 Goals of physical therapy

- Pain reduction: PT can reduce pain by improving circulation, stimulating endorphin release, and using methods such as TENS or heat/cold therapy.

- Improved mobility and function: By strengthening muscles, improving flexibility, and correcting gait abnormalities, PT restores movement and prevents muscle atrophy and joint stiffness.

- Prevention of complications: PT prevents complications, such as muscle wasting, contractures, and joint instability, commonly seen in long-term neuropathic pain.

- Balance and coordination: PT helps improve balance and proprioception, reducing the risk of falls and promoting functional independence [20].

4.1.2 Physical therapy techniques

- Strengthening: Focuses on strengthening muscles, especially in the quadriceps, hamstrings, and calves, to reduce joint strain.

- Stretching and flexibility: Targets improved range of motion, reducing muscle tightness and joint stiffness.

- Aerobic conditioning: Low-impact activities such as walking or cycling improve overall fitness and reduce pain.

4.1.3 Modalities

- TENS: Uses electrical currents to block pain signals.

- Heat and cold therapy: Reduces muscle spasms, inflammation, and pain through the application of heat or cold.

- Ultrasound therapy: Uses sound waves to promote healing and reduce deep tissue inflammation.

- Manual therapy:

- Joint mobilization: Helps improve flexibility and alleviate pain through controlled joint movements.

- Soft tissue mobilization: Reduces muscle tightness and spasms through massage techniques.

- Neuromuscular re-education: Helps retrain the nervous system to improve balance and movement, focusing on gait and proprioception exercises.

Treating LLNP with physical therapy can be challenging due to the heightened pain sensitivity associated with neuropathic conditions. It requires careful tailoring of exercises to avoid exacerbating pain while ensuring effectiveness. Psychological factors such as anxiety or depression can also affect patient engagement, requiring a holistic approach that may involve addressing emotional barriers.

Through targeted exercises, modalities, and manual therapy, PT can enhance mobility and quality of life, especially when combined with other pharmacological and interventional treatments. A patient-specific approach is essential for maximizing effectiveness and ensuring successful outcomes [21].

4.2 Pharmacological treatment

Pharmacological treatment is generally the first line for managing post-traumatic neuropathic pain (PTNP), especially when the pain is severe or difficult to control with non-pharmacological methods alone. A multimodal approach is often used, combining different classes of drugs to maximize efficacy and minimize side effects. Below is a detailed overview of the primary classes of medications used in the pharmacological management of PTNP [22, 23].

4.2.1 First-line medications

The first-line pharmacological treatments for PTNP typically include antidepressants and anticonvulsants, as these medications have been shown to be effective in modulating neuropathic pain mechanisms, particularly in terms of central sensitization and abnormal nerve firing.

4.2.1.1 Antidepressants

Certain antidepressants are particularly effective in treating neuropathic pain, even in the absence of a mood disorder. These medications target neurotransmitters such as serotonin and norepinephrine, which are involved in pain modulation.

Tricyclic antidepressants (TCAs) block the reuptake of norepinephrine and serotonin, which enhances the activity of these neurotransmitters in the pain-processing pathways in the brain and spinal cord. They also have an anticholinergic effect and can block sodium channels, which contributes to their analgesic effect.

Serotonin-norepinephrine reuptake inhibitors (SNRIs) block the reuptake of both serotonin and norepinephrine, which play key roles in descending pain modulation. By increasing the levels of these neurotransmitters in the spinal cord, SNRIs can reduce the transmission of pain signals [23].

4.2.1.2 Anticonvulsants

Anticonvulsants are often used as first-line agents because they target mechanisms involved in abnormal neuronal firing, which is a hallmark of neuropathic pain.

Gabapentinoids: Both gabapentin and pregabalin bind to the alpha-2-delta subunit of voltage-gated calcium channels. Examples: gabapentin (neurontin), pregabalin (Lyrica) [24].

4.3 Second-line medications

If first-line medications are insufficient or cause intolerable side effects, second-line treatments are considered. These include opioids, topical treatments, and local anesthetics.

4.3.1 Opioids

While opioids are not typically the first choice for neuropathic pain due to concerns about tolerance, dependence, and side effects, they may be appropriate for patients with severe PTNP who have not responded adequately to other treatments.

Opioids primarily bind to mu-opioid receptors in the brain and spinal cord, blocking pain signals. In the case of tramadol and tapentadol, these medications also inhibit the reuptake of serotonin and norepinephrine, contributing to their analgesic effects.

4.3.2 Topical treatments

Topical treatments can be highly effective for localized neuropathic pain and often have fewer systemic side effects compared to oral medications.

Lidocaine patches: Lidocaine is a local anesthetic that works by blocking sodium channels, which prevents the transmission of pain signals along nerve fibers.

Capsaicin cream (8%): Capsaicin is derived from chili peppers and works by depleting substance P, a neuropeptide involved in pain transmission, from sensory nerve terminals.

4.3.3 Topical gabapentinoids

Topical gabapentinoids, like gabapentin gel, are emerging as a novel treatment for localized neuropathic pain. Though not yet widely available, these gels may offer an alternative to oral medications, with potentially fewer systemic side effects (**Figure 2**).

4.4 Adjunctive medications

These medications are not typically used as primary treatments but may be prescribed in conjunction with other drugs for more comprehensive pain management.

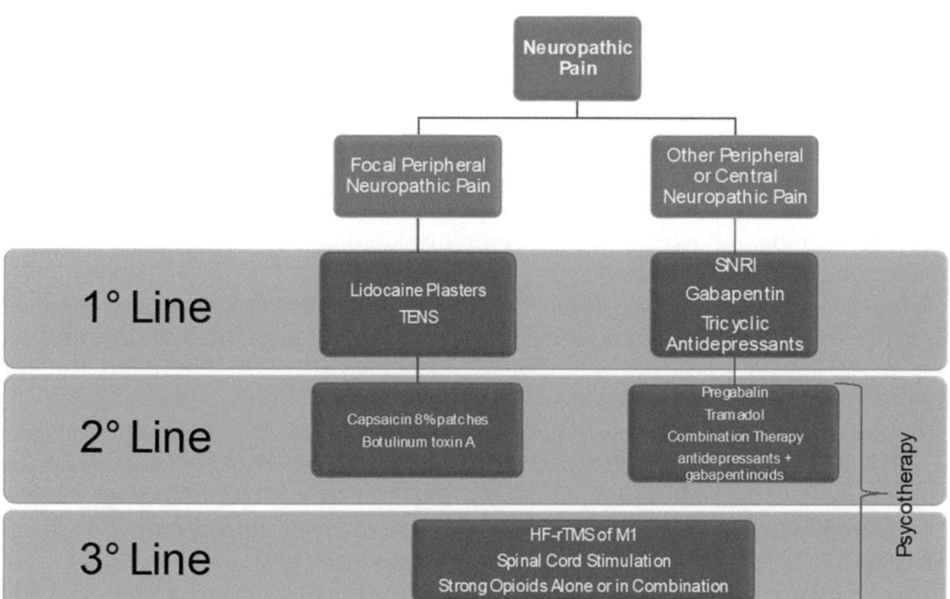

Figure 2.
Flowchart for pharmacological treatment (Moisset et al.).

4.4.1 Anti-seizure medications

In some cases, other antiepileptic drugs (AEDs) beyond gabapentinoids are considered for neuropathic pain.

Carbamazepine: Frequently used for trigeminal neuralgia, carbamazepine stabilizes hyperexcitable nerve membranes. It is usually not first-line for PTNP but may be used in certain situations where the pain is localized to a specific nerve distribution.

4.4.2 Baclofen (muscle relaxant)

Baclofen is a GABA-B receptor agonist that inhibits presynaptic release of excitatory neurotransmitters in the CNS. It is sometimes used for muscle spasms associated with PTNP, especially in cases involving spinal cord injury [1, 23].

4.5 Nerve block

A nerve block involves the injection of local anesthetic or other agents around a specific nerve or group of nerves to reduce pain transmission. In the case of post-traumatic neuropathic pain (PTNP) affecting the lower limb, ultrasound-guided nerve blocks are used to block the pain signals transmitted from the injured nerves to the brain. This can provide temporary or, in some cases, long-lasting relief [25].

4.5.1 Mechanism of action

Nerve blocks work by interrupting the transmission of pain signals along the nerves. Local anesthetics, such as lidocaine, bupivacaine, or ropivacaine, are commonly used in nerve block procedures. These anesthetics work by binding to sodium channels on nerve fibers, preventing the propagation of action potentials that transmit pain. In addition to local anesthetics, nerve blocks can sometimes include steroids or anti-inflammatory agents to reduce inflammation around the nerve and improve the duration of pain relief [26].

4.5.2 Types of nerve blocks for lower limb neuropathic pain

Several specific nerve blocks may be employed depending on the source and distribution of pain in the lower limb:

Sciatic nerve block: The sciatic nerve, which provides sensation and motor function to the lower limb, is often targeted when neuropathic pain is felt in the thigh, lower leg, or foot. A sciatic nerve block can be performed at different points along the nerve's course, depending on the location of pain.

Femoral nerve block: This block targets the femoral nerve, which supplies the anterior and medial aspects of the thigh, as well as the hip and knee. A femoral nerve block is commonly used for knee or hip pain, including after surgical procedures or trauma.

Lumbar plexus block: In cases of more widespread lower limb neuropathic pain, a lumbar plexus block, also known as a psoas compartment block, may be used to target a broader range of nerves that supply the lower extremities. It is often employed for pain relief following hip or pelvic trauma.

Saphenous nerve block: The saphenous nerve, which is a branch of the femoral nerve, can be blocked when the pain is localized to the medial aspect of the lower leg or foot, such as in cases of post-traumatic pain from knee surgery or fractures (**Figure 3**) [27].

	Indications	Key Anatomy	Nerve stimulation response	Tips
Femoral Nerve Block	Analgesia on Femour, anterior thight and knee	Femoral nerve lateral to femoral artery, below fascia iliaca	Quadriceps muscle contraction	If Femoral nerve not seen, track the iliac fascia medially towards Femoral nerve
Sciatic Nerve Block	Analgesia below the knee	Sciatic nerve under gluteus maximum muscle	Twitch of foot or calf	Needle should go in proximity of the nerve sheet either at lateral or medial aspect of Sciatic Nerve
Popliteal Block	Analgesia on ankle and foot	Presence of common epineural scheet of sciatic nerve	Twitch of foot or toes	Injection can be made more proximally at either medial or lateral aspect of Sciatic Nerve in proximity to epidural sheet
Saphenous Block	Supplement to popliteal and sciatic blocks	Femoral artery below sartorius muscle, nerve often not seen	Paresthesia of the medial aspect of the lower leg	If identification of the nerve is difficutl try to track it more proximally

Figure 3.
Lower limb nerve blocks (kind concession of NYSORA).

4.5.3 Indications for nerve blocks

Nerve blocks are typically indicated when PTNP is localized to a specific nerve or group of nerves, and when conservative pharmacological treatments have proven ineffective.

They are often used as:

Diagnostic tools to determine whether a particular nerve is the source of pain.

Therapeutic treatments for pain relief, providing both short-term and long-term symptom controls.

Part of a multidisciplinary pain management strategy, including physical therapy or rehabilitation.

4.5.4 Procedure

Technique: Nerve blocks are typically performed using ultrasound guidance to ensure precise placement of the needle near the nerve, while avoiding intraneural injections that can cause nerve fiber disruption and neuromas. The local anesthetic is injected slowly around the nerve, dissecting adherences and causing temporary blockage of the nerve's ability to transmit pain signals.

Duration: The effects of a nerve block can vary. Local anesthetics typically provide relief for several hours to days. When combined with steroids or other medications, the antalgic/anti-inflammatory effect can last longer.

4.5.5 Outcomes and benefits

Pain relief: Nerve blocks provide temporary yet significant pain relief, helping to identify the source of pain in preparation for other interventional treatments.

Reduced need for systemic medications: By targeting the source of pain directly, nerve blocks can reduce the need for systemic pain medications like opioids, helping to minimize side effects and improve patient quality of life.

4.5.6 Risks and side effects

Temporary numbness or weakness: Patients will experience temporary numbness and possibly muscle weakness.

Infection or bleeding: As with any procedure involving injections, there is a small risk of infection or bleeding at the injection site.

Nerve injury: Although rare, there is a risk of nerve injury due to improper needle placement. This risk is significantly reduced by proper ultrasound guidance.

Allergic reaction: Some patients may have an allergic reaction to the local anesthetic or corticosteroids used in the block.

Nerve blocks are typically indicated when PTNP is attributable to a specific nerve or group of nerves, and when conservative pharmacological treatments have proven ineffective. They are often used as diagnostic tools to determine whether a particular nerve is the source of pain.

The overall benefit of nerve blocks is to obtain pain relief reducing the need for medications while identifying the exact target for therapeutic procedures such as adipose fat transfer or surgery [26, 27].

4.6 Adipose fat transfer

Adipose fat transfer (AFT) is emerging as a promising approach for the minimally invasive management of post-traumatic neuropathic pain. Adipose tissue is rich in stem cells, growth factors, stromal and vascular cells, and anti-inflammatory mediators. Together, these properties offer a potential pathway for both pain relief and tissue regeneration (**Figure 4**) [10, 28].

4.6.1 Mechanisms of action

AFT harnesses adipose-derived stem cells (ADSCs), stromal vascular fraction, and vascular cells secreting stimulating growth factors such as vascular endothelial growth factor (VEGF) and nerve growth factor (NGF). These factors support the repair and regeneration of injured tissues including nerves. At the same time, fat grafts act as a cushioning layer, dissecting the nerve from the scar adherences and allowing for decreased mechanical pressure from scar tissue and nerve gliding. This effect is particularly beneficial for pain resulting from scar adhesions.

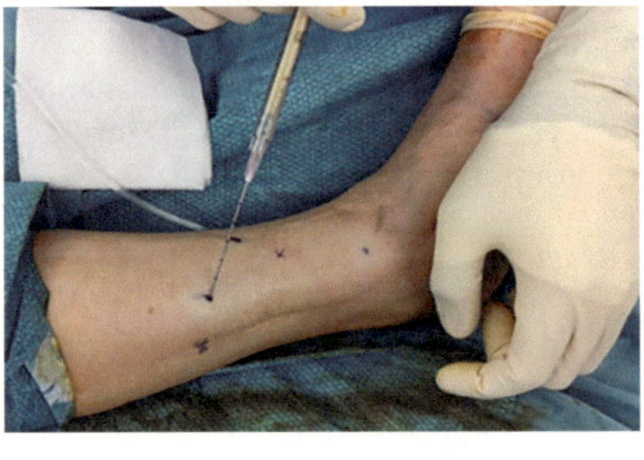

Figure 4.
Adipose fat transfer (Pietramaggiori et al.).

Adipose tissue itself secretes other cytokines such as adiponectin and interleukin-10. Their anti-inflammatory properties contribute to resolve chronic inflammation.

4.6.2 Procedural steps

The donor site for fat tissue, typically the abdomen or flanks, is thoroughly prepped and draped for the procedure. A tumescent solution, consisting of 0.5 L of NaCl and 0.5 mg of epinephrine, is injected into the subcutaneous tissue using an infiltration cannula (Gems tumescent Infiltrator, 2.1 mm 14G, Tulip Medical, USA). For each zone, approximately 200 ml of the solution was administered, targeting the lower abdomen, the area beneath the umbilicus, and the flanks. Lidocaine is generally not added to the solution to avoid potential lipotoxic effects. After allowing 10 to 15 minutes for the epinephrine to take effect, fat is harvested using an 18G blunt cannula, which is connected to a 20 cc luer-lock syringe, pre-filled with 5 ml of Ringer's solution.

The harvested adipose tissue is rinsed several times (3–5) with Ringer's solution until it becomes yellow and clear, indicating no blood contamination. Following fat extraction, 20 cc of 1% lidocaine and epinephrine is injected into the donor site to minimize post-operative discomfort. The processed fat is then transferred into 1 cc syringes and injected into the target subcutaneous area using an 18G blunt cannula (Gems spoon tip injector, 2.1 mm, Tulip Medical, USA). The injection is done using a fanning technique to help dissect adhesions beneath scar tissue and reconstruct the subcutaneous tissue layer. To minimize tissue damage, bleeding, and prevent the formation of cysts, no sharp cannulas are used, and the fat is injected in small aliquots while retracting the cannula (**Figure 5**).

The average amount of fat transferred is 15 cc, depending on the size of the affected area (typically 10–20 cm^2). After the fat injection, a double-layer bandage is applied: a cotton layer in contact with the skin to help warm the lymph, followed by an elastic bandage to reduce swelling and prevent shear forces. Patients are instructed to avoid prolonged standing position for 5 days to decrease edema [10, 29, 30].

4.6.3 Clinical applications

Scar-related neuropathic pain: following trauma or surgery, scar tissue may affect the nerves by causing entrapments or adhesions. AFT acts as a biological interface

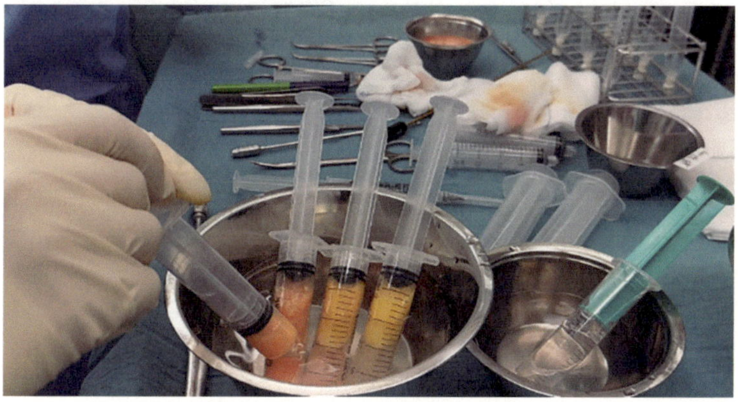

Figure 5.
Fat preparation.

that cushions and separates the nerves from the scar tissue, reducing pain due to nerve-scar adhesions.

Neuroma management: Neuromas, painful nerve growths resulting from direct nerve injury, can be alleviated by AFT. The fat graft provides an anti-inflammatory interface reducing the pressure and tension on the nerve.

Post-surgical pain syndromes: AFT has shown promise in managing chronic neuropathic pain after surgeries such as knee arthroplasties, ankle surgeries, neurosurgery, or amputations, where nerve branches are entrapped in scar tissue. By promoting tissue healing and regeneration, AFT addresses both the mechanical and inflammatory aspects of post-surgical pain [10, 29, 30].

4.6.4 Outcomes and evidence

Clinical studies have demonstrated significant efficacy of AFT in reducing pain and improving function. In a study of patients with post-traumatic neuropathic pain and allodynia, over 80% of those treated with AFT reported significant (>50%) and long-lasting pain relief. Moreover, patients experienced less reliance on analgesics and increased ability to work, demonstrating the long-term effectiveness of this treatment in addressing both pain and tissue regeneration [10].

4.6.5 Innovations and research

Recent advancements in AFT, such as the use of stromal vascular fraction (SVF)-enriched fat grafting, may enhance the regenerative potential of adipose tissue by concentrating stem cells and growth factors. Additionally, improved imaging-guided injection techniques have increased the precision and efficacy of the procedure, minimized complications, and optimized outcomes [31].

Ongoing research is exploring different harvesting and injection techniques and the combinations of AFT with other regenerative therapies, such as platelet-rich plasma (PRP), exosomes, and adipose-derived stem cells to further enhance the regenerative potentials and therapeutic outcomes.

Adipose fat transfer (AFT) represents a novel and promising approach to managing post-traumatic neuropathic pain. By leveraging the regenerative properties of adipose tissue, AFT not only alleviates pain but also promotes tissue regeneration. As the technique evolves, it holds great potential as a minimally invasive and effective option for managing complex pain conditions.

4.7 Selective denervation

Selective denervation is a precise, minimally invasive procedure focused on interrupting pain signals along specific nerve pathways, particularly useful for treating localized neuropathic pain not responding to conventional or less invasive treatments. This technique is especially beneficial for patients with chronic pain following trauma or surgery, where traditional approaches have failed [11, 32].

4.7.1 Mechanisms and objectives

Targeted injured nerve branch ablation: The primary mechanism of selective denervation is the targeted disruption of terminally injured nerve branches responsible for transmitting pain signals, thus providing focused pain relief while preserving the function of surrounding, unaffected nerves. By interrupting only those nerve fibers involved in pain transmission, this approach minimizes collateral damage to sensory and motor functions, ensuring that other functions, like movement and sensation, are preserved [11, 32, 33].

Neuroma prevention: Combining denervation with adjunctive therapies such as adipose fat transfer (AFT) or muscle burial, selective denervation helps mitigate the formation of painful neuromas. The soft tissue environment created by the fat grafts supports nerve healing and reduces the risk of scar tissue formation, thus promoting better outcomes and preventing the recurrence of nerve pain [33].

4.7.2 Procedural steps

Pre-operative planning: Before the denervation procedure, diagnostic nerve blocks are performed to identify which nerve branches are responsible for the pain and the exact, most distal level where the procedure should take place. Imaging techniques such as high-resolution ultrasound and targeted nerve blocks are used to ensure precise localization of the level of the surgical procedure.

Neuroma/Injured nerve branches Ablation: Once the target nerves are identified, they are surgically resected using minimally invasive techniques.

Adjunctive measures: To further improve outcomes, fat grafting, muscle embedding, or targeted muscle reinnervation may be used to guide nerve regrowth and prevent recurrence of pain. These soft tissue interventions reduce the risk of scar and adherence formation and provide a more supportive environment for nerve healing [11].

4.7.3 Applications and indications

Selective denervation is effective for various chronic pain conditions, particularly post-traumatic where scarring affects directly nerve integrity. Common applications include the following:

Chronic knee pain: Selective denervation has shown significant success in managing post-surgical knee pain, particularly following procedures like total knee replacement. By targeting specific nerve branches responsible for joint and surrounding tissue innervation, this technique offers relief for patients with persistent pain after surgery.

Ankle and foot neuropathies: Peripheral nerve injuries around the ankle and foot, such as post-surgical injury to the peroneal nerve, are classic indications for selective denervation.

Neuromas: Neuromas, or painful nerve growths that develop after nerve injury, can be effectively managed with selective denervation. By removing the source of nerve irritation, the technique provides relief for patients with painful neuromas following trauma or surgery.

4.7.4 Case studies and evidence

In a clinical case series, patients undergoing selective denervation for knee pain reported a significant reduction in pain, with an average reduction of 70% on the visual analog scale (VAS). Functional improvements, such as increased mobility and reduced reliance on mobility aids, were also noted. Combining selective denervation with adipose fat transfer (AFT) has been shown to improve long-term outcomes by

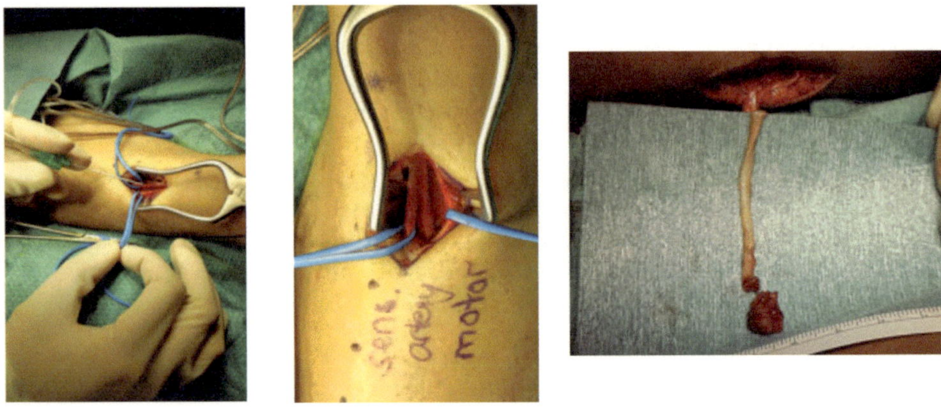

Figure 6.
Selective denervation of deep peroneal nerve (case from Pietramaggiori et al.).

reducing scar adhesion and promoting better tissue healing, enhancing the overall success of the procedure [10, 11].

While selective denervation offers highly targeted pain relief, it requires meticulous planning and technical expertise. One of the main challenges of this procedure is the precise identification of the pain-producing nerve branches, as improper selection can lead to incomplete pain relief or unnecessary sacrifice of functional structures. Additionally, potential risks include sensory deficits, incomplete pain relief, and the recurrence of pain due to factors such as nerve regeneration or neuroma formation. These risks are decreased using ancillary techniques such as AFT, muscle burial, and targeted muscle reinnervation (**Figure 6**).

5. Advantages and challenges

The appeal of minimally invasive surgical treatments lies in their ability to deliver targeted pain relief with minimal disruption to patients' daily lives.

Due to lack of specialized training, multidisciplinary approaches such as a radiologist specialized in ultrasound diagnostics working with the surgeon or inadequate procedural technique can result in suboptimal results.

5.1 Radiofrequency ablation

Radiofrequency ablation (RFA) is a minimally invasive procedure used to temporarily alleviate chronic neuropathic pain. RFA uses heat generated by radiofrequency energy to target and destroy nerve tissue, which interrupts the transmission of pain signals [34].

5.1.1 Mechanism of action

RFA works by applying controlled heat to specific nerves using a small, needle-like electrode. The radiofrequency energy heats the tissue to a temperature of about 70–80°C, causing the nerve fibers to be damaged and unable to transmit pain signals to the brain. This disruption of nerve function can provide long-term pain relief (up to several months).

By disrupting the pain signal transmission from the injured or damaged nerve, RFA can temporarily reduce or eliminate chronic pain [35].

5.1.2 Indications for radiofrequency ablation

RFA is often recommended for patients with chronic neuropathic pain who do not respond to conservative treatment and cannot undergo surgery or other minimal invasive procedures. After an ultrasound guided block is performed on the targeted nerve, the patient should report a temporary but significant pain improvement.

5.1.3 Procedure

The procedure is typically performed under local anesthesia and sedation to ensure comfort.

A needle-like electrode is inserted near the nerve or nerve root suspected to be causing pain under ultrasound guidance to position the needle close to the target.

Once the needle is in place, a small amount of radiofrequency energy is passed through the electrode to deliver heat, causing partial nerve ablation. This procedure usually takes around 15–30 minutes per nerve treated in skilled hands.

5.1.4 Outcomes and benefits

RFA can provide significant and long-lasting relief for patients with chronic neuropathic pain. The duration of relief varies, but most patients experience relief for several months to a year.

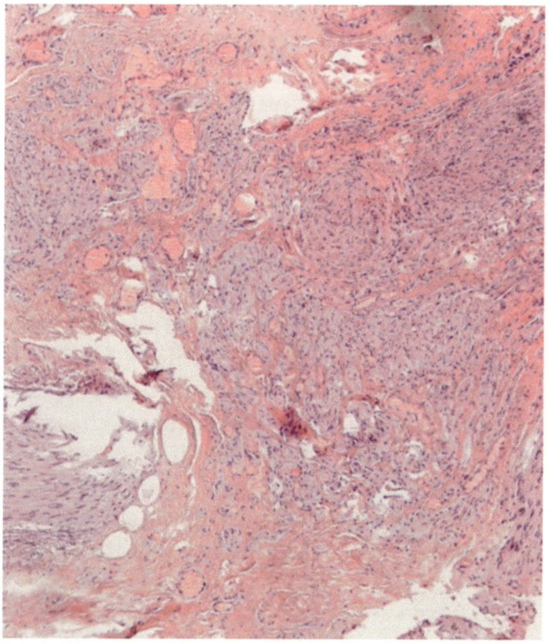

Figure 7.
Post-radiofrequency neuroma: Histology section.

By reducing or eliminating pain, RFA can greatly improve a patient's mobility, sleep, and overall quality of life. It can also reduce the need for systemic medications, including opioids, which lowers the risk of side effects or addiction.

RFA is performed as an outpatient procedure with minimal downtime.

5.1.5 Risks and side effects

Patients experience numbness or tingling in the treated area. Though rare, there is a risk of infection at the needle insertion site.

The major risk is of damaging healthy nerve branches, which could potentially result in weakness, numbness, allodynia, and neuroma formation.

In our experience, the risk of neuroma in continuum formation is high making all further treatments more difficult. We recommend leaving RFA as last option for neuropathic pain treatment (**Figure** 7) [34, 35].

6. Conclusions

Minimally invasive treatments have fundamentally transformed the management of post-traumatic neuropathic pain (PTNP), offering patients an effective alternative when traditional, less invasive therapies have failed to provide relief. These treatments are designed to precisely target the pain pathways responsible for chronic discomfort, without the need for invasive surgery. By minimizing the risks of complications and reducing recovery times, these interventions empower patients to regain control of their lives, improving overall health and well-being.

By utilizing the regenerative properties of adipose tissue, AFT bridges the gap between alleviating pain and promoting healing, offering a dual benefit to patients. This technique harnesses stem cells, growth factors, and anti-inflammatory mediators from fat tissue, addressing both the biochemical and structural causes of neuropathic pain.

In addition to AFT, selective denervation has become an invaluable tool for treating patients with refractory pain syndromes. This procedure allows for the precise interruption of pain signals by targeting specific nerve pathways responsible for the transmission of pain. With its ability to selectively address localized pain without disrupting surrounding tissue or function, selective denervation offers a targeted solution for patients suffering from chronic, persistent pain that has not responded to other treatments.

As medical technology and research continue to advance, the potential for these minimally invasive techniques to alleviate the burden of PTNP will continue to expand. Innovations in imaging, precision medicine, and regenerative therapies are improving the effectiveness, safety, and accessibility of these treatments, providing hope for a growing number of patients. Over time, these advances will not only provide more options for pain relief but will also significantly enhance the quality of life for those suffering from PTNP, ultimately transforming the landscape of pain management and offering new possibilities for managing this challenging condition.

Author details

Giorgio Pietramaggiori[1*], Federico Ricci[2], Franco Bassetto[2] and Saja Scherer[1]

1 Global Medical Institute, Lausanne, Switzerland

2 Department of Plastic and Reconstructive Surgery, University Hospital Padua, Padua, Italy

*Address all correspondence to: dr.pietramaggiori@global.surgery

References

[1] Treede RD, Jensen TS, Campbell JN, Cruccu G, Dostrovsky JO, Griffin JW, et al. Neuropathic pain. Neurology. 2008;**70**(18):1630-1635

[2] Keene DJ, Knight R, Bruce J, Dutton SJ, Tutton E, Achten J, et al. Chronic pain with neuropathic characteristics after surgery for major trauma to the lower limb: Prevalence, predictors, and association with pain severity, disability, and quality of life in the UK WHiST trial. The Bone and Joint Journal. 2021;**103-B**(6):1047-1054

[3] Baron R, Binder A, Wasner G. Neuropathic pain: Diagnosis, pathophysiological mechanisms, and treatment. The Lancet Neurology. 2010;**9**(8):807-819

[4] Nakagawa R, Yamaguchi S, Kimura S, Sadamasu A, Yamamoto Y, Sato Y, et al. Association of Anxiety and Depression with Pain and quality of life in patients with chronic foot and ankle diseases. Foot and Ankle International. 2017;**38**(11):1192-1198

[5] Phillips CJ. The cost and burden of chronic pain. Reviews in Pain. 2009;**3**(1):2-5

[6] Dieleman JP, Kerklaan J, Huygen FJPM, Bouma PAD, Sturkenboom MCJM. Incidence rates and treatment of neuropathic pain conditions in the general population ☆. Pain. 2008;**137**(3):681-688

[7] Hooten WM. Chronic pain and mental health disorders. Mayo Clinic Proceedings. 2016;**91**(7):955-970

[8] Finnerup NB, Kuner R, Jensen TS. Neuropathic pain: From mechanisms to treatment. Physiological Reviews. 2021;**101**(1):259-301

[9] Ji RR, Nackley A, Huh Y, Terrando N, Maixner W. Neuroinflammation and central sensitization in chronic and widespread pain. Anesthesiology. 2018;**129**(2):343-366

[10] Pietramaggiori G, Ricci F, L'Erario S, Bassetto F, Scherer S. Minimally invasive scar release by autologous adipose tissue transfer for post-traumatic neuropathic pain. Regenerative Therapy. 2024;**25**:302-307

[11] Pietramaggiori G, Sapino G, De Santis G, Bassetto F, Scherer S. Chronic knee and ankle pain treatment through selective microsurgical approaches: A minimally invasive option in the treatment algorithm for refractory lower limb pain. Journal of Reconstructive Microsurgery. 2020;**37**(03):234-241

[12] Gao N, Li M, Wang W, Liu Z, Guo Y. The dual role of TRPV1 in peripheral neuropathic pain: Pain switches caused by its sensitization or desensitization. Frontiers in Molecular Neuroscience. 2024;**17**:1-14

[13] Bin Ibrahim MZ, Wang Z, Sajikumar S. Synapses tagged, memories kept: Synaptic tagging and capture hypothesis in brain health and disease. Philosophical Transactions of the Royal Society B: Biological Sciences. 2024;**379**(1906):1-16

[14] da Silva MDV, Martelossi-Cebinelli G, Yaekashi KM, Carvalho TT, Borghi SM, Casagrande R, et al. A narrative review of the dorsal root ganglia and spinal cord mechanisms of action of neuromodulation therapies in neuropathic pain. Brain Sciences. 2024;**14**(6):589

[15] Monteiro BP, Otis C, Nitulescu R, Troncy E. Quantitative sensory testing

in canine musculoskeletal pain: Findings from a systematic review, meta-analysis feasibility assessment, and limitations. The Veterinary Journal. 2024;**304**:106102

[16] Aguiar ROC, Umans H. Imaging considerations in differentiating plantar plate pathology and webspace neuroma. Foot and Ankle Clinics. 2024;**29**(4):571-590

[17] Leone CM, Truini A. Understanding neuropathic pain: The role of neurophysiological tests in unveiling underlying mechanisms. Journal of Anesthesia, Analgesia and Critical Care. 2024;**4**(1):1-9

[18] Granzer-Corno L, Rana R, Dick BD, Sankar T. Different scale, different pain? Discordant pain measurements after surgery for trigeminal neuralgia. World Neurosurgery. 2025;**194**:123481

[19] Ranzatto AD d S, Chaves TC, Martins MN, Motta DP, Nogueira LC, Meziat-Filho N, et al. Pain intensity scales: A cross-sectional study on the preferences and knowledge of physiotherapists and participants with musculoskeletal pain. Musculoskeletal Science and Practice. 2024;**73**:103162

[20] Akyuz G, Kenis O. Physical therapy modalities and rehabilitation techniques in the management of neuropathic pain. American Journal of Physical Medicine and Rehabilitation. 2014;**93**(3):253-259

[21] Ruan QZ, Chang J, Pak D, Supra R, Yazdi C, Kollenburg L, et al. Literature review: Mechanism, indications, and clinical efficacy of peripheral nerve stimulators in lower extremity pain. Current Pain and Headache Reports. 2024;**28**(6):469-479

[22] Moisset X. Neuropathic pain: Evidence based recommendations. La Presse Médicale. 2024;**53**(2):104232

[23] Shkodina AD, Bardhan M, Chopra H, Anyagwa OE, Pinchuk VA, Hryn KV, et al. Pharmacological and non-pharmacological approaches for the Management of Neuropathic Pain in multiple sclerosis. CNS Drugs. 2024;**38**(3):205-224

[24] Pickering G, Kotlińska-Lemieszek A, Krcevski Skvarc N, O'Mahony D, Monacelli F, Knaggs R, et al. Pharmacological pain treatment in older persons. Drugs and Aging. 2024;**41**(12):959-976

[25] Sperling PK, Launa N, Ghaffari A, Rømer H, Sørensen MPB, Rahbek O, et al. Neuropathic pain after orthopaedic surgery with continuous peripheral nerve block. Danish Medical Journal. 15 Feb 2024;**71**(3):A09230581. DOI: 10.61409/A09230581

[26] On'Gele MO, Weintraub S, Qi V, Kim J. Local anesthetics, local anesthetic systemic toxicity (LAST), and liposomal bupivacaine. Anesthesiology Clinics. 2024;**42**(2):303-315

[27] El-Boghdadly K, Albrecht E, Wolmarans M, Mariano ER, Kopp S, Perlas A, et al. Standardizing nomenclature in regional anesthesia: An ASRA-ESRA Delphi consensus study of upper and lower limb nerve blocks. Regional Anesthesia and Pain Medicine. 2023;**49**(11):782-792

[28] Beugels J, Hommes JE, Balthasar AJR, van der Hulst RRWJ, Piatkowski de Grzymala AA. Autologous fat transfer as a treatment for peripheral neuropathic pain without apparent cause. Plastic and Reconstructive Surgery - Global Open. 2018;**6**(8):e1905

[29] Coleman S. Structural fat grafting. Aesthetic Surgery Journal. 1998;**18**(5):386-388

[30] Klinger M, Caviggioli F, Klinger FM, Giannasi S, Bandi V, Banzatti B, et al. Autologous fat graft in scar treatment. Journal of Craniofacial Surgery. 2013;**24**(5):1610-1615

[31] Gentile P, Orlandi A, Scioli MG, Di Pasquali C, Bocchini I, Curcio CB, et al. A comparative translational study: The combined use of enhanced stromal vascular fraction and platelet-rich plasma improves fat grafting maintenance in breast reconstruction. Stem Cells Translational Medicine. 2012;**1**(4):341-351

[32] Chin KWTK, Engelsman AF, van Gulik TM, Strackee SD. Selective denervation of the wrist for chronic pain: A systematic literature review. Journal of Hand Surgery (European Volume). 2019;**45**(3):265-272

[33] Madersbacher H. Denervation techniques. BJU International. 2000;**85**(S3):1-6

[34] Abd-Elsayed A, Kennedy K. The art of radiofrequency ablation. Annals of Palliative Medicine. 2024;**13**(3):471-476

[35] Kwon HJ, Kim CS, Kim DH, Shin JW, Choi D, Choi SS. Effectiveness of the Cooled Radiofrequency Ablation of Genicular Nerves in Patients with Chronic Knee Pain Due to Osteoarthritis: A Double-Blind, Randomized, Controlled Study. Medicina (Kaunas). 24 May 2024;**60**(6):857. DOI: 10.3390/medicina60060857

Chapter 6

Perspective Chapter: Trimalleolar Fracture

Wael Abdelkarim Aldahshan, Ahmed Mohamed Abd-alkhalek, Ahmed Sayed Elshamy and Mohammed Ahmed Abd Elfattah

Abstract

A trimalleolar fracture is an ankle fracture involving the posterior malleolus, which ranges from small avulsions to large intra-articular fragments, with impacted small fragments causing subluxation of the talus. Proper evaluation, including detailed radiographic imaging, is essential for accurate classification and treatment planning. A trimalleolar ankle fracture is inherently unstable, with possible syndesmotic disruption. Computed tomography is the gold standard for diagnosis, staging, and surgical planning. However, the management of trimalleolar ankle fractures is controversial in terms of approaches, fixation methods, postoperative rehabilitation, and weight-bearing protocols. The author generated a grading system based on CT, demonstrating four grades that facilitate management, are relevant for prognosis, and can be applied in research and clinical settings. This chapter aims to provide a comprehensive review of trimalleolar ankle fractures, highlighting the mechanisms of injury, diagnostic approaches, grading system, surgical treatment options, and complications.

Keywords: trimalleolar ankle fracture, posterior malleolus, posterolateral approach, posteromedial approach, trimalleolar fracture classification

1. Introduction

Ankle fractures are a significant concern, occurring in 187 per 100,000 adults annually. They exhibit a bimodal distribution, with the highest incidence in young males between 15 and 24 years of age and in older females aged 75–84. Isolated malleolus fractures account for 70%, bimalleolar for 20%, and trimalleolar for 7%. Posterior malleolar fractures are found in 40% of rotational ankle fractures but can also occur as an isolated fracture [1–6].

While recent efforts have been directed towards managing trimalleolar fractures, it is essential to note that controversies persist regarding them, underscoring the urgent need for further research [7–9].

It is essential to differentiate between a pilon and a trimalleolar fracture accurately. This precision in diagnosis is a key factor in effectively managing these complex injuries. A Pillon fracture is a fracture of the distal end of the tibia associated with comminution and intra-articular extension. A trimalleolar fracture is an ankle fracture involving the posterior malleolus, ranging from small avulsions to large intra-articular fragments, with impacted small fragments causing subluxation of the talus.

2. Relevant anatomy

The ankle is a modified hinge joint that allows dorsiflexion and plantar flexion in the sagittal plane, and two rotations occur in the axial and coronal planes [10].

The ankle joint is formed of the distal tibia, fibula, and the superior dome of the talus, creating a saddle-shaped mortise joint that provides stability through its bony structure. The ligamentous structure formed by the lateral ligamentous complex, medial deltoid ligament, syndesmotic complex and posterior ligaments provides static stability [11].

The distal tibia is formed by five surfaces: the inferior, anterior, posteriorlateral, and medial surfaces. The medial surface extends distally at an obtuse angle to create the medial malleolus. It is thick at the base anteroposteriorly but flat and narrow transversely. The malleolus's lateral surface articulates with the talus's comma-shaped articular surface. The inferior articular surface aligns with the talus dome, being concave in the anteroposterior direction and slightly convex transversely [11].

The posterior malleolus has distinct features that provide stability to the ankle. The bony surface is continuous. The posterior surface of the tibial shaft is smooth and slightly convex in the proximal segment. The distal segment has an oblique sulcus directed downwards and inward on the medial malleolus for the tendon of the tibialis posterior. The posterior ligamentous structures form a labrum, which is formed by binding the superficial posterior inferior tibiofibular ligament, and the transverse ligament stabilises the talar translation [11].

The lateral malleolus is pyramidal and presents lateral, medial, and posterior surfaces. The lateral and medial surfaces meet at the anterior border. The posterior surface is bordered laterally by the oblique fibular crest and medially by extending the posterior border of the fibular shaft. The lateral malleolus extends outward and descends 1 cm further than the medial malleolus [11].

The stability at the distal tibiofibular joint results from the syndesmotic ligaments. Which can be divided into segments by location and attachments, including the anterior inferior tibiofibular ligament, the posterior-inferior tibiofibular ligament (PITFL), the interosseous ligament, and the transverse ligament [12, 13].

The Posterior Inferior Tibiofibular Ligament (PITFL) contributes 42% of syndesmosis stability (Ogilvie-Harris DJ, 1994). It has superficial and deep components. The superficial component of the PITFL spans across the posterior aspect of the ankle, from the posterior aspect of the lateral malleolus to the posterior malleolus of the tibia [14, 15].

The deep component is called the transverse ligament. It originates above the digital fossa of the lateral malleolus and inserts on the lower part of the posterior border of the tibial articular surface in a superomedial direction. Acting as a true labrum, the transverse ligament deepens the articular tibial surface, increasing the tibial concavity [16].

In posterior malleolar injuries, the transverse ligament and the PITFL are often attached to the posterior fracture fragment [17]. Therefore, it is crucial to preserve both ligaments during surgical procedures.

The anteroinferior tibiofibular ligament runs from the lateral surface of the tibia to the fibula and is quadrilateral. This ligament can be avulsed with its tibial attachment at the tubercle of Chaput, resulting in the Chaput fracture [18].

The interosseous ligament runs obliquely downward from the tibia towards the fibula and is the distal condensation of the interosseous membrane between the tibia and fibula. It makes up the most substantial portion of the syndesmosis [18].

3. Mode of trauma and descriptive anatomy of the fracture

In the Supination-External Rotation (SER) type of the Lauge-Hansen classification, the fracture pattern includes an anterior tibiofibular ligament sprain, a lateral short oblique fibula fracture (extending from anteroinferior to posterosuperior), and a posterior tibiofibular ligament rupture or avulsion of the posterior malleolus. This is often followed by a transverse fracture of the medial malleolus or a deltoid ligament disruption [18, 19].

In contrast, the pronation-external rotation type typically starts with a transverse fracture of the medial malleolus or deltoid ligament disruption. This is followed by anterior tibiofibular ligament disruption and a lateral short oblique or spiral fracture of the fibula (extending from anterosuperior to posteroinferior) above the joint level. Finally, it involves a posterior tibiofibular ligament rupture or avulsion of the posterior malleolus [18, 19].

This indicates that external rotation is a key factor in posterior malleolar fractures.

Weber et al. [20] have noted that there are typically two primary posterior fragments, which may be impacted at the posteromedial plafond. The injury mechanism is believed to involve vertical shearing, occurring with the foot in a hyperflexed position under partial axial load. As a result, this type of fracture cannot be classified within the Lauge-Hansen system [21].

The size of the posterior malleolus fracture varies, ranging from an extra-articular ship fracture to large articular fragments of up to 40% of the sagittal diameter of the articular surface. Usually, it is triangular-shaped, with its base lateral. A medial malleolar fracture usually presents as a transverse or short oblique fracture at the level of the tibiotalar joint. The posteriorly dislocating talus may impact the posterior edge of the tibial plafond, detaching additional osteochondral fragments, which may block anatomic reduction and prevent restoration of normal joint relationships and stability [20].

In another scenario, the entire posterior tibial lip is fractured, including the posterior colliculus of the medial malleolus. This results in a larger triangular posteromedial fragment and a smaller rectangular posterolateral fragment. Additionally, osteochondral fragments may become detached from the posteromedial tibial plafond. This leads to a significantly larger defect in the posteromedial area compared to the posterolateral tibial plafond, causing posteromedial subluxation of the talus.

Biomechanically, the tibiotalar contact area decreases significantly when the fragment size exceeds 33%. Additionally, posterior subluxation increases notably between 25% and 40%, leading to more significant stress on the remaining joint [22–26].

4. Classification

Haraguchi et al. identified three major fracture patterns: Type I: Wedge-shaped posterior fragment extending through the tibial plafond and exiting posteromedially.

Type II: Transverse fracture line from the fibular notch of the tibia into the medial malleolus. Type III: "Shell fractures," consisting of single or multiple superficial tibial bone fragments from the posterior malleolar lip [27].

Mason and Molloy classify posterior malleolus ankle fractures based on the mechanism of injury and severity into three types: Type 1: Avulsion fractures of the posterior malleolar fragment caused by pulling forces from the posterior inferior tibiofibular ligament (PITFL), typically occurring with a plantar-flexed ankle (a stage III supination-external rotation injury). Type 2: Divided into two subtypes: Type 2A: Involves fractures in the Volkmann area of the posterior tibia from talus rotation on the tibial plafond (Haraguchi's type I). Type 2B: Results from increased rotational force, leading to fractures extending through the medial component of the tibia (Haraguchi's type II). Type 3: Complete separation of the posterior tibial component via a coronal plane fracture, often associated with a high oblique fibula fracture [9].

Bartoníček et al. postulated a more specific CT-based classification system that considers the stability of the tibiotalar joint and the integrity of the fibular notch. Type 1: extraincisural fragment with an intact fibular notch. Type 2: posterolateral fragment extending into the fibular notch. Type 3: posteromedial two-part fragment involving the medial malleolus. Type 4: large posterolateral triangular fragment (involving more than one-third of the notch). Type 5: irregular, osteoporotic fragments [28]. This classification system of the posterior malleolus can guide further operative or non-operative treatment but fails to fully characterise the kind of trimalleolar fracture [29].

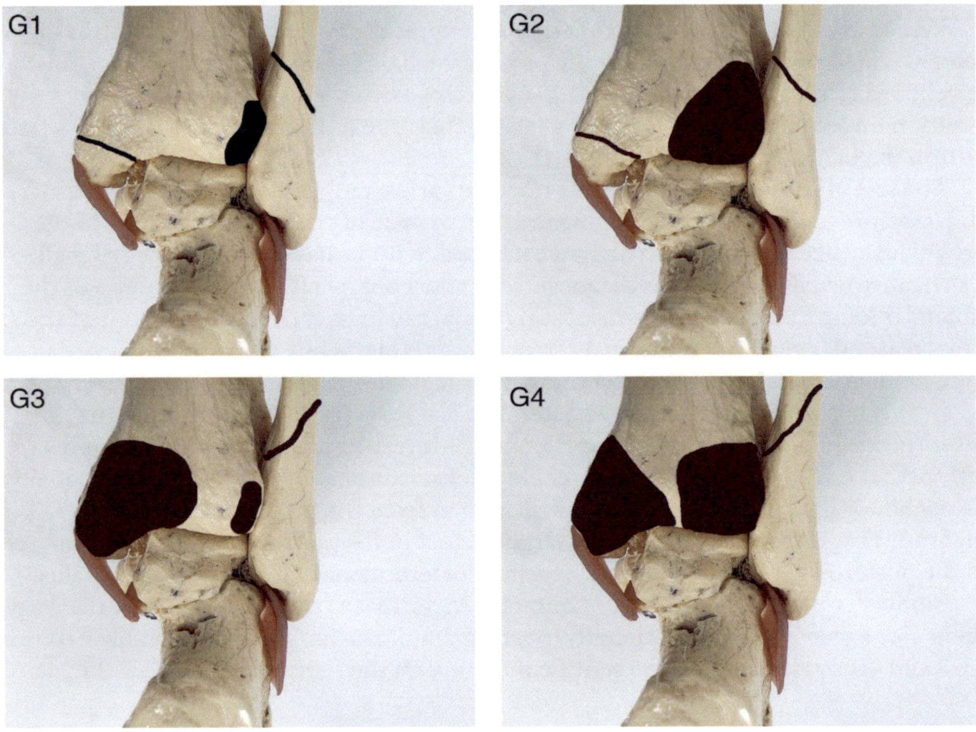

Figure 1.
Author grading of the trimalleolar fracture; G1; Transverse or short oblique medial malleolus transvers + lateral malleolus + shill avulsion posterior malleolus. G2; Medial malleolus + lateral malleolus + triangular posterolateral fragment. G3; Lateral malleolus + posteromedial triangular fracture ± small posterolateral fragment. G4; Lateral malleolus + rectangular posterolateral + triangular posteromedial.

The author generated a grading system based on CT, demonstrating four grades that facilitate management, are relevant for prognosis, and can be applied in research and clinical settings.

Author (Dahshan) grading of the trimalleolar fracture (**Figure 1**).

G1

Transverse or short oblique medial malleolus transvers + lateral malleolus + shill avulsion posterior malleolus avulsion of PITFL.

G2

Transvers or short oblique medial malleolus + lateral malleolus + triangular postero-lateral fragment > 25% of articular surface or > 2 mm articular step-off

G3

Lateral malleolus + posteromedial triangular fracture of medial malleolus (malleolus spur sign) ± small posterolateral fragment

G4

Lateral malleolus + rectangular posterolateral > 25% of the articular surface or > 2 mm articular step-off + triangular posteromedial with fragment impaction.

5. Radiographic evaluation

Despite the significant effort put into guidelines for requesting X-rays to minimise exposure, such as the Ottawa ankle rules, the authors strongly recommend considering the medicolegal aspects. At a minimum, three views should be obtained: a true anteroposterior (AP) view, a lateral view, and a mortise view (AP with 15° internal rotation). These views are essential for assessing the ankle joint by examining the medial malleolus, lateral malleolus, and syndesmosis, evaluating the medial clear space, tibiofibular clear space, talar tilt and posterior malleolus. Some X-ray signs, such as the double contour, misty mountains, and spur signs, show a posterior malleolar fracture and indicate CT (**Figure 2**).

- CT scan is the gold standard for diagnosing and managing ankle fractures, particularly trimalleolar ones. Axial, sagittal, coronal, and 3D imaging are crucial for a thorough preoperative assessment. CT also helps evaluate the fracture's size, shape, and site, identify any trapped loose fragments, and aid in planning the appropriate reduction method (**Figure 3**).

6. Management

6.1 Initial management

The question is: Would early management of a trimalleolar fracture in the ER be the same as management of an ankle fracture, or should it be like management of a Pilon fracture?

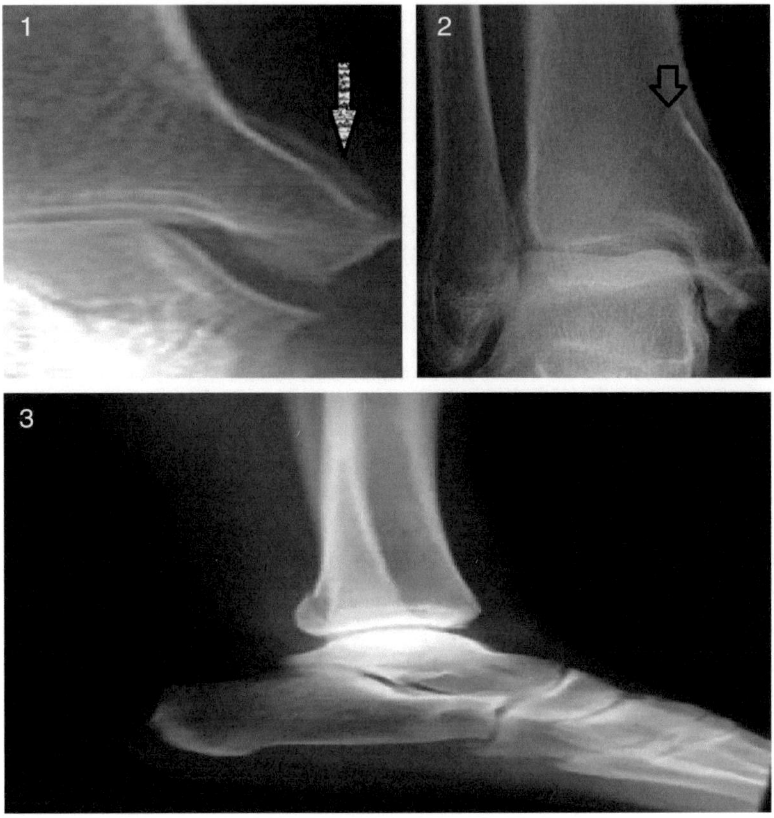

Figure 2.
1: The X-ray shows a posterior malleolus fracture manifested by 1, with a double contour sign. 2: Misty Mountains sign. 3: Spur signs.

The author's preferred method is to perform closed reduction in the ER under conscious sedation and use an open below-knee slab or ankle-foot orthosis with cold packs for 10 minutes every hour for 48 hours and leg elevation. Anticoagulants with analgesia are essential. Patient education and consent should be completed.

The radiology work should be completed during this period. The surgeon should start the operative planning early to avoid skin problems and subsequent surgery delays. Planning includes choosing the appropriate approaches and methods of reduction and fixation, considering skin condition, bone quality, fracture grading, and the functional demand of the patients.

External fixation is used as a staging procedure in open contaminated fractures (3%) with poor soft tissue or unstable reduction to prevent redislocation and minimise skin complications [30, 31].

6.2 Conservative treatment

Conservative treatment plays a minimal role in trimalleolar fractures due to high-energy trauma causing such fractures, related displacement due to the second fracture, or an additional ligamentous disruption (a fracture equivalent) leading to an unstable ankle and requiring surgical stabilisation. However, conservative treatment may be

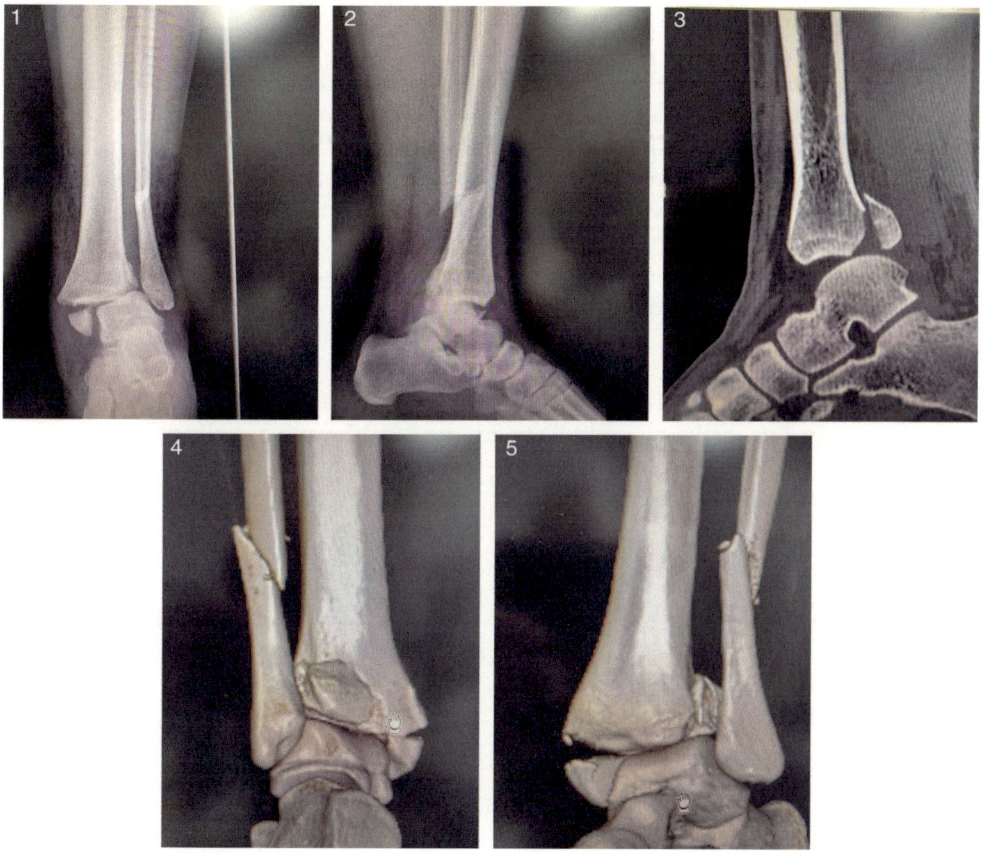

Figure 3.
A 37-year-old male with a trimalleolar fracture of G2. 1 and 2: Preoperative radiographs show the ankle fracture without a clear view of the posterior malleolus. 3: CT scans show the posterior malleolus fracture, size and site. 4 and 5: The 3-D reconstruction reveals the involvement of the posterolateral segment.

considered for stable medial malleolus fractures, stable lateral malleolus fractures with posterior malleolar fractures with <25% joint involvement or < 2 mm step-off.

The conservative treatment consisted of a close reduction below the knee, cast under anaesthesia, non-weight-bearing for four weeks, and full weight-bearing by weeks six to eight. Regular radiographs were conducted to monitor joint congruency [32].

Nineteen to thirty-eight percent of patients demonstrate loss of reduction, radiologic malunion, limited range of motion, and subsequently require conversion to internal fixation [32, 33].

6.3 Operative treatment

However, the functional outcome of trimalleolar fractures is found to be worse compared to uni- and bimalleolar fractures [34], and conditions such as diabetes, smoking, and vascular diseases raise the risk of wound complications after surgery that may result in amputation below the knee [35]; the surgeon must do his best to achieve good outcomes. A step-off of the posterior malleolus must be reduced, and the fragment should be fixed anatomically, achieving joint stability and restoring the syndesmosis stability to prevent redislocation and osteoarthritis [36–38].

6.4 Timing of surgery

There is debate regarding the timing of surgery for trimalleolar ankle fractures, ranging from a few hours to several days of delay to reduce soft tissue swelling [39]. However, the emergency indications include unsatisfactory closed reduction, severe soft tissue injury, compartment syndrome, and open fractures with or without concomitant vascular or nerve injury [40].

Some studies concluded no difference regarding postoperative wound infections, postoperative length of stay, complications, and functional outcomes in patients with closed ankle fractures treated with ORIF during the first eight hours and over six days [41–44]. Other studies found a significant increase in wound complications when surgery was delayed [39, 45].

Clinically, it depends on the skin condition around the incisional site; if it is not good, the surgical procedure should be postponed until proper healing.

6.5 The author's scheme for management

G1

Transverse or short oblique medial malleolus transvers + lateral malleolus + shill avulsion posterior malleolus avulsion of PITFL.: ORIF of the fibula, syndesmotic fixation and medial malleolus.

G2

Transverse or short oblique medial malleolus + lateral malleolus + triangular posterolateral fragment >25% of the articular surface or > 2 mm articular step-off: ORIF of the posterior malleolus, then fibula using a posterolateral approach. (Avoid neurovascular).

G3

Lateral malleolus + posteromedial triangular fracture of the medial malleolus (malleolus spur sign) + small posterolateral fragment: ORIF of the posterior malleolus (medial fragment) using a posteromedial approach (between flexor hallucis longus (FHL) and FDL and NV) and double plating. (With the risk of neurovascular injury).

G4

Lateral malleolus + rectangular posterolateral >25% of the articular surface or > 2 mm articular step-off + triangular posteromedial with fragment impaction: combine both a posterolateral and a posteromedial approach with double plating. Or a posteromedial approach with double plating (with the risk of neurovascular injury).

6.6 Surgical techniques

The posterior malleolus can be fixed via percutaneous, arthroscopic-assisted or open-approach fixation. Percutaneous screw fixation of the posterior malleolus can be performed from anterior to posterior after achieving closed reduction with ligamentotaxis. This approach has some advantages, as it is minimally invasive and facilitates fragment fixation while the patient remains supine. Nevertheless, it has disadvantages, such as the complexity of the reduction technique and the difficulty in extracting

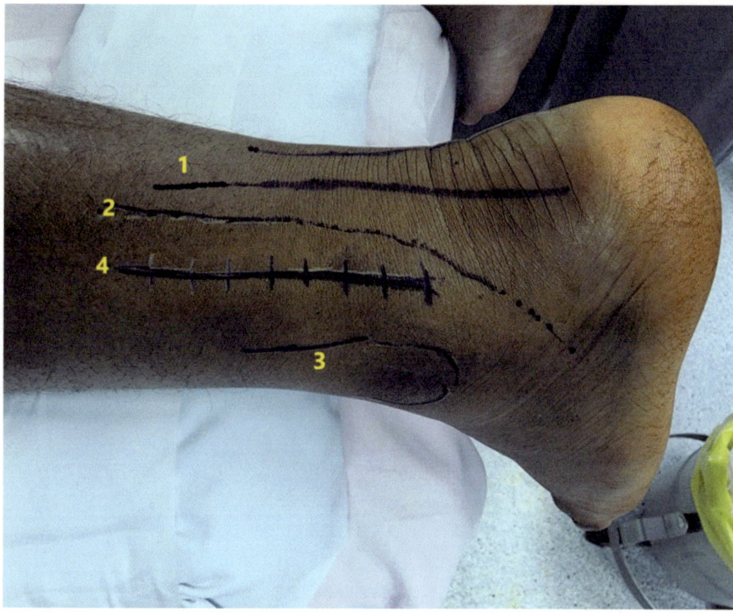

Figure 4.
Preoperative preparation: the patient is in a prone position, and there are skin markings of 1; the Achilles tendon, 2; sural nerve, 3; fibula and 4; the incision mark, located between the lateral edge of the Achilles tendon and the fibula.

intra-articular loose body fragments. Additionally, this method is not appropriate for all grades of trimalleolar fractures. The arthroscopic-assisted method is still being trialled. It is also less popular and requires a special grade of fracture and skilled hands.

Open reduction and internal fixation through posterolateral or posteromedial approaches seem superior to percutaneous anterior-to-posterior fixation [36, 46]. The prone position with a hang-free ankle and foot effectively addresses the posterior malleolus using the posterolateral or posteromedial approaches (**Figure 4**).

6.7 Posterolateral approach

This approach's advantages include direct access to and visualisation of the posterior fragment, which allows evaluation of the chondral surface and inspection for intra-articular bony pieces. Also, it avoids approaching the neurovascular bundle on the medial aspect of the ankle. Through this approach, the fibula can be reduced and plated [18].

Under GA or spinal anaesthesia and complete aseptic condition, with a high thigh tourniquet and in a prone position with a hanged ankle, the talus reduced spontaneously. A longitudinal incision is made midway between the tip distal fibula and the Achilles tendon, extending proximally about 10 cm; a scissor is used to identify the sural nerve, which crosses the incision from superomedial to inferolateral. To avoid nerve damage, retract it laterally. The plan between the peroneal muscles and the flexor hallucis longus (FHL) can be identified through an incision through the peroneal tendon sheath and repeated flexion/extension of the great toe to identify FHL. The posterior tibia is exposed by dissecting and retracting the FHL, medially protecting the posteromedial neurovascular bundle (**Figure 5**).

Special care was employed in managing the peroneal artery and its side branches during the dissection of FHL from the interosseous membrane, especially the

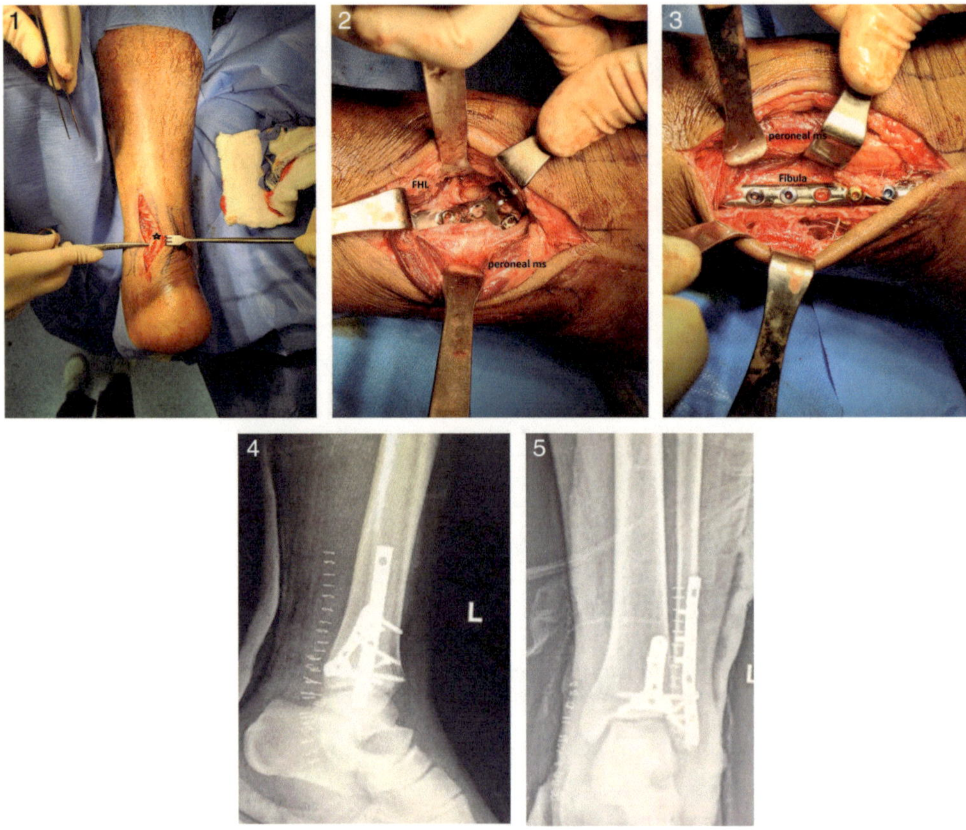

Figure 5.
1: Identification of the sural nerve, which crosses the incision from superomedial to inferolateral. 2: The plan between the peroneal muscles and FHL, after reduction and fixation of the posterior malleolus with T buttress plate. 3: Plan between the peroneal muscles and fibula after reduction and fixation of the fibula by lag screw and 1/3 plate. 4, 5: Postoperative X-ray.

transverse communicating branch. The PITFL could be identified as usually intact and should be respected [47]. Then, the tibiotalar joint can be inspected.

If the distal fibular fracture was proximal, it was mobilised through the same interval between the flexor hallucis longus and the peroneal muscles. If it was a low fracture, posterior subcutaneous dissection to the posterolateral border of the fibula was carried out [20].

This approach's disadvantage is that it cannot address the medial malleolar component, which should be addressed with a traditional medial incision. There is also a possibility of sural nerve injury or peroneal artery injury.

6.8 Posteromedial approach

A longitudinal incision is made midway between the medial malleolus and the Achilles tendon, extending about 10–12 cm proximally. The fascia is opened to expose the superficial layer over the flexor hallucis longus. This layer is incised laterally to the extent permitted by the incision. Caution is exercised during this process, as the posteromedial neurovascular bundle is medial to the flexor hallucis longus [48]. Identify FHL (the only fleshy muscle at this site and extension/flexion of the great toe) to develop a plane between it laterally and FDL medially. The neurovascular bundle can be retracted medially with FDL or laterally with FHL, according to the surgeon's preference.

Another option is to develop a plane between the FHL medially and the peroneal tendons laterally, exposing the posterior malleolus. Thus, the FHL tendon protects the neurovascular bundle. Releasing the FHL tendon from its retinaculum at the posterior talus allows muscle mobilisation.

The medial posteromedial approach provides access to the posteromedial edge of the tibia while limiting access to its posteromedial surface, particularly where the tibialis posterior tendon fully enters its groove. This technique particularly benefits fractures involving a sizeable posteromedial fragment with a medial apex. The incision is made along the posteromedial edge of the tibia, revealing the tibialis posterior tendon within its sheath, which is then opened longitudinally [48].

6.9 Reduction and fixation

The reduction and fixation of the posterior malleolus should be started before the fibula. This will allow more rooming, leading to easy reduction and fixation. Other advantages include achieving the appropriate fibular length, allowing for visualisation of the fracture without implant interference on radiographs, and stabilising the large fragment of medial malleolar fractures [48].

First, the fracture line between the posterolateral and posteromedial main fragments must be identified. Then, incise the periosteum and lift the two fragments. Hinge the lateral fragment using the posterior tibiofibular ligament and the medial fragment on the posterior tibial tendon sheath.

The posteromedial fragment should be reduced first because the elevated posterolateral fragment provides a better view of the posteromedial corner and because of the risk of medial translation of the posteromedial fragment when the posterolateral fragment is compressed and fixed with temporary k wire [20, 48].

During the reduction and fixation of the posteromedial fragment, and because the tibialis posterior may limit the space, it is advised not to elevate the tendon off the fragment but rather to place the fixation at the periphery of the fragment to minimise the disturbance of its vascularity and to eliminate the potential of hardware interference with the tendon [20]. Then, the posterior malleolar fragment is debrided and meticulously freed from medial soft tissue attachments. The capsule is incised inferiorly and checks the articular surface. The posterior malleolar fragment is anatomically reduced and provisionally secured with a K wire [49].

Posterior talar subluxation is an essential indication for posterior malleolus reduction to restore ankle congruity [18].

In his meta-analysis, Wang 2023 concluded that plate fixation resulted in a better alignment of articular step-off or gap compared to "A to P" screw fixation for the posterior malleolus in trimalleolar ankle fractures. But screw fixation allowed a shorter surgical time than plate fixation. However, when comparing the two methods, no significant differences were observed in AOFAS scores, the incidence of arthritis, infections, sural nerve injuries, or overall complications [50].

But in 2024, Ting concluded that plate fixation is a favourable alternative to screw fixation in posterior malleolar fractured patients. Although plate fixation was at risk of longer surgery time, postoperative adhesions of the flexor hallucis longus muscle belly and more blood loss, it provided better postoperative functional outcomes, shorter healing, weight-bearing and off-bed ambulation time and less pain compared to screw fixation [51].

The author's preferred fixation method depends on the fracture's size. For large fragments, fixation is better achieved using a plate or two screws with washers (to avoid fragment rotation) and may use the ACL C guide to get the trajectory of the screws. However, a buttress plate is recommended if the fragment is small or friable. Preoperative CT evaluation is crucial as it determines the fracture size and guides the selection of the most appropriate fixation method.

After fixation of the posterior malleolus, reduction and fixation of the fibula can be done through the interval between the FHL and peroneal muscle in proximal fractures; in contrast, in distal fractures, posterior subcutaneous dissection of the posterolateral border of the fibula was carried out for reduction and fixation (**Figure 5**) [20]. The lateral malleolar fracture is reduced and fixed using a plate. The stability of the syndesmosis is checked, and a syndesmosis screw is routinely applied if there is instability. The medial malleolar fracture is approached separately, either in a prone or supine position, according to the surgeon's preference [52].

7. Postoperative care

A splint or orthosis should be used for 4–6 weeks. However, after the first 3 weeks, range-of-motion exercises may be initiated. Partial weight-bearing is permitted after 6 weeks with physiotherapy, but full weight-bearing activities are generally restricted for about 10–12 weeks postoperatively.

This guideline should be adjusted based on factors like bone quality, fixation stability, patient reliability, comorbid conditions, and the need to protect soft tissues such as syndesmosis.

Patients who start bearing weight early tend to return to work sooner than those who delay [53–55]. Early weight-bearing helps stabilise the ankle joint and prevents harmful movements [56]. However, for obese and diabetic patients, it is advisable to have a more extended period of non-weight-bearing or partial weight-bearing. Premature weight-bearing is a significant factor contributing to the loss of fracture reduction in this specific patient population [57, 58].

8. Complication

Overall complication rates following ORIF of ankle fractures vary in the literature, ranging from 1 to 40%. These complications can be divided into early and late [59–61].

8.1 Early complications include

8.1.1 Superficial or deep infection

Postoperative wound infection is one of the most common complications following ankle fracture surgery [62]. The overall rate reported in the literature varies between 1.4% and 13.0%. Specifically, the prevalence of superficial infections ranges from 3.0% to 10.0%, while deep infections occur at rates between 1.0% and 6.8% up to 20% in diabetic patients [63–65].

The patient complains of increased pain, fever, swelling, redness, pus, and an unpleasant odour in the wound. Investigation shows high C-reactive protein levels and ESR. Bacterial culture confirms the diagnosis. The most frequently identified bacteria are *Staphylococcus aureus* and *Staphylococcus epidermidis*.

The author recommends using antibiotics and appropriate follow-up care to manage superficial wound infections. Aggressive treatment through open debridement and irrigation is essential in cases of deep infections. If the fracture is not united and the implant demonstrates stable fixation, the implant can be retained; however, if there is any sign of loosening and the fracture is not united, the implant should be removed to ensure optimal recovery and use a temporary fixation. If the fracture is united and the implant is stable, removing the implant is advised to eradicate the infection.

8.1.2 Neurovascular injury

In posterolateral appraisal, the sural nerve and peroneal artery are liable to injury. Injury to the sural nerve causes a painful neuroma or numbness along the lateral border of the foot. In the posteromedial approach, the posterior tibial nerve and artery are susceptible to injury [63].

8.2 Late complications include

8.2.1 Posttraumatic OA

Treatment involves reducing activities, administering anti-inflammatory medications, providing intra-articular injections, and utilising modified footwear or braces. Salvage procedures such as ankle arthrodesis or ankle arthroplasty should be considered in advanced cases.

8.2.2 Malunion

The surgeon must thoroughly review the closed treatment reduction images or the intraoperative and postoperative radiographs to confirm acceptable reduction and no step-off.

Patients with ankle fractures require careful monitoring to detect malunions. This allows for the early restoration of anatomic osseous and articular alignment, potentially preventing or postponing traumatic arthrosis. Therefore, secondary reconstruction should be prioritised in treating a malunited ankle fracture, while other options like supramalleolar osteotomy or arthrodesis should only be explored if this approach is unsuccessful.

8.2.3 Residual pain

This pertains to chondral injuries and soft tissue impingement [66], along with posttraumatic neuromas [67], arthrofibrosis [68], malreduction, loss of reduction, and malunion [63].

8.2.4 Implant irritation

Peroneal tendonitis can occur due to irritation caused by the posteriorlateral plating of the fibula, particularly when the plate is placed distally. Additionally, posterior tibial tendonitis may start if screws are placed at the posterior medial malleolus. Therefore, it is advisable to position the plate at the periphery of the fracture.

8.2.5 Non-union

Non-union ankle fractures are uncommon. The periosteum may intervene within a medial malleolus, necessitating the removal of the interposed material, bone grafting, and subsequent stabilisation. Generally, most non-union can be effectively treated with cancellous grafting and stable internal fixation [19].

Author details

Wael Abdelkarim Aldahshan[1,2*], Ahmed Mohamed Abd-alkhalek[3], Ahmed Sayed Elshamy[4] and Mohammed Ahmed Abd Elfattah[5]

1 Orthopedic Surgery, Al-Azhar University, Egypt

2 Orthopedic Consultant, Prince Fahd Bin Sultan Hospital, KSA

3 Medical Intern, Al-Azhar University, Egypt

4 Faculty of Medicine, Orthopaedic Surgery, Al-Azhar University, Egypt

5 Faculty of Medicine for Girls, Orthopaedic Surgery, Al-Azhar University, Egypt

*Address all correspondence to: drwaelaldahshan@hotmail.com

References

[1] Alluri R et al. Radiographic detection of marginal impaction in supination-adduction ankle fractures. Foot & Ankle International. 2017;**38**(9):1005-1010. DOI: 10.1177/1071100717709565

[2] Boraiah S et al. High association of posterior malleolus fractures with spiral distal tibial fractures. Clinical Orthopaedics and Related Research. 2008;**466**(7):1692-1698. DOI: 10.1007/s11999-008-0224-5

[3] Jung KJ et al. Concomitant ankle injuries associated with tibial shaft fractures. Foot & Ankle International. 2015;**36**:1209-1214. DOI: 10.1177/1071100715588381

[4] Kempegowda H et al. Posterior malleolar fractures associated with tibial shaft fractures and sequence of fixation. Journal of Orthopaedic Trauma. 2016;**30**(10):568-571. DOI: 10.1097/BOT.0000000000000629

[5] Court-Brown CM et al. Epidemiology of adult fractures: A review. Injury. 2006;**37**:691-697. DOI: 10.1016/j.injury.2006.04.130

[6] Jaskulka RA et al. Fractures of the posterior tibial margin: Their role in the prognosis of malleolar fractures. The Journal of Trauma. 1989;**29**(11):1565-1570. DOI: 10.1097/00005373-198911000-00018

[7] Irwin T et al. Posterior malleolus fracture. The Journal of the American Academy of Orthopaedic Surgeons. 2013;**21**(1):32-40. DOI: 10.5435/JAAOS-21-01-32

[8] Solan MC, Sakellariou A. Posterior malleolus fractures: Worth fixing. Bone Joint Journal. 2017;**99**(11):1413-1419. DOI: 10.1302/0301-620X.99B11.BJJ-2017-1072

[9] Lyndon W, Mason WJ. Pathoanatomy and associated injuries of posterior malleolus fracture of the ankle. Foot & Ankle International. 2017;**38**(11):1229-1235. DOI: 10.1177/1071100717719533. Epub 2017 Jul 31

[10] Inman V. The Joints of the Ankle. Baltimore: Williams & Wilkins; 1976

[11] Sarrafian SK, Sarrafian's AS. Anatomy of the Foot and Ankle: Descriptive, Topographic, Functional. Baltimore: Williams & Wilkins; 2012

[12] Clanton T et al. Biomechanical analysis of the individual ligament contributions to syndesmotic stability. Foot & Ankle International. 2016;**38**(1):66-75. DOI: 10.1177/1071100716666277

[13] Lilyquist M et al. Cadaveric analysis of the distal tibiofibular syndesmosis. Foot & Ankle International. 2016;**37**(8):882-890. DOI: 10.1177/1071100716643083

[14] Jan B. Anatomy of the tibiofibular syndesmosis and its clinical relevance. Surgical and Radiologic Anatomy. 2003;**25**:379-386. DOI: 10.1007/s00276-003-0156-4

[15] Golano P et al. Anatomy of the ankle ligaments: A pictorial essay. Knee Surgery, Sports Traumatology, Arthroscopy. 2010;**18**(5):557-569. DOI: 10.1007/s00167-010-1100-x

[16] Golanò P et al. Arthroscopic anatomy of the posterior ankle ligaments. Arthroscopy. 2002;**18**(4):353-358. DOI: 10.1053/jars.2002.32318

[17] Miller AN et al. Posterior malleolar stabilisation of syndesmotic injuries is equivalent to screw fixation. Clinical Orthopaedics and Related Research. 2010;**468**(4):1129-1135. DOI: 10.1007/s11999-009-1111-4

[18] Christian Bergman MM. Anatomy, classification, and management of Ankle Fractures Involving the posterior malleolar fragment: A literature review. Foot & Ankle Orthopaedics. 2019;**4**(4):1-11. DOI: 10.1177/2473011419887724

[19] Charles L, Saltzman RB. Mann's Surgery of the Foot and Ankle. 2-Volume Set. Philadelphia: Elsevier; 2013. eBook ISBN: 9781455748617

[20] Weber M. Trimalleolar fractures with impaction of the posteromedial tibial plafond: Implications for talar stability. Foot & Ankle International. 2004;**25**:716-727. DOI: 10.1177/107110070402501005

[21] Gardner MJ et al. The ability of the Lauge-Hansen classification to predict ligament injury and mechanism in ankle fractures: An MRI study. Journal of Orthopaedic Trauma. 2006;**20**(4):267-272. DOI: 10.1097/00005131-200604000-00006

[22] Hartford JM et al. Tibiotalar contact area. Contribution of posterior malleolus and deltoid ligament. Clinical Orthopaedics and Related Research. 1995;**320**:182-187

[23] Macko VW et al. The joint-contact area of the ankle. The contribution of the posterior malleolus. The Journal of Bone and Joint Surgery. American Volume. 1991;**73**(3):347-351

[24] Raasch WG et al. Assessment of the posterior malleolus as a restraint to posterior subluxation of the ankle. The Journal of Bone and Joint Surgery. American Volume. 1992;**74**(8):1201-1206

[25] Scheidt KB et al. Posterior malleolar ankle fractures: An in vitro biomechanical analysis of stability in the loaded and unloaded states. Journal of Orthopaedic Trauma. 1992;**6**(1):96-101

[26] Fitzpatrick DC et al. Kinematic and contact stress analysis of posterior malleolus fractures of the ankle. Journal of Orthopaedic Trauma. 2004;**18**(5):271-278. DOI: 10.1097/00005131-200405000-00002

[27] Haraguchi N et al. Pathoanatomy of posterior malleolus fractures of the ankle. The Journal of Bone and Joint Surgery. American Volume. 2006;**88**(8):1835. DOI: 10.2106/JBJS.E.00856

[28] Bartoníček J et al. Anatomy and classification of the posterior tibial fragment in ankle fractures. Archives of Orthopaedic and Trauma Surgery. 2015;**135**:505-516. DOI: 10.1007/s00402-015-2171-4

[29] Patrick Pflüger K-FB. Current management of trimalleolar ankle fractures. EFORT Open Reviews. 2021;**6**(8):692-703. DOI: 10.1302/2058-5241.6.200138

[30] Bennett A. Open fractures. Journal of Orthopaedic Trauma. 2013;**27**:9-14. DOI: 10.1016/j.mporth.2013.01.001

[31] Court-Brown CM et al. Open fractures in the elderly: The importance of skin ageing. Injury. 2015;**46**:189-194. DOI: 10.1016/j.injury.2014.07.021

[32] Willett K et al. Ankle injury management (AIm) trial collaborators. Close contact casting vs surgery for initial treatment of unstable ankle fractures in older adults: A randomised clinical trial. JAMA. 2016;**316**:1455-1463. DOI: 10.1001/jama.2016.14719

[33] Makwana NK, Bhowal B. Conservative versus operative treatment for displaced ankle fractures in patients over 55 years of age: A prospective, randomised study. Journal of Bone and Joint Surgery (British). 2001;**83**:525-529. DOI: 10.1302/0301-620x.83b4.11522

[34] Verhage SM, Schipper I. Long-term functional and radiographic outcomes in 243 operated ankle fractures. Journal of Foot and Ankle Research. 2015;**8**:45. DOI: 10.1186/s13047-015-0098-1

[35] Ovaska MT, Madanat R. Predictors of postoperative wound necrosis following primary wound closure of open ankle fractures. Foot & Ankle International. 2016;**37**:401-406. DOI: 10.1177/1071100715609182

[36] Verhage SM, Hoogendoorn JM. When and how to operate the posterior malleolus fragment in trimalleolar fractures: Systematic literature. Review Archives of Orthopaedic and Trauma Surgery. 2018;**138**(9):1213-1222. DOI: 10.1007/s00402-018-2949-2

[37] Gardner MJ, Brodsky A. Fixation of posterior malleolar fractures provides greater syndesmotic stability. Clinical Orthopaedics and Related Research. 2006;**447**:165-171. DOI: 10.1097/01.blo.0000203489.21206.a9

[38] Langenhuijsen J, Heetveld M. Results of ankle fractures with involvement of the posterior tibial margin. Journal of Trauma. 2002;**53**:55-60. DOI: 10.1097/00005373-200207000-00012

[39] Saithna A. The influence of timing of surgery on soft tissue complications in closed ankle fractures. European Journal of Orthopaedic Surgery and Traumatology. 2009;**19**:481-484. DOI: 10.1007/s00590-009-0455-5

[40] Rammelt S. G. R. Ankle fractures. Unfallchirurg. 2008;**111**:421-437. DOI: 10.1007/s00113-008-1460-6

[41] Naumann MG, Sigurdsen U. Associations of timing of surgery with postoperative length of stay, complications, and functional outcomes 3-6 years after operative fixation of closed ankle fractures. Injury. 2017;**48**:1662-1669. DOI: 10.1016/j.injury.2017.03.039

[42] Breederveld RS, Straaten J. Immediate or delayed operative treatment of fractures of the ankle. Injury. 1988;**19**:436-438. DOI: 10.1016/0020-1383(88)90142-8

[43] Singh RA, Trickett R. Early versus late surgery for closed ankle fractures. Journal of Orthopaedic Surgery (Hong Kong). 2015;**23**:341-344. DOI: 10.1177/230949901502300317

[44] Miller AG, Margules A. Risk factors for wound complications after ankle fracture surgery. Journal of Bone & Joint Surgery. 2012;**94-A**:2047-2052. DOI: 10.2106/JBJS.K.01088

[45] Sukeik M, Qaffar M. Ankle fractures: Impact of swelling on timing of surgery, length of hospital stay and the economic burden. Orthopaedic Proceedings. 2011;**93-B**(Supp II):124. DOI: 10.1016/J.INJURY.2010.07.419

[46] Deborah Carr CV. Posterior-based approaches to open reduction internal fixation of Bimalleolar and Trimalleolar fractures: A systematic review and meta-analysis. The Journal of Foot & Ankle Surgery. Apr 2020;**59**(2):373-378. DOI: 10.1053/j.jfas.2019.09.004

[47] Mingo-Robinet J, J. M. Posterolateral approach in trimalleolar ankle fractures: Surgical technique. Revista Española de Cirugía Ortopédica y Traumatología.

2012;**56**(4):313-318. DOI: 10.1016/j.recot.2012.02.003

[48] Mason LW, A. K. Posterior malleolar ankle fractures. An effort at improving outcomes. JBJS Open Access. 2019;**4**(2):e0058. DOI: 10.2106/JBJS.OA.18.00058

[49] Franzone JM, Vosseller JT. Posterolateral approach for open reduction and internal fixation of a posterior malleolus fracture—Hinging on an intact PITFL to disimpact the Tibial plafond: A technical note. Foot and Ankle International. 2013;**34**(8):1177-1181. DOI: 10.1177/1071100713481455

[50] Jie Wang H-BJ-G. Plate versus screws fixation for the posterior malleolar fragment in trimalleolar ankle fractures. Injury. 2023;**54**(2):761-767. DOI: 10.1016/j.injury.2022.10.032

[51] Tu T-Y, Huang S-T, Chou Y-J. Comparison of plate versus screw internal fixation in the treatment of posterior malleolar fracture: A systematic review and meta-analysis. Foot and Ankle Surgery. 2024;**30**(3):191-218. DOI: 10.1016/j.fas.2023.12.004

[52] Yang Y, He W, Zhou H, Xia J, Li B, Tao Y. Combined posteromedial and posterolateral approaches for 2-parts posterior malleolar fracture fixation. Foot and Ankle Surgery. 2020;**41**(10):1234-1239. DOI: 10.1177/1071100720937637

[53] Black JD et al. Early weight bearing in operatively fixed ankle fractures: A systematic review. Foot (Edinburgh, Scotland). 2013;**23**:78-85. DOI: 10.1016/j.foot.2013.05.002

[54] Kubiak EN et al. Early weight bearing after lower extremity fractures in adults. The Journal of the American Academy of Orthopaedic Surgeons. 2013;**21**:727-738. DOI: 10.5435/JAAOS-21-12-727

[55] Simanski CJ et al. Functional treatment and early weight bearing after an ankle fracture: A prospective study. Journal of Orthopaedic Trauma. 2006;**20**:108-114. DOI: 10.1097/01.bot.0000197701.96954.8c

[56] Starkweather MP et al. Early protected weight bearing after open reduction internal fixation of ankle fractures. The Journal of Foot and Ankle Surgery. 2012;**51**:575-578. DOI: 10.1053/j.jfas.2012.05.022

[57] Rizvi AA et al. Perioperative management of diabetes and hyperglycemia in patients undergoing orthopaedic surgery. The Journal of the American Academy of Orthopaedic Surgeons. 2010;**18**:426-435. DOI: 10.5435/00124635-201007000-00005

[58] Chaudhry S et al. Ankle injuries and fractures in the obese patient. The Orthopedic Clinics of North America. 2011;**42**:45-53. DOI: 10.1016/j.ocl.2010.07.003

[59] SooHoo NF et al. Complication rates following open reduction and internal fixation of ankle fractures. The Journal of Bone and Joint Surgery. American Volume. 2009;**91**(05):1042-1049. DOI: 10.2106/JBJS.H.00653

[60] Ebraheim NA et al. Ankle fractures involving the fibula proximal to the distal tibiofibular syndesmosis. Foot & Ankle International. 1997;**18**(08):513-521. DOI: 10.1177/107110079701800811

[61] Leyes M et al. Complications of open reduction and internal fixation of ankle fractures. Foot and Ankle Clinics. 2003;**8**(01):131-147. DOI: 10.1016/s1083-7515(02)00162-6

[62] Schepers TVL. Increased rates of wound complications with locking

plates in distal fibular fractures. Injury. 2011;**42**(10):1125-1129. DOI: 10.1016/j.injury.2011.01.009

[63] Ovaska M. Complications in ankle fracture surgery. Acta Orthopaedica. Supplementum. 2015;**86**(358):1-32. DOI: 10.3109/17453674.2014.100227

[64] Zalavras CG et al. Infection following operative treatment of ankle fractures. Clinical Orthopaedics and Related Research. 2009;**467**(07):1715-1720. DOI: 10.1007/s11999-009-0743-8

[65] Scheperst DV. The timing of ankle fracture surgery and the effect on infectious complications: A case series and systematic review of the literature. International Orthopaedics. 2013;**37**:489-494. DOI: 10.1007/s00264-012-1753-9

[66] Kannus P et al. Increasing number and incidence of low-trauma ankle fractures in elderly people: Finnish statistics during 1970-2000 and projections for the future. Bone. 2002;**31**(03):430-433. DOI: 10.1016/s8756-3282(02)00832-3

[67] Redfern DJ et al. Investigation of incidence of superficial peroneal nerve injury following ankle fracture. Foot & Ankle International. 2003;**24**(10):771-774. DOI: 10.1177/107110070302401006

[68] Utsugi K et al. Intra-articular fibrous tissue formation following ankle fracture: The significance of arthroscopic debridement of fibrous tissue. Arthroscopy. 2007;**23**(01):89-93. DOI: 10.1016/j.arthro.2006.07.055

Chapter 7

Posterior Malleolar Fractures

Christopher Lenz

Abstract

Posterior malleolar fractures (PMF) often occur with the ankle fractures. They usually lead to poorer outcomes. PMF can impact ankle stability and the joint surface. Over time, our approach to these complex fractures has evolved. In the past, we fixed fragments based on their size (25–30% of the joint surface) and displacement. Now, our understanding of PMF has improved, along with the diagnostic and treatment methods. This book chapter reviews our current knowledge of PMF. It covers topics such as epidemiology, classification, pathophysiology, diagnostic imaging, treatment strategies, and outcomes.

Keywords: ankle fractures, ankle joint, stability, posterior malleolar fractures, Volkmann tubercle, treatment

1. Introduction

Ankle fractures are a common orthopaedic injury, making up around 9% of all fractures [1]. These injuries can range from simple to complex patterns, posing significant challenges for surgeons. When the posterior malleolus is involved, the fracture becomes even more complex, requiring careful consideration of patient positioning, surgical approach, and implant choice, making the procedure more demanding. In 1822, Cooper first described the posterior malleolar fracture (PMF) in a chronic ankle fracture-dislocation [2]. The term “trimalleolar fracture” was introduced by Henderson in 1932, describing the involvement of the fibula, medial malleolus, and posterior malleolus in ankle fractures [3].

These fractures usually result from rotational injury mechanisms, with various factors influencing the injury pattern, such as bone quality, impact, duration, and mechanism of injury, as well as external factors like footwear. The fracture morphology is highly heterogeneous, and there is no consensus on optimal treatment.

Posterior malleolar fractures (PMFs) are crucial in the treatment and prognosis of ankle fractures due to their variability in size, location, number of fragments, and displacement. Clinically, PMFs are significant because they affect ankle ligaments, the syndesmotic complex, joint congruency, stability, and load distribution across the ankle joint.

Studies have shown that trimalleolar fractures have worse outcomes than isolated fibular or bimalleolar fractures [4–6].

To provide thorough insights, it is essential to discuss terminology. As mentioned, the term “trimalleolar fracture” was introduced in 1932 [3]. However, there is no clear consensus on the right terms, and it remains inconsistent. The term “Volkmann

IntechOpen

fracture" actually refers to fractures of the posterior tibial lip, whereas Volkmann described an anterolateral distal tibia fracture [7]. The term lacks specificity regarding fragment morphology, size, and associated injuries. Destot introduced the term "malléole postérieure" [8]. Therefore, "posterior malleolar fracture" seems accurate but still nonspecific. It makes sense to use a comprehensible classification to adequately address the specific fracture and its characteristics.

2. Anatomy and biomechanics

The ankle joint is an ultracongruent joint, a complex ginglymoid joint stabilized by its bony congruency and multiple ligaments, including the syndesmotic complex. The bony congruency is important to understand, as the talus is narrow in the axial plane and widens from posterior to anterior. This means the most stable joint position, in terms of bony congruency and stability, is in dorsiflexion, when the foot is fixed on the ground without any forces acting on the ankle. The posterior malleolus, also known as the posterior tibial lip, forms the posterior part of the distal tibia. In the sagittal plane, the distal articular joint surface is concave and extends distally, forming the posterior malleolus, or Volkmann tubercle, a term commonly used in German.

The Volkmann tubercle provides attachments for the posterior inferior tibiofibular ligament (PITFL), also known as the posterior syndesmosis, which runs obliquely to its insertion at the posterior distal fibula. The distal syndesmotic complex also consists of the anterior inferior tibiofibular ligament (AITFL), the interosseous ligament (IOL), and the interosseous membrane (IOM). The PITFL provides 42% of syndesmotic stability [9], emphasizing the importance of the anatomic structure of the ligament itself and its attachment area at the posterior malleolus.

Biomechanically, many approaches have been used to define and determine the impact of injuries to the posterior malleolus. Early biomechanic studies showed that the posterior malleolus contributes approximately 25–30% to ankle joint stability and load bearing. Furthermore, a fragment size of 33% has been considered crucial in terms of peak stresses acting on the articular surface, with a higher risk of developing posttraumatic ankle joint arthritis [10, 11]. This fact has been crucial in determining the treatment approach to PMF. Fragments involving less than 25–33% and with less than 2 mm of fracture dislocation on the lateral X-ray have been considered for non-operative treatment [12–15]. With a growing body of evidence and more frequent use of CT imaging, knowledge has increased, and more detailed classification systems have arisen. Thus, the three-dimensional fracture morphology has become clearer, and several factors have become essential in considering the proposed best way to address PMF. These factors include not only fragment size and dislocation but also the involvement of the incisura, the presence of intercalary fragments, impaction of the distal joint surface, and stability of the syndesmotic complex. In conclusion, the goals of treatment aim to restore the distal joint surface and the fibular notch, including posterior containment of the talus and reduction of the distal fibula, and stability of the PITFL by strong bone-to-bone fixation of the PMF.

3. Epidemiology and pathomechanism

Considering all ankle fractures, around 7–44% are accompanied by PMF [4, 16]. In more complex ankle fractures, the prevalence is higher, as they involve more crucial structures, such as the syndesmotic complex, and more severe ligament injuries.

A typical mechanism of injury is a rotational force transmitted through the ankle joint complex, classified by Lauge-Hansen as Pronation-Abduction or Pronation-External Rotation injury mechanisms [17]. However, it can also occur during Supination-External Rotation. Lauge-Hansen classified ankle fractures into several stages, representing fracture patterns by their mechanism of injury. The first word describes the foot position when the injury starts, and the second word describes the direction of the force, usually a rotational force [17].

High-energy trauma, such as falls from heights, work accidents, or motor vehicle accidents, can cause more complex injury patterns. These injuries are often accompanied by severe soft tissue damage and complex, multifragmentary fracture patterns. In rare cases, a PMF can occur as an isolated fracture.

4. Classification systems

Several attempts have been made to classify PMF. A good classification system in traumatology should be simple and practical. It must cover the full range of fracture types while being comprehensive. High reproducibility is also important, so different observers can apply it consistently. The system should guide treatment strategies and connect to outcomes and prognosis.

The oldest classification was by Nelson and Jensen [18]. They distinguished "classical" from "minimal" based on the percentage of the involved articular surface. They recommended surgical fixation for classical fractures and introduced the "one-third rule." It is surprising that many surgeons still use this outdated approach for fracture treatment. This rule is now obsolete and should be discarded.

In 1990, the AO classified PMF into Type 1 to Type 3, which includes extra articular, small articular, and large articular fragments, respectively [19]. Today, we need to evaluate the exact morphology of fractures. Modern classification systems are CT-based and do not rely on conventional X-rays. The most common and reliable systems were published by Haraguchi et al. in 2006 and Bartoníček in 2015. Haraguchi analysed CT scans of 57 patients and proposed three types of PMF (**Figure 1**).

Type I (67% of cases): posterior oblique fracture of the distal tibia (triangular fragment).
Type II (19%): PMF with medial extension involving the posterior part of the medial malleolus.
Type III (14%): shell-like fracture of the cortical and subcortical bone of the distal posterior tibia.

Bartoníček et al. proposed a classification system with four fracture patterns. They focused on the fibular notch and its involvement (**Figure 2**).

Type I (8% of cases): characterized by an extraincisural fragment.
Type II (52%): a posterolateral fragment.
Type III (28%): 2-part fragment at the posteromedial aspect of the tibia.
Type IV (9%): a large posterolateral fragment involving 33–50% of the fibular incisura.
Type V (3%): irregular osteoporotic fracture.

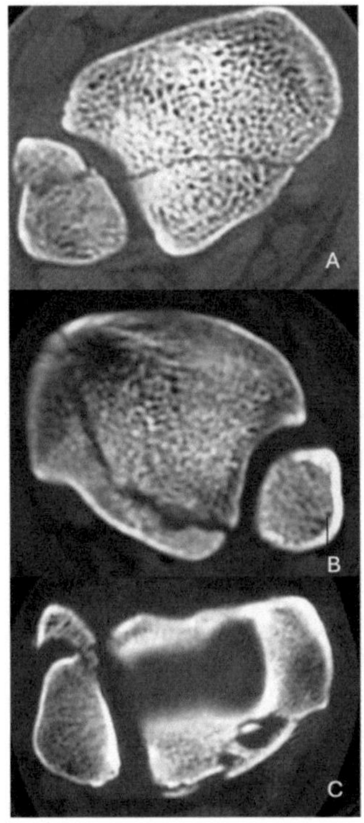

Figure 1.
Axial CT scans showing fracture examples according to the classification of Haraguchi [20]: (A) posterolateral type, (B) medial-extension type, (C) small-shell type.

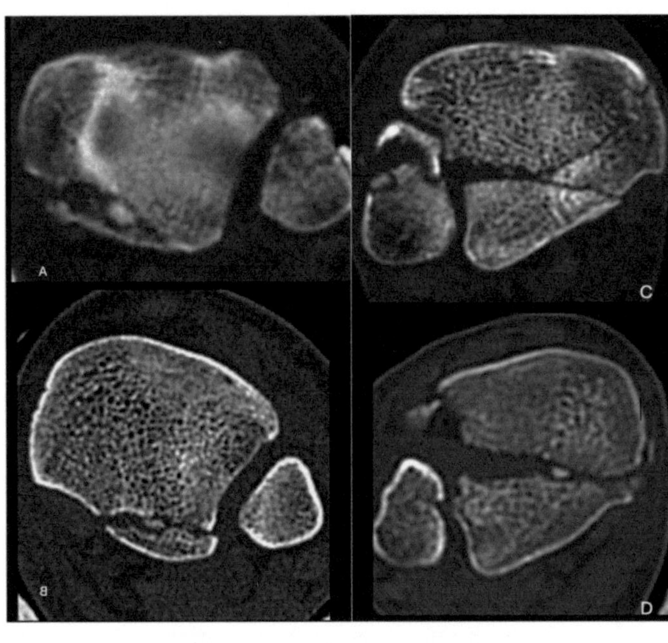

Figure 2.
Axial CT scans showing fracture examples according to the classification of Bartoníček [21]: (A) extraincisural fragment with intact fibular notch, (B) posterolateral fragment extending into the fibular notch, (C) posteromedial two-part fragment involving the medial malleolus, (D) large posterolateral triangular fragment.

Emerging systems emphasize the functional impact of the fracture, including ligamentous injuries and syndesmotic stability. Adding simple descriptive terms can help fully describe the fracture pattern. It is crucial to have a complete understanding of the fracture before planning surgery and osteosynthesis.

5. Diagnostics and imaging

The initial trauma assessment follows general guidelines for trauma surgery. Key findings that influence decisions include pain, swelling, deformity, and instability. Standard anteroposterior (AP), lateral, and mortise views can show fractures. However, simple X-rays often miss details of the pilon fracture (PMF). They may not capture the number of fragments, fracture path, impaction, size, displacement, or intercalary fragments. The author strongly recommends a CT scan for every PMF. If standard X-rays cannot rule it out, a CT scan is needed. CT is the gold standard for PMF evaluation. It provides detailed views of all relevant aspects. Three-dimensional reconstructions also help with surgical planning. MRI scans can assess related soft-tissue injuries such as ligament tears and cartilage damage, but they are usually not needed. For stability, MRI lacks enough information. Clinical and intraoperative evaluations are more important.

6. Management and treatment

In most cases, PMF needs surgery because of its key role in the ankle joint. However, nonoperative treatment is an option for isolated, nondisplaced fractures. A thorough assessment, including CT scans, is needed to confirm these conditions.

The percentage of articular surface involvement is no longer a reliable factor for decision-making. There are no evidence-based guidelines or treatment algorithms to follow. Many surgeons evaluate the PMF during surgery after stabilizing the fibula. Often, they use ligamentotaxis to reduce the posterior malleolus fragment, especially the PITFL. If this is confirmed during surgery, no additional fixation is needed. Other surgeons prefer to fix the PMF if the fragment can be secured with a screw or plate and screw construct. There is no high-level evidence indicating which method yields better results. The best treatment approach remains controversial, with many factors and methods debated, and little evidence supporting one over the other.

6.1 Patient positioning and surgical approach

The type of ankle fracture affects the surgical approach. The prone position is best for accessing the posterior tibia. This method also allows for reducing and fixing the fibula. However, it requires skill, especially if the surgeon usually works on the fibula in isolated fractures, while the patient is supine or in lateral decubitus. The same goes for the medial malleolus. It can be accessed in the prone position but is trickier than the fibula. The lateral decubitus position also offers good access to the posterior tibia and fibula. If necessary, the leg can be externally rotated to reach the medial malleolus. Sometimes, changing the patient's position during surgery can help with access to the malleoli. The author usually prefers the prone position for fractures of the posterior malleolus and fibula. For trimalleolar fractures, position the patient in lateral decubitus on their belly, with support at their back. When addressing the medial malleolus, remove the back support and gently rotate the patient to the supine position. This method saves time and avoids needing new drapes or surgeon wear.

Once the patient positioning decision has been made, the posterolateral approach is the most common and best approach to adequately address the PMF. The most important landmarks for this approach are the tip of the fibula and the Achilles tendon. The incision is made midway between these landmarks. The sural nerve must be identified and handled with care and preserved during surgery. In a cadaver study by Jowett et al., the sural nerve was identified in 83% of cases using the posterolateral approach [22].

After preparation on the fascia of the peroneal tendons and muscle, you can develop two soft tissue windows anterior and posterior to the peroneal muscle to address the fibula and posterior malleolus, respectively. This will result in more soft tissue trauma, morbidity and possibly swelling, which may compromise wound healing. Therefore, a single window approach should be preferred. This involves creating a plane between the flexor hallucis longus (FHL) muscle and the peroneal muscle. The peroneal tendons and muscle can be retracted laterally and posteriorly and the muscle belly of the FHL can be dissected away from the tibia to allow access to the bone. The posterior malleolus fragment is mobilized from medial to lateral to avoid injury and damage to the PITFL, which inserts into the posterior aspect of the fibula and Volkmann's tubercle. From a lateral approach, it is often possible to visualize the PMF through the fibular fracture. This provides a perfect view of the articular surface to control a perfect reduction. In most cases, intercalary fragments or cartilage lesions can also be seen and treated accordingly.

There are fractures that extend well into the medial posterior tibia or even the medial malleolus. In these cases, a traditional or modified posteromedial approach (TPA or MPA, respectively) may be the best choice to adequately address the fragments and achieve anatomical reduction and strong fixation. Several studies have analysed the approach, its use, and risks. Grillo et al. found TPA to be a valid alternative for surgical access and visualization of 77% of the distal tibial plafond [23]. The MPA appears to be a valid alternative that allows high-quality operative fracture management [24].

The choice of approach is the first important step towards high-quality fracture treatment and ultimately a good outcome. In the context of high-quality treatment, arthroscopic fracture treatment is also important. There are several studies that present different techniques of fracture management in combination with arthroscopic assistance [25, 26]. However, it is more costly and time-consuming, and there are no high-quality comparative studies that have analysed whether arthroscopic assistance can significantly improve outcomes. Nevertheless, it may be a useful adjunct in the management of ankle fractures [27].

6.2 Fixation techniques and implants

The choice of implant, reduction technique, and fixation technique must take into account the morphology and intraoperative assessment in terms of reduction, ligamentotaxis and stability, and containment of the joint. Another decision is whether the fibula or the PMF should be addressed first. If the PMF is fixed first, it is easier to allow fluoroscopic imaging as there is no fibular implant to interfere with imaging. However, this can usually be tolerated and adequate visualization is possible. If the fibula is fixed first, it is easier to reduce the PMF because of the restoration of length and the effect of ligamentotaxis. On the other hand, reduction of the PMF also facilitates reduction of the fibula, so it seems appropriate to start with the fracture that appears easier to reduce. The author usually finds it advantageous to address the fibula first. When adequate fluoroscopy is critical, perhaps in more complex multi-fragmentary PMFs, the fibula can be temporarily stabilized with a lag screw and/or reduction clamp. This will allow adequate fluoroscopic imaging but will also assist in the reduction of the PMF.

In general, indirect reduction, direct reduction with anteroposterior screw fixation, direct posterior screw fixation, or plate and screw constructs are techniques that have been described and used by many surgeons.

Indirect reduction in prone position is achieved by dorsiflexion of the ankle and the reduction can be held with a pointed reduction clamp. Adequate reduction should be confirmed with lateral fluoroscopy. One or two partially threaded screws can be used from anterior to posterior to achieve adequate fixation (**Figures 3** and **4**). A small anterior approach is recommended to respect the fracture line while protecting the extensor tendons, the anterior tibial neurovascular bundle, and the superficial peroneal nerve. This method is best suited for single large fragments without intercalary fragments.

Direct posterolateral reduction and fixation are used in the majority of cases (**Figures 5–7**). The procedure is described in the previous section. After mobilization

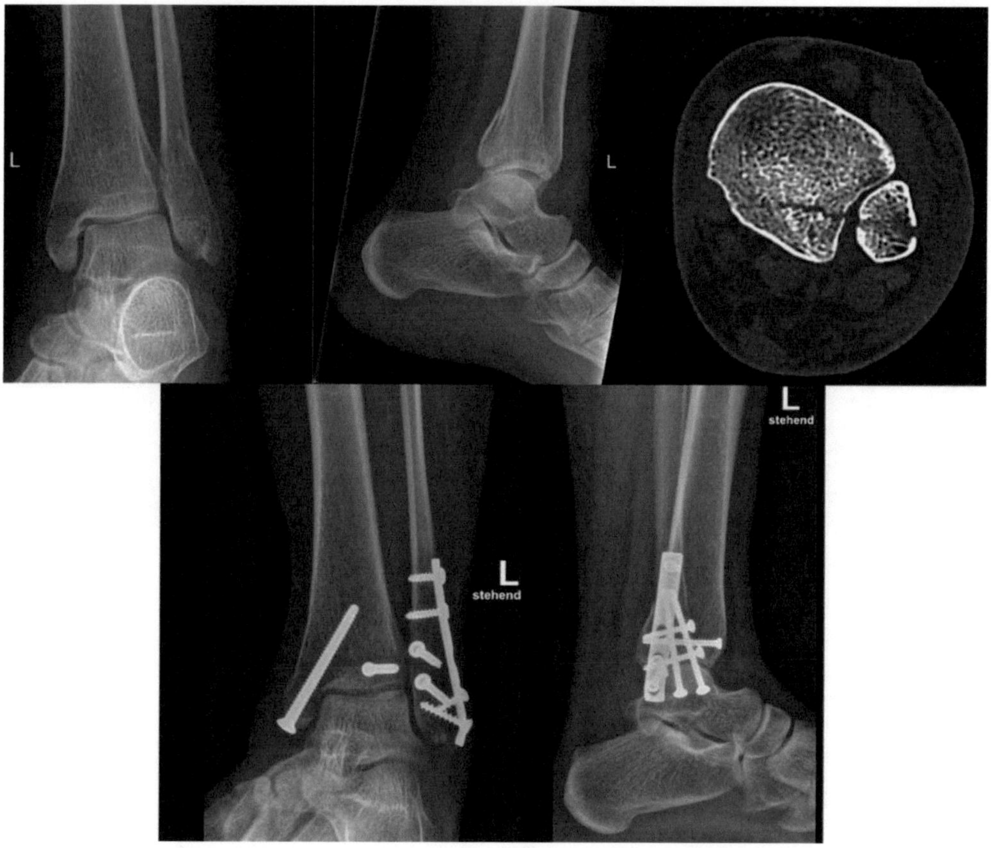

Figure 3.
Haraguchi type I and Bartoníček type II fracture with indirect reduction of the PMF and anteroposterior screw fixation without indication for further syndesmotic stabilization.

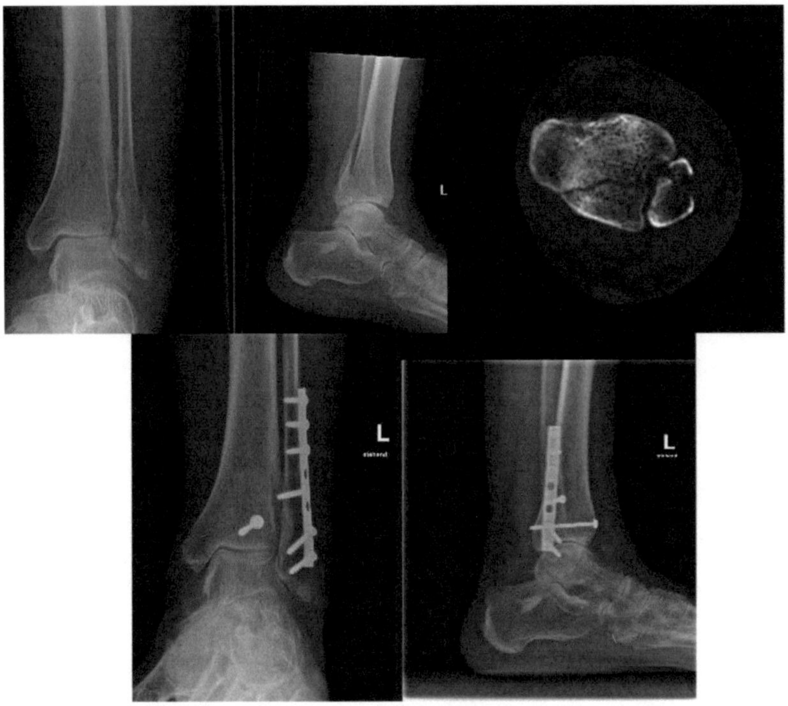

Figure 4.
Multifragmentary Haraguchi type I and Bartoníček type II fracture with indirect reduction of the PMF and anteroposterior screw fixation without indication for further syndesmotic stabilization.

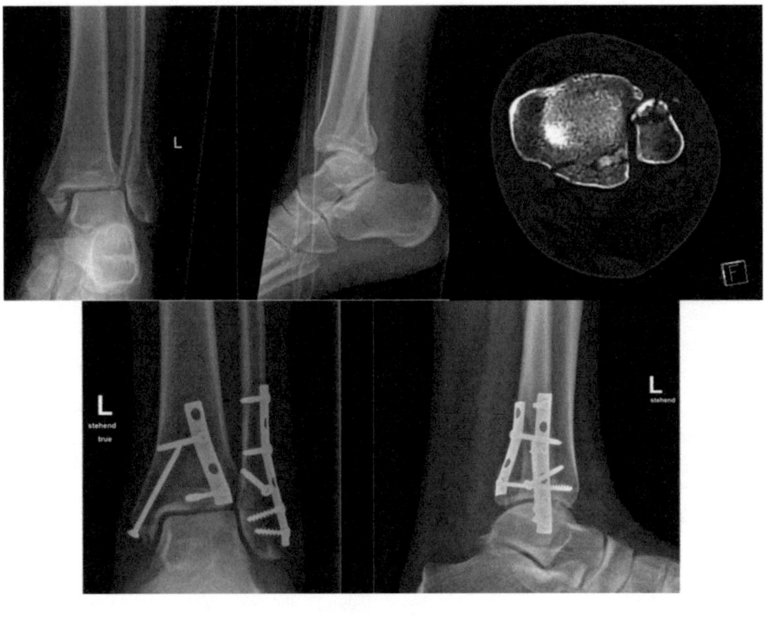

Figure 5.
Multifragmentary Haraguchi type I and Bartoníček type II fracture with intercalary fragment which has been removed, direct reduction of the PMF, and dorsal buttress plate/screw fixation. Again without indication for further syndesmotic stabilization.

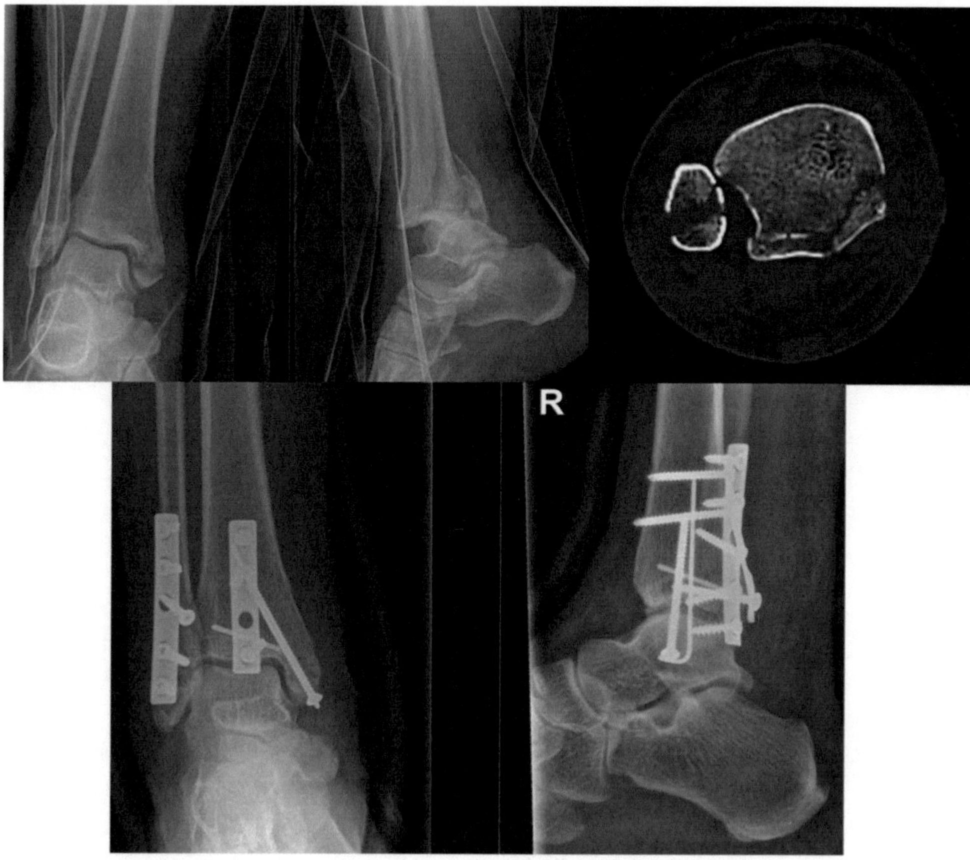

Figure 6.
Multifragmentary Haraguchi type II and Bartoníček type III fracture, direct reduction of the PMF and dorsal buttress plate/screw fixation, plus additional single screw to fix the postermedial fragment. The syndesmotic complex was sufficiently stabilized and needed no further fixation.

of the posterolateral fragment, intercalary fragments and fracture debris or fragments that are not amenable to fixation can be removed. Reduction is achieved using direct and indirect techniques. The metaphyseal proximal fracture line is the best reference for guiding reduction. Once an anatomical reduction is achieved, it can be maintained with reduction clamps and K-wires. The preferred method of fixation is a posterior buttress plate and screws, as this has been shown to provide the strongest fixation [28–30]. There is no need for expensive and bulky locking plates, and one-third tubular plates and standard cortex screws are sufficient in most cases. In osteoporotic bone and multifragmentary fractures, locking plates may be a better choice. Several biomechanical studies have demonstrated superior fixation strength of plate/screw constructs compared to anterior-posterior and posterior-anterior screw fixations (**Figure 8**).

Direct posteromedial reduction and fixation may be an approach to consider for Bartoníček type 3 or Haraguchi type 2 fractures. Reduction and fixation are achieved in a similar way to the posterolateral approach.

The use of syndesmotic fixation is rarely required. In most cases, stability of the syndesmotic complex is restored after anatomical reduction and internal fixation of the fracture. There are few studies available, but it seems to be rarely necessary to apply additional dynamic or static syndesmotic stabilization during this procedure [31–33].

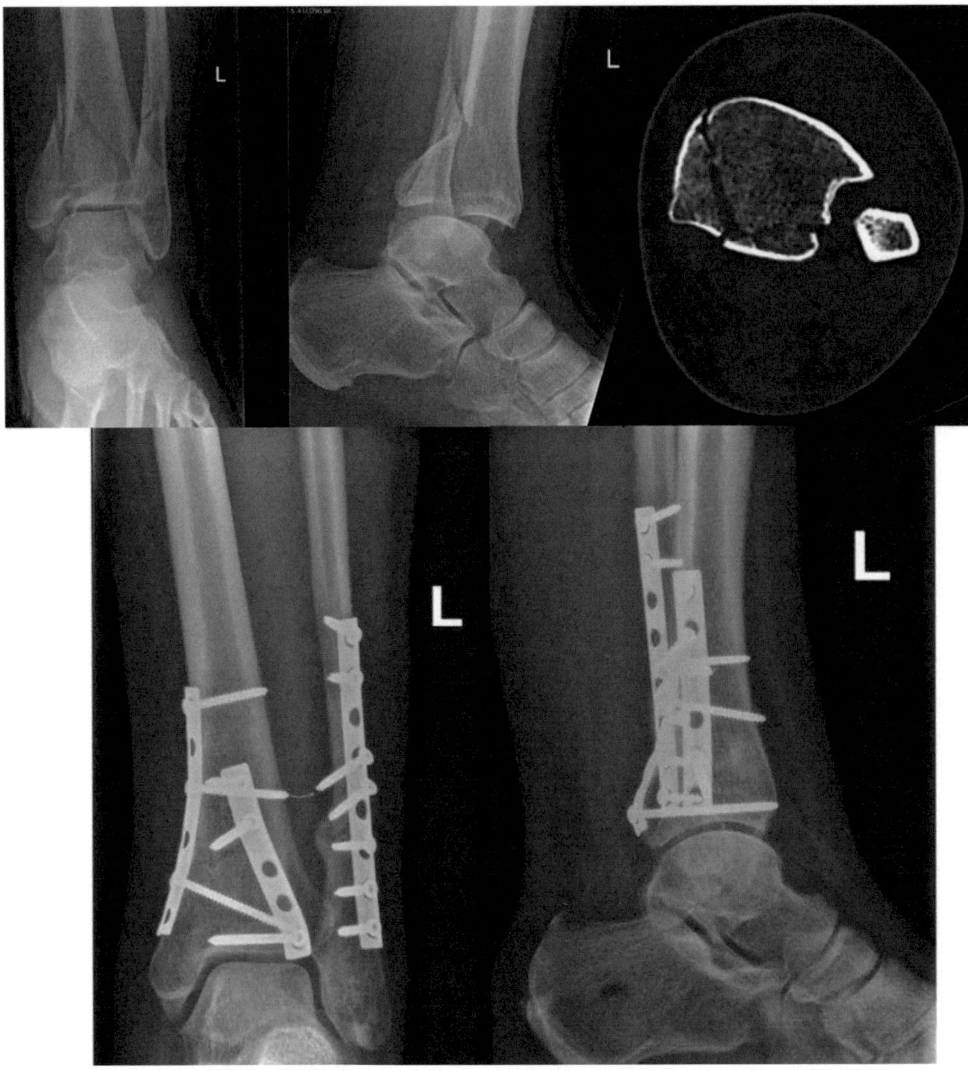

Figure 7.
Haraguchi type II and Bartoníček type III fracture with large fragment and shearing fracture of the medial malleolus. Direct reduction of the PMF and dorsal and medial buttress plate/screw fixation was performed without indication for further syndesmotic stabilisation.

6.3 Postoperative care and treatment

A splint or cast is applied immediately after surgery. The patient is instructed to keep the operated leg elevated for 1 or 2 days, depending on the level of soft tissue swelling. As soon as the swelling is reduced to a reasonable extent and the wounds are unremarkable, mobilization is started under physiotherapeutic supervision and instruction, with non-weight-bearing or partial weight-bearing (10–20% of body weight). Protected weight-bearing is recommended for at least 6 weeks. Patients are encouraged and instructed to begin gentle early ROM exercises approximately 2 weeks after surgery, once the stitches have been removed from the healed skin incisions. After 6 weeks, patients gradually progress to full weight-bearing in a walker or brace, depending on clinical and radiological assessment 6 weeks after surgery.

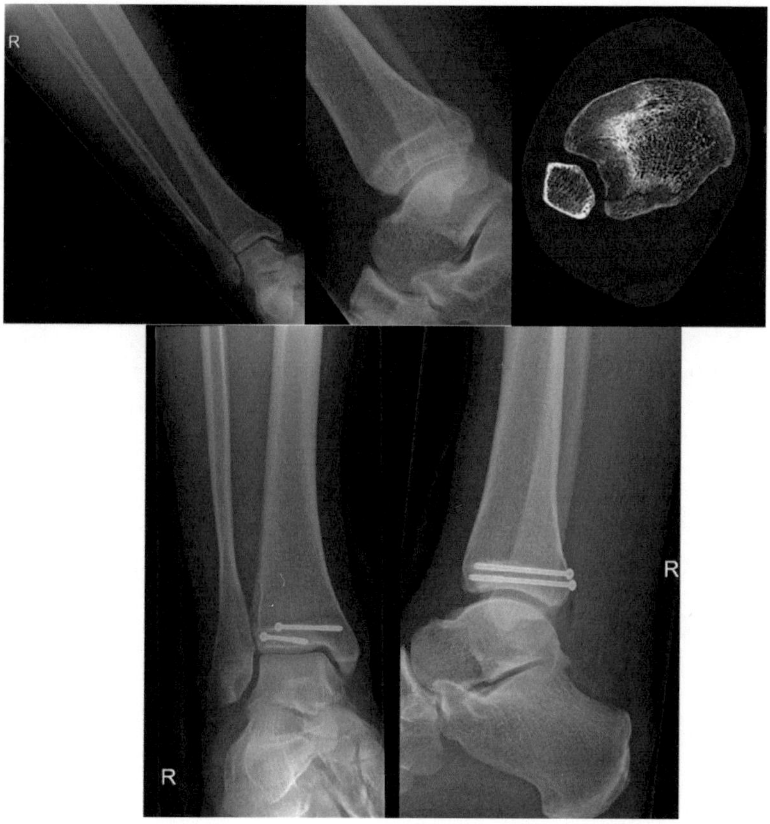

Figure 8.
Haraguchi type I and Bartoníček type II fracture and high fibula fracture. Direct reduction of the PMF and posterior-anterior screw fixation was chosen because of only mild instability and good bone quality in a young, male patient. The syndesmotic was stable after fixation.

7. Complications and outcomes

Initial assessment and treatment are already a crucial part of fracture management, influencing outcome and risk of complications. It is a challenge for the practitioner in the field and for emergency care (early closed reduction, splints, RICE protocol, etc.). The importance of definitive fracture treatment has been thoroughly outlined.

The many factors and the importance of adequate fracture management have been described in this chapter. Basically, the outcome of PMF depends significantly on the quality of reduction, joint stability and containment, and ligamentous integrity. Neumann et al. published a retrospective series with a follow-up of 7 years [34]. They found favourable results when the principles of preoperative assessment and fracture management were implemented. Chang et al. suggest that anatomical reduction of the posterior malleolus correlates with the improved functional outcomes and lower rates of osteoarthritis. Meijer et al. evaluated outcomes in a Dutch patient population with a follow-up of 24 years [35]. Both the Neumann et al.'s and Meijer et al.'s studies found improved clinical scores with a better range of motion. Even when favourable results are reported, one-third of patients still have some residual pain and 42% have a tendency for the ankle to swell with exercise [34].

8. Future considerations and conclusion

Key areas of debate in the management of posterior malleolar fractures include the threshold for surgical intervention, the optimal fixation approach, whether there is a minimum fragment size that requires fixation, and the role of minimally invasive techniques. Emerging evidence suggests potential benefits in refining surgical indications with the use of individualized imaging and minimally invasive techniques, especially arthroscopic assisted fracture treatment [36]. Future research is needed to clarify optimal management strategies, particularly with regard to minimally invasive approaches and the biomechanical significance of smaller fragments. Posterior malleolar fractures present a complex challenge in orthopaedic trauma. Correct diagnosis, classification, and individualized treatment strategies are essential to optimise patient outcomes. Continued research into fixation techniques, imaging modalities, and long-term outcomes will help to refine treatment protocols and improve prognostic models for these fractures.

Conflict of interest

The author declares no conflict of interest.

Author details

Christopher Lenz
Ortho Clinic Zurich, Zurich, Switzerland

*Address all correspondence to: christopher.lenz@hirslanden.ch

References

[1] Court-Brown CM, Caesar B. Epidemiology of adult fractures: A review. Injury. 2006;**37**:691-697. DOI: 10.1016/j.injury.2006.04.130

[2] Cooper AP. A Treatise on Dislocations, and on Fractures of the Joints. London, UK: Longman, Hurst, Reese, Orme, and Brown, E. Cox and Son; 1822. pp. 238-357

[3] Henderson MS. Trimalleolar fracture of the ankle. The Surgical Clinics of North America. 1932;**12**:864

[4] Jaskulka RA, Ittner G, Schedl R. Fractures of the posterior tibial margin: Their role in the prognosis of malleolar fractures. The Journal of Trauma. 1989;**29**(11):1565-1570

[5] McDaniel WJ, Wilson FC. Trimalleolar fractures of the ankle: And end result study. Clinical Orthopaedics and Related Research. 1977;**122**:37-45

[6] Mingo-Robinet J, López-Durán L, Galeote JE, Martinez-Cervell C. Ankle fractures with posterior malleolar fragment: Management and results. The Journal of Foot and Ankle Surgery. 2011;**50**(2):141-145

[7] von Volkmann R. Beitràge zur Chirurgie. Leipzig: Breitkopf und Härtel; 1875

[8] Destot E. Traumatismes du Pied et Rayons X. Malleoles, Astragale, Calcaneum, Avant-Pied. Paris: Masson et Cie; 1911. pp. 1-10

[9] Ogilvie-Harris DJ, Reed SC, Hedman TP. Disruption of the ankle syndesmosis: Biomechanical study of the ligamentous restraints. Arthroscopy. 1994;**10**(5):558-560

[10] Macko VW, Matthews LS, Zwirkowski P, Goldstein SA. The joint-contact area of the ankle: The contributions of the posterior malleolus. The Journal of Bone and Joint Surgery. American Volume. 1991;**73**(3):347-351

[11] Hartford JM, Gorczyca JT, McNamara JL, Mayour MB. Tibiotalar contact area: Contribution of posterior malleolus and deltoid ligament. Clinical Orthopaedics and Related Research. 1995;**320**:182-187

[12] Weber BG. Die Verletzung des Oberen Sprunggelenkes. Aktuelle Probleme in der Chirurgie. Vol. 1. New Jersey: Huber; 1966

[13] Müller M, Allgöwer M, Schneider R, Willenegger H. Manual of Internal Fixation. Techniques Recommended by the AO-ASIF Group. 1st-3rd ed. Berlin: Springer; 1991

[14] Heim U. Trimalleolar fractures: Late results after fixation of the posterior fragment. Orthopedics. 1989;**12**(8):1053-1059

[15] Heim D, Niederhauser K, Simbrey N. The Volkmann dogma: A retrospective, long-term, single-center study. European Journal of Trauma and Emergency Surgery. 2010;**36**:515-519

[16] Court-Brown CM, McBirnie J, Wilson G. Adult ankle fractures: An increasing problem? Acta Orthopaedica Scandinavica. 1998;**69**(1):43-47

[17] Lauge-Hansen N. Fractures of the ankle: II. Combined experimental-surgical and experimental-roentgenologic investigations. Archives of Surgery. 1950;**60**(5):957-985

[18] Nelson MC, Jensen NK. The treatment of trimalleolar fractures of the ankle. Surgery, Gynecology & Obstetrics. 1940;**71**:509-514

[19] Müller ME, Koch P, Nazarian S, Schatzker J. The comprehensive classification of fractures of long bones. Berlin, Heidelberg: Springer-Verlag; 1990

[20] Haraguchi N, Haruyama H, Toga H, Kato F. Pathoanatomy of posterior malleolar fractures of the ankle. The Journal of Bone and Joint Surgery. American Volume. 2006;**88**(5):1085-1092

[21] Bartoníček J, Rammelt S, Tuček M, Nanka O. Posterior malleolar fractures of the ankle. European Journal of Trauma and Emergency Surgery. 2015;**41**(6):587-600. Epub 2015 Aug 8

[22] Jowett AJ, Sheikh FT, Carare RO, Goodwin MI. Location of the sural nerve during posterolateral approach to the ankle. Foot & Ankle International. 2010;**31**(10):880-883

[23] Grillo JE, Cano DP, Íñiguez LT, Vidal CM, Reinales ÁF, Oliva XM. Traditional postero-medial ankle approach for Bartonícek type III in Volkmann fractures: Is it useful? Foot and Ankle Surgery. 2024;**15**:S1268-7731(24)00268-6. DOI: 10.1016/j.fas.2024.12.005

[24] Pino F, Lagos L, Urbina C, Vargas F, Parra M, Bravo F, et al. Reduction quality in posterior malleolar fractures using a modified posteromedial ankle approach. Foot & Ankle Orthopaedics. 2024;**9**(4):24730114241290201. DOI: 10.1177/24730114241290201

[25] Warburton C, Perez OF, Cohen JL, Steinlauf SD. Reduction of the posterior malleolar component of trimalleolar fractures using dry arthroscopic visualization and manipulation by working through the medial malleolus fracture. Foot & Ankle Orthopaedics. 2024;**9**(2):24730114241258098. DOI: 10.1177/24730114241258098

[26] Martin KD, Tripp CT, Huh J. Outcomes of posterior arthroscopic reduction and internal fixation (PARIF) for the posterior malleolar fragment in trimalleolar ankle fractures. Foot & Ankle International. 2021;**42**(2):157-165. DOI: 10.1177/1071100720955149

[27] Chan KB, Lui TH. Role of ankle arthroscopy in management of acute ankle fracture. Arthroscopy. 2016;**32**(11):2373-2380. DOI: 10.1016/j.arthro.2016.08.016

[28] De Vries JS, Wijgman AJ, Sierevelt IN, Schaap GR. Long-term results of ankle fractures with a posterior malleolar fragment. The Journal of Foot and Ankle Surgery. 2005;**44**(3):211-217

[29] Li YD, Liu SM, Jia JS, Zhou JL. Choice of internal fixation methods for posterior malleolus fracture in both biomechanics and clinical application. Beijing Da Xue Xue Bao. Yi Xue Ban. 2011;**43**(5):718-723. Chinese

[30] Hartwich K, Lorente Gomez A, Pyrc J, Gut R, Rammelt S, Grass R. Biomechanical analysis of stability of posterior antiglide plating in osteoporotic pronation abduction ankle fracture model with posterior tibial fragment. Foot & Ankle International. 2017;**38**(1):58-65

[31] Gardner MJ, Brodsky A, Briggs SM, Nielson JH, Lorich DG. Fixation of posterior malleolar fractures provides greater syndesmotic stability. Clinical Orthopaedics and Related Research. 2006;**447**:165-171. DOI: 10.1097/01.blo.0000203489.21206.a9

[32] Miller AN, Carroll EA, Parker RJ, Helfet DL, Lorich DG. Posterior malleolar stabilization of syndesmotic injuries is equivalent to screw fixation. Clinical Orthopaedics and Related Research. 2010;**468**(4):1129-1135. DOI: 10.1007/s11999-009-1111-4. Epub 2009 Oct 2

[33] Behery OA, Narayanan R, Konda SR, Tejwani NC, Egol KA. Posterior malleolar fixation reduces the incidence of trans-syndesmotic fixation in rotational ankle fracture repair. The Iowa Orthopaedic Journal. 2021;**41**(1):121-125

[34] Neumann AP, Rammelt S. Ankle fractures involving the posterior malleolus: Patient characteristics and 7-year results in 100 cases. Archives of Orthopaedic and Trauma Surgery. 2022;**142**(8):1823-1834. DOI: 10.1007/s00402-021-03875-3. Epub 2021 Apr 9

[35] Meijer DT, Gevers Deynoot BDJ, Stufkens SAS, Sierevelt IN, Goslings JC, Kerkhoffs GMMJ, et al. What factors are associated with outcomes scores after surgical treatment of ankle fractures with a posterior malleolar fragment? Clinical Orthopaedics and Related Research. 2019;**477**(4):863-869

[36] Wright DJ, Bariteau JT, Hsu AR. Advances in the surgical management of ankle fractures. Foot and Ankle Orthopaedics. 2019;**4**(4):2473011419888505

Chapter 8

Fractures of the Talus: Diagnosis, Management Strategies, and Clinical Outcomes

Sedeek M. Mosaid, Khaled Elawady, Ashok Marudanayagam and Rohit Rambani

Abstract

Talus fractures are rare but one of the most complex and challenging injuries in orthopedic trauma due to their anatomy, weight-bearing and limited blood supply. These fractures are often high-energy injuries and can lead to complications. This chapter will cover the anatomy, vascular supply, classification systems, mechanism of injury and clinical evaluation of talar fractures. Radiological imaging, especially computed tomography (CT), is crucial for diagnosis and surgical planning in these cases. The chapter will discuss various fracture patterns, head, neck, body and lateral processes, and modern operative techniques. The fracture type, soft tissue condition and the need for anatomical reduction will determine the surgical approach. The chapter will discuss complications and their management to guide clinicians in providing the best care and improving the outcomes for these patients.

Keywords: talus fracture, surgical fixation, posttraumatic arthritis, complications, fracture classification, avascular necrosis

1. Introduction

Talus fractures occur infrequently while presenting distinct management difficulties. The talus has a complex anatomy and limited blood supply, which leads to serious long-term complications such as avascular necrosis and posttraumatic arthritis. These injuries represent less than 1% of all fractures and typically result from high-energy trauma [1].

A precise diagnostic and management strategy is needed to achieve the best results. As high-speed trauma becomes more frequent, especially among younger patients, complex talar fractures also occur more commonly in specialized centers. The talus is a crucial part of the hindfoot and ankle, articulating with the tibia, fibula, calcaneus and navicular bones. The position, with more than 60% of its surface covered with articular cartilage and no muscle or tendon attachments, makes it vulnerable. The blood supply is mainly from the posterior tibial, the dorsalis pedis and the perforated peroneal arteries; therefore, it is easily disrupted in fractures [2, 3].

Maintaining this blood supply and proper reduction of the talus is critical in managing these fractures. Talar fractures are classified by where they occur—the neck, body, head, lateral and posterior processes. The most common is a talar neck fracture [3].

Hawkin classification has been used for decades to predict the risk of avascular necrosis based on the degree of fracture displacement and whether any surrounding joints are involved. More recent approaches have shown that CT scans can be beneficial in assessing of the fracture classification and guiding surgical planning [4, 5].

Surgical intervention, often involving open reduction and internal fixation, is typically required for displaced fractures, while nonoperative management is usually reserved for nondisplaced fractures [3].

1.1 Anatomy

The talus is the second largest bone in the hindfoot and serves as a crucial joint component that links the lower leg to the foot.

This bone serves as an essential component of weight-bearing mechanics because it relays axial loads from the leg to the foot and operates similarly to a keystone within an archway [6].

The talus bone stands out among human bones because it lacks muscle attachments which makes its stabilization primarily dependent on surrounding ligaments and joint structures [6].

The talus displays a notable feature because of its wide surface area, which consists mainly of articular cartilage covering approximately 70% of the bone. The cartilage layer enables almost frictionless movement between the adjoining bones. This feature enables effective joint movement and reduces wear when performing dynamic actions, such as walking, running, and jumping [7].

Anatomically, the talus can be categorized into three primary components: the body, the neck, and the head.

The body is the main, central part and is roughly trapezoidal in shape with a convex upper surface that forms the talar dome. This dome is wider at the front than at the back, which aids in stability in dorsiflexion [3, 6].

The talar neck is a narrower portion of the talus that connects the head of the bone to its body. It acts as a bridge between these two components, making it a crucial link.

Anatomical angles of the talar neck are crucial for biomechanics. It has a varus angle (between 10° and 44°) and a plantarflexed neck-body angle (ranging between 5° and 50°). These angles help determine how forces are transmitted through the foot and influence ankle joint stability [3, 8].

The talus neck is the weakest portion of the talus due to its porosity for vascular ingrowth and small cross-sectional area. This makes it particularly susceptible to fractures [9].

The talus head has a convex configuration, fully covered by articular cartilage, which enables it to articulate with the navicular bone. The head's rounded shape is critically important in absorbing the forces associated with movement.

The talar head is supported by the "spring" or calcaneonavicular ligament. This ligament acts as a strong and flexible support like a rope or spring, holding the structural arrangement of the foot arch [3, 10].

The talus bone possesses distinct lateral and posterior processes. The posterior process is especially important because it creates a channel through which the flexor hallucis longus tendon passes to control the movement of the hallux (big toe).

These small "handles" or "extensions" improve ankle joint stability and function by facilitating tendon movement while securing joint stability [3, 10].

The talus has seven joint articulations. The upper three are the tibial plafond, medial malleolous and fibula. The three lower are between the talus and calcaneus, which are the anterior, middle, and posterior facets. A considerable bony sulcus known as sulcus tali isolates the posterior from the anterior and middle facets. This sulcus creates the tarsal canal, which broadens laterally to create the sinus tarsi. The anterior surface of the talar head articulates with the navicular bone [3].

1.2 Blood supply

Blood supply to the talus is unique and critical; given the lack of musculotendinous attachments on the talus, blood is derived from a vascular sling around its neck and perforating branches. Vascular orientation and retrograde flow to the talar body have traditionally been attributed to high avascular necrosis (AVN) of the talar body with displaced talar neck fractures [10, 11]; however, an extensive antegrade supply has recently been discovered through quantitative magnetic resonance imaging (MRI) studies [12].

The blood supply to the talus comes mainly from three key arteries. The posterior tibial artery (PTA) is the most important contributor. It supplies most of the talar body and dome areas, which bear significant weight.

PTA gives rise to the tarsal canal artery, contributing to the deltoid branches. In neck fractures, the only vascular supply that remains after the fracture is usually the deltoid branches located at the deep part of the deltoid ligament. Therefore, avoiding surgical dissection of the deltoid ligament is necessary to preserve these branches [3, 13].

The artery of tarsal canal continues along the sulcus tali on the inferior surface of the talus and anastomoses with the tarsal sinus artery (a branch of the peroneal artery)—the posterior tubercle branches from the PTA supply to the posterior process.

The anterior tibial artery (ATA) supplies the head and neck, and it continues as the dorsalis pedis artery on the dorsum of the foot.

The peroneal artery is the third major source, contributing by forming the tarsal sinus artery, which is anastomosis with the tarsal canal artery is complete in only 60% of individuals and serves as a backup supply to the head and neck of the talus [3, 14].

2. Epidemiology of talus fractures

Talus fractures are relatively uncommon compared with other types of bone fractures. Men are more likely than women to have talar fractures; the typical patient age is early to mid-30s, with a wide variation. Talus fractures account for 3–5% of foot and ankle injuries [10].

Talar neck fractures are the most common type, constituting approximately 45–50% of all talus fractures. Given the underlying high-energy injury, the associated fracture rate reaches as high as 64%. Open fractures account for 18–25% of talar neck fractures. Subtalar dislocations occur in 15% of talar injuries [10, 15].

Fractures of the talar body are rarer than neck injuries, accounting for 13–23% of all talar fractures. Fractures of the talar head, including osteochondral injuries, remain uncommon and seem to constitute 3–10% of all talar fractures. There appears to be a greater incidence in conjunction with dislocation of the talus. Fracture of the lateral process is frequently encountered as a delayed presentation. Its frequency is difficult to determine, but one study noted that it accounts for 0.86% of all ankle injuries [8, 10, 16].

3. Classification

Talus fractures can be classified anatomically as head, neck, body and process fractures.

The Hawkins classification system is well known for determining the types of talar neck fractures, a system developed many years ago. It classifies fractures based on the level of displacement and the risk for avascular necrosis (AVN). Initially, the Hawkins classification recognized three types of fractures: type I to type III [4, 17]. This was later expanded to type IV by Canale and Kelly [18]. Type I involves vertical fractures of the talar neck where the talus has minimal displacement, and the fracture line enters the subtalar joint between the middle and posterior facets. In these cases, the talus is in its anatomical position within the ankle, and the subtalar joint remains aligned. Hawkins suggested that only one out of the three main blood vessels to the talus is injured in these cases, and he reported no cases of AVN associated with these injuries. Type II fractures are associated with vertical displacement where the subtalar joint is subluxated or dislocated, but the talus is still in the mortise position within the ankle. Hawkins noted that two of three primary blood supply vessels to the talus were disrupted. Type III fractures are like type II, in addition to ankle dislocation. The rate of AVN is high due to the severing of all three principal blood vessels to the injured talus [4, 17].

In 1978, Canale and Kelly included Type IV, which involves a talar neck fracture accompanied by body dislocation from the ankle or subtalar joint and additional dislocation or subluxation of the talus head from the talonavicular joint [18].

In their systematic review, Halvorsen et al. identified an upward trend in avascular necrosis corresponding to each Hawkins type. The incidence was 5.7% for Hawkins type 1, 18.4% for Hawkins type 2, and 44.7% for Hawkins type 3. However, this percentage decreased to 12% for type 4 fractures, which the authors suggested might be due to the rarity of the injury [19].

Talar body fractures have various classifications. The commonly used Sneppen's classification [20] divided these fractures into five types based on the fracture pattern:

Type I: Osteochondral or transchondral fractures of the talar dome.

Type II: Coronal, sagittal, or horizontal shear fractures of the talar body.

Type III: Posterior tubercle fractures.

Type IV: Lateral process fractures.

Type V: Crush fractures of the entire talar body.

Fortin et al. [8] proposed a classification of talar body fractures based on the fracture's location and extent:

Type I: Fractures of the body proper or cleavage of any plane.

Type II: Talar process or tubercle fractures.

Type III: Compression or impaction fractures of the articular surface of the body.

According to the Arbeitsgemeinschaft für Osteosynthesefragen (AO) classification system, the talar body fractures are divided into three distinct groups: C1 (osteochondral defect of the superior dome of the body), C2 (coronal split of body talus with both tibiotalar and subtalar joints), and C3 (comminuted talar body) [21, 22].

The circumferential blending of the head with the neck makes distinguishing talar body fractures from neck fractures challenging [22].

To address this, Inokuchi et al. [23] proposed a classification system based on the position of the inferior fracture line in relation to the lateral processes of the talus. If the fracture line extends anterior to the lateral process, it will be described as a neck fracture; if it goes within the lateral process, it will be a body fracture [23].

Talar body fractures are intra-articular fractures involving the tibiotalar and subtalar joints. In contrast, talar neck fractures are extra-articular, or, at best, partially intra-articular, involving the medial facet of the subtalar joint [22].

There is no widely used classification system for talar head fractures, and in clinical practice, these injuries are often described based on the observed pattern. However, the Orthopaedic Trauma Association (OTA) classification system does include all talar fractures, including those of the head. This system differentiates between extra-articular avulsion fractures, partial articular injuries, and complete articular or crush injuries. The head is classified as 81-A, the neck as 81-B, and the body as 81-C [3, 24].

The lateral process of the talus is a wedge-shaped prominence extending from the body of the talus. It constitutes a component of the subtalar joint, articulating laterally with the fibula and inferiorly with the calcaneum. Fractures of the lateral process are frequently observed in snowboarders [25].

The Hawkins classification system is one of the first systems developed and often used to classify lateral process fractures. It includes type I—a simple fracture of the lateral process; type II—a comminuted fracture of the lateral process further subdivided into type IIa with less than 2 mm of displacement and type IIb with greater than 2 mm displacement; and type III—chip or avulsion fracture of the tubercle laterally [26].

Recently, Wang et al. based on CT scans of patients, created an exhaustive classification system of fractures of the lateral process of talus. They divided fractures into two types based on the existence of associated injuries and developed type I into three subtypes and type II into five. They concluded that the system is more reliable and reproducible, making it a valuable tool for decision-making regarding treatment options [5].

4. Mechanism of injury

4.1 Fracture head of talus

The injury mechanism involves a sudden dorsiflexion force applied to a fully plantarflexed foot, resulting in a compressive force through the talar head.

Additionally, talar head fractures may occur in isolation from a direct blow to the talar head. Another possible mechanism is hyperdorsiflexion, which compresses the talar head against the anterior tibial edge. Impaction fractures of the talar head can also occur alongside subtalar dislocations [8].

4.2 Fracture neck of talus

The primary mechanism is forced dorsiflexion of the foot, resulting in the narrow talar neck to collide with the strong anterior tibial crest, typically resulting in fractures in the frontal plane. As forces persist, the interosseous talocalcaneal ligament and the ligamentous structures of the posterior ankle and subtalar joints experience disruption. Eventually leading to subluxation or dislocation of the body from the subtalar and tibiotalar articulations [3, 27]. With forced supination of the hindfoot, the neck may encounter the medial malleolus, causing medial neck comminution and rotational displacement of the head. Additionally, hindfoot supination can lead to concomitant medial malleolus fractures, with a reported incidence of 28%. The most common contemporary mechanisms are motor vehicle accidents and falls from heights. Producing talar neck fractures with forced dorsiflexion alone is challenging in the laboratory [3, 28].

Peterson and colleagues were able to create these fractures in their experiments only after they restricted movement in the ankle joint by applying vertical pressure through the calcaneus, which pushed the talus against the front of the tibia. This combined action explains why these fractures are common in car accidents or falls, where the foot is fixed and cannot move out of the way [29].

4.3 Fracture body of the talus

Mechanism of injury leading to fracture of the body of the talus is axial compression, where the talus is squeezed between the tibial plafond and the calcaneum. These fractures are most often seen as a result of high-energy impacts. One common scenario is a fall from a height, where the person lands with a forceful impact on the foot or in motor vehicle or motorcycle collisions [30].

Medial-side talar body fracture is commonly associated with supination trauma, whereas a lateral-side fracture is due to pronation or pronation-external rotation trauma.

Lateral process fractures occur usually following an axial force in excessive dorsiflexion and eversion [25, 30].

4.4 Clinical assessment

When initially assessing patients with talus injuries, it is essential to adhere to the Advanced Trauma Life Support (ATLS) protocol, giving priority to injuries that threaten life or limb.

The examination should include a survey for other orthopedic injuries, especially ipsilateral extremity injuries, which accompany talus fractures. Particular attention should also be directed to the thoracolumbar spine because spine fractures have been found to be associated with talar neck and body fractures [8, 31].

A comprehensive evaluation of the affected foot should encompass an assessment of the neurovascular condition and the integrity of the skin at the fracture site.

Patients with talar neck fractures show noticeable midfoot and hindfoot swelling. The degree of gross deformation will depend on the fracture displacement and any accompanying subtalar and ankle joint subluxation or dislocation [8, 31].

Displaced talar neck fractures often lead to significant stretching of the dorsal soft tissue. In cases where the talus is severely deformed and dislocated, there may be a risk to the integrity of the skin and the neurovascular status of the limb, and posterior displacement of the body can lead to bowstringing of the flexor tendons and neurovascular bundle. Therefore, closed reduction under sedation should be attempted to avoid skin necrosis and vascular compromise.

These injuries present significant challenges for treatment in the emergency department and frequently necessitate the use of general anesthesia. It is advisable to avoid multiple attempts at closed reduction, as these can increase soft tissue damage. In such instances, an open reduction is required.

Approximately 50% of type III Hawkins fractures present as open injuries, with an associated infection rate reaching up to 38%. Consequently, it is crucial that these open fractures receive urgent intervention [8, 31].

4.5 Radiologic evaluation

The radiographic evaluation (X-ray) for characterizing talar neck fractures involves an ankle series (anteroposterior (AP), lateral, and mortise) and a foot series (AP, lateral, and oblique). The Canale view can also aid in visualizing the talar neck by positioning the foot in maximal equinus on the X-ray cassette, pronating the foot 15°, and directing the X-ray beam 75° cephalad from the horizontal [10, 32].

Although plain radiographs are the gold standard for initial screening of bony injuries in the foot and ankle, their sensitivity for detecting any talar injury is only 74%, with displacement being the primary factor influencing radiographic sensitivity.

Notably, the most overlooked fractures are the talar dome osteochondral fracture, lateral process fracture, and posterior process fracture [10, 33].

Given these observations, computed tomography (CT) is considered the gold standard for diagnosis. Therefore, CT should be routinely used for monitoring ankle injuries that exhibit swelling and pain disproportionate to radiographic findings [10, 33].

Several authors advocate that a CT scan is pivotal in the surgical fixation of a talus fracture and must be done after a closed reduction. While radiographs may reveal the fracture's profile, CT scans offer supplementary insights by depicting the degree of comminution and joint surface involvement, which assists in the preoperative surgical plan [10, 34].

Considering the high diagnostic accuracy of CT imaging, additional imaging is usually unnecessary. However, MRI can be helpful in the diagnosis of cases of unresolved posttraumatic pain due to peritalar soft tissue injuries and osteochondral injuries, including those of the head or dome of the talus [10, 35].

4.6 Treatment

4.6.1 Talar head fractures

The primary objectives of treating talar head fractures are to ensure the congruity and stability of the talonavicular joint and to preserve the length and height of the medial column. With these principles in mind, satisfactory outcomes can be achieved through various management strategies. Nonoperative management is effective for undisplaced fractures with stable joints, which can be treated by casting the foot and ankle in a neutral position for 6 weeks. Partial weight-bearing is recommended for approximately 8–10 weeks until radiographic evidence confirms fracture union [36]. However, even in the absence of imaging-evident displacement, the predominantly articular nature of the bone might necessitate stable fixation of fractures in the weight-bearing and load-transferring areas of the head [10].

Open reduction and internal fixation are performed for displaced fractures or those with joint instability. Small-fragment subchondral cancellous lag screws, headless compression screws, or bioabsorbable implants can be placed using dorsal or medial approaches. Removing comminuted fragments may help restore talonavicular joint motion [3].

Typically, a medial approach to the talonavicular joint is used, sparing the posterior attachment of the tibial tendon to the navicular bone. Dissection must also be performed cautiously over the anterior aspect of the talar head to prevent the disruption of its blood supply [37, 38].

Articular impaction is common, usually occurring on the medial talar head and distraction through the talonavicular joint aids visualization and fragment disimpaction. It may require the filling of the metaphyseal voids. Crushed cancellous allograft chips or synthetic bone void fillers can support these fragments and maintain articular reduction. Postoperatively, weight bearing is prohibited for 6–8 weeks after surgery. Early range-of-motion exercises can be initiated if fixation is stable and the patient is reliable [8, 38].

Rapid healing usually occurs due to the abundant blood supply to the talar head and low incidence of osteonecrosis.

The prognosis is favorable if no severe comminution and anatomic reduction is performed [8, 38].

The main goal when managing talar neck fractures is obtaining an anatomic reduction, which requires attention to rotation, length, and neck angulation [8].

Cadaveric biomechanical studies have shown that an accurate reduction of talar neck fractures optimizes results. One of the cadaveric studies noted that displacements as minor as 2 mm could change the contact mechanics of the subtalar joint. The most significant dorsal and medial or varus displacement changed the weight-bearing load pathway, resulting in a contact stress decrease in the anterior and middle facets but increased localization in the posterior facet [8, 39].

Additionally, Daniels et al. showed that removing a medially based wedge of bone from the talar neck led to the inability to evert the hindfoot with the new position featuring an internal rotation of the calcaneus, varus heel, and forefoot adduction. These altered hindfoot mechanics due to a talar neck fracture likely contribute to the development of subtalar arthritis [40].

4.6.2 Type I fractures

The role of nonoperative management in talar neck fractures is limited to patients who have nondisplaced fractures.

Care must be taken to obtain appropriate radiographs, including a Canale view and CT, to ensure no displacement or malrotation.

Patients should undergo frequent and meticulous monitoring for displacement. They will remain non-weight-bearing in a well-molded cast for a duration of 8 weeks, followed by a period of mobilization in a cast for an additional 6 weeks [8].

However, this type of fracture is particularly challenging to treat. CT is critical for diagnosis because plain radiography may not capture all fractures. Even rotational deformities may not be visible on the CT scans. Surgical intervention is indicated if any doubt of displacement is noted on radiography or CT, or if the fracture was previously reduced after some displacement, or if there is any uncertainty about the patient's commitment to follow-up appointments [41].

4.6.3 Type II fractures

Displaced talar neck fractures should be initially managed with a prompt reduction to reduce the risk of soft tissue damage. This is often possible in an emergency room. However, it is important to avoid multiple forceful attempts at reduction. The foot is positioned in a plantarflexed position to bring the head of the talus in line with the talar body. The heel can then be moved into inversion or eversion depending on whether the subtalar displacement is medially or laterally displaced. Closed reduction methods are extremely difficult or impossible to achieve anatomic fracture reduction. Even when anatomic reduction is claimed to be achieved, immobilization in significant plantarflexion is typically necessary to maintain position. Therefore, operative treatment of all types of fractures has been recommended [8, 42].

A variety of approaches have been described for talar neck fractures. The medial approach is frequently employed in practice. The anteromedial approach is from the tip of the medial malleolus to the first metatarsal and uses an interval between the tibialis anterior and posterior muscles. This approach allows access to the medial talar neck and the anterior tibiotalar joint region. The long saphenous vein is retracted and protected, and the dissection is carried on to the superomedial talar neck with minimal soft tissue dissection along the neck itself [31, 43].

The incision can be altered accordingly if a medial malleolar osteotomy is planned preoperatively. Stripping of dorsal neck vessels should also be avoided, and deltoid branches on the deep deltoid ligament should be preserved. A drawback of the medial approach is that it gives less exposure than the lateral aspect of the neck, making it challenging to assess rotation and medial neck shortening. Medial neck comminution or impaction may be underestimated [31, 43].

The anterolateral approach involves making an incision between the peroneus brevis and tertius muscles, extending from the distal syndesmosis, located at the anterolateral corner of the ankle, to the fourth metatarsal. During this procedure, the superficial peroneal nerve is safeguarded, and the sinus tarsi fat pad and the origin of the extensor digitorum brevis are lifted to reveal the superolateral talar neck and lateral process [31].

To optimize access to the talar neck and anterior body, dual anteromedial and anterolateral surgical exposures are recommended.

A sufficiently wide skin bridge must be present between the two incisions. Notably, the use of dual surgical exposure has never been shown to increase the risk of osteonecrosis [15, 44].

High-energy talar neck fractures often have some degree of comminution, with tensile failure typically occurring laterally and compressive failure medially.

As a result, the lateral fracture is often simple, and the medial neck fracture is comminuted. A common mistake in these cases is not recognizing the dorsal and medial comminution of the talar neck. Aligning the cortical margins of the fracture in these cases can lead to varus and extension malalignment. For this reason, a dual incision approach is highly recommended. This technique allows for the reduction of maneuvers while simultaneously visualizing both aspects of the fracture and prevents rotational and angular malreductions. Confirming the reduction of the medial and lateral cortices through direct visualization and fluoroscopy (AP or Canale view) before proceeding with fixation is crucial. After reduction is achieved, comminution may leave a cortical deficiency in the dorsal and medial neck. In these cases, local bone grafts or allografts can be used in these areas to provide mechanical support [15, 45, 46].

Using a lamina spreader, soft tissue elevators, and joysticks helps with visualization, fragment manipulation and reduction. Once the fracture is reduced, it can be provisionally stabilized with K-wires. Fixation can be achieved with dual minifragment plates, plating and positional screws or screws alone [3, 35]. Two screws, positioned medially and laterally, can be placed just beneath the articular surface of the head and aimed posteriorly into the body. Lag screws may be used unless there is considerable comminution of the neck, particularly on the medial side, which can cause neck shortening or malalignment when the fracture is compressed [8].

Another option is the posterolateral approach, where an incision is made lateral to the heel cord at the interval between the flexor hallucis longus and peroneal muscles, allowing safe access to the entire posterior talar process of the foot. Caution must be taken during exposure so as not to damage the peroneal artery or the branches [8]. The posterolateral approach is often combined with an initial anteromedial or anterolateral approach for provisional fracture reduction and stabilization. if anatomic reduction can be achieved with closed manipulation, posterior-anterior screw fixation can be done through a single posterior approach as an option, as This method is restricted to straightforward fracture patterns that can be fixed with screws, as it does not provide a clear view of the talar neck [34, 47].

The advantage of using posterior to anteriorly directed screws is that the fixation crosses the fracture perpendicularly, which may increase the strength of the fixation [48].

Nonetheless, Attiah et al. performed a biomechanical study and reported that there was no difference in fixation strength to the yield point with anterior to posterior screws, posterior to anterior screws, and a medial-side plate with a lateral screw; they concluded that anterior plate fixation provided equivalent stability to posterior screw fixation [49].

The potential drawbacks of posterior-anterior screws are the technical challenges of intraoperative positioning, risk of articular cartilage damage, neurovascular structure damage, subtalar joint or lateral trochlear surface penetration, and restriction of ankle plantarflexion due to screw head impingement. These potential drawbacks can be minimized by using smaller-diameter countersunk screws directed along the talar axis [8].

Screw fixation is typically reserved for simple fracture patterns where anatomic reduction is achievable, and there is no comminution that might cause fracture collapse and malalignment [47]. The surgical approach and fracture pattern should guide the direction of screw placement. The size of the screw depends on the size of the fracture fragment, and it is crucial to either countersink the screw heads or use headless screws to prevent impingement, as biomechanical studies have shown no difference in strength [43, 47].

Lateral and medial plating is becoming a popular and effective way of talar neck fixation, especially in comminuted cases. Plates can be augmented with independent screw fixation as needed [47].

However, Charlson et al. in their biomechanical study concluded that while plate fixation may offer significant advantages in controlling the anatomic alignment of comminuted talar neck fractures, it does not confer any biomechanical superiority over axial screw fixation [50].

A smaller implant footprint allows for fragment-specific fixation and more fixation points in a three-dimensional complex bone with limited surface area for implant application. Plates can be placed on the most comminuted column of the talus, medial, lateral or both. They provide a solid buttress as a bridging strut, resisting collapse and shortening [10, 47].

In dual plating, the lateral plate extends from just in front of the lateral process to the junction of the lateral head and neck, while the medial plate extends from the plantar side to the medial talar body cartilage, reaching the medial head-neck junction [31].

To prevent medial shortening and varus malunion, particularly when the neck shortens by more than 2 mm, it is advisable to contour minifragment plating on the lateral surface of the talus during surgery [51].

The minifragment locking plate system allows for selection between locking and nonlocking screws to stabilize reductions in both medial and lateral columns. When applying the medial plate, careful planning is required to avoid impingement within the medial tibiotalar joint gutter.

Nevertheless, the availability of minifragment locking plates in various thicknesses effectively mitigates this issue. These plates offer multiple fixation points and benefit from the buttressing effect of screws engaging with the plate, which is particularly advantageous in areas with comminuted fractures [47].

4.6.3.1 Timing of open reduction and internal fixation

In the past, immediate treatment and stabilization were advised for talus fractures due to the risk of osteonecrosis associated with talar neck fractures. However, this approach has recently evolved [10, 35].

Fracture dislocations that cannot be reduced require an urgent closed and potentially open reduction. Once the reduction is achieved, most orthopaedic specialists do not consider emergency surgery necessary for displaced talar neck fractures [52].

There was no noticeable rise in complications with the delay from injury to surgical fixation [53]. Definitive treatment should be carried out as soon as a skilled surgical team can safely perform the procedure, with particular attention to the condition of the soft tissue. If there is considerable swelling, the surgery can be postponed until the soft tissue quality allows for safe surgical dissection and primary incision closure [22].

4.6.4 Type III fractures

The displacement of the talar body from the ankle and subtalar joints creates significant treatment challenges. Therefore, open reduction becomes urgently necessary to relieve the neurovascular bundle and medial skin pressure from the displaced body and minimize the potential risk for osteonecrosis [8].

A considerable number of these injuries involve medial malleolar fractures, which assist in exposure. If the malleolus is intact, a medial malleolar osteotomy is usually required to help expose and reposition the body. Approximately 50% of these fractures are open, requiring immediate and thorough irrigation and debridement [8].

4.6.5 Type IV fractures

Type IV injuries are managed similarly to type III injuries, requiring prompt open reduction and internal fixation. The talar body and fragments of the head are aligned and securely fixed. The stability of the talonavicular joint is evaluated, and if it is found to be unstable, pinning the joint should be considered. This injury is significant because osteonecrosis can develop in the talar body and head fragment [8, 42].

4.7 Talar body fractures

The management principles for talar body fractures are analogous to those for neck fractures. Fractures that are undisplaced and involve stable joints may be managed non-operatively with a non-weight-bearing short-leg cast for approximately 8 weeks, until radiographic evidence of healing is confirmed [3].

Open reduction and internal fixation (ORIF) is necessary for all displaced fractures. The morphology of talar body fractures varies significantly, and the fracture pattern dictates the surgical approach. Depending on the fracture's orientation and location relative to the plafond and the extent of subtalar involvement, the surgeon must decide between anterior or posterior approaches, a combination of both, or a malleolar osteotomy [37].

Intraoperative visualization of the talar dome is often required for body fractures to ensure the articular surfaces are anatomically reduced. Standard dual anteromedial and anterolateral approaches are typically sufficient to view the anterior half of the talar dome; however, visualizing the posterior dome often necessitates additional procedures, such as medial malleolar or fibular osteotomy [37, 54].

The posteromedial approach to the talar body is advantageous for addressing and stabilizing fractures of the posterior talar body and posterior process, especially when the fracture line is oriented in the coronal plane. The patient is positioned prone, and an incision is made just medial to the Achilles tendon, ensuring the Achilles paratenon remains intact while retracting the flexor hallucis longus and other posterior structures medially. This technique provides access to the tibiotalar and subtalar joints [54, 55].

Achieving adequate exposure is the primary challenge in properly reducing talar body fractures, and traditional surgical approaches may not provide sufficient exposure, particularly in complex cases. Medial malleolar osteotomy is the most frequently performed osteotomy for reducing complex talar body fractures, with most surgeons agreeing that the osteotomy should target the intersection between the tibial plafond and the medial malleolus's articular facet. Failing to exit at this point can result in limited exposure (too medial) or damage to the weight-bearing cartilage on the tibial plafond (too lateral) [56, 57].

van Bergen et al. [57] conducted a study using radiological and computed tomography (CT) to determine the optimal orientation for an oblique medial malleolar osteotomy to expose the talar dome surgically. The study found that an osteotomy directed at an average angle of 30° relative to the tibia's longitudinal axis (or about 57° relative to the tibial plafond) is perpendicular to the tibial articular surface at the intersection of the plafond and medial malleolus. This orientation allows for precise exposure while minimizing the risk of cartilage damage or incongruent reduction, and the authors point out that to obtain optimal compression and maintain a congruent joint surface following reduction, lag screws must be placed perpendicular to the osteotomy plane [57].

A femoral distractor can be used to view the body of the talus fragments.

The talar dome fragments can be reduced from posterior to anterior and lateral to medial. K-wires may be used as joysticks to stabilize mobile fragments. The subtalar joint is assessed from the lateral approach for residual step-offs or fracture distraction. Body fractures can occur in the coronal or sagittal planes or as crush injuries [30, 58].

A fracture along the sagittal plane can be stabilized by inserting screws from the medial to the lateral side. These screws should be deeply countersunk into the cartilage, or alternatively, headless screws can be utilized. For lateral comminuted fractures, plate fixation is necessary to prevent collapse and subsequent malunion. Minifragment implants may be positioned just below the articular margin of the tibiotalar cartilage [58].

4.8 Role for arthroscopy

Arthroscopic reduction and internal fixation (ARIF) is a minimally invasive technique that offers excellent visibility of fractures in both the frontal and sagittal planes. Additionally, arthroscopy can serve as a supplementary method, aiding in open reduction procedures for percutaneous screw fixation [59].

ARIF facilitates anatomical reduction and fixation with interfragmentary screws under direct vision and avoids any minimal displacement, which proves that it might adversely alter foot biomechanics [39, 59]. Moreover, less interruption of the soft tissues minimizes the risk of further talar revascularization. Arthroscopy provides easy access for fracture fixation in the posterolateral to the anteromedial plane, which is biomechanically strong [59, 60].

However, it is unsuitable as the sole method of fracture visualization and reduction for large displaced fragments or complex fracture dislocations. Additionally, associated soft tissue involvement in these fractures increases the risk of saline leakage and compartment syndrome [30, 60].

The selection of an arthroscopic technique is determined by the fracture's characteristics. Anterior arthroscopy is generally recommended for fractures affecting the anterior two-thirds of the talus and for longitudinal fractures. Conversely, posterior arthroscopy is best suited for fractures involving the posterior one-third of the talus [30, 60].

Cellier et al. [61] conducted a systematic review of 12 studies involving 22 patients. The studies showed favorable outcomes with no reported complications, infections, or avascular necrosis. The majority of cases were Hawkins type II neck fractures and Sneppen type II body fractures. Hawkins type IV or complex comminuted fractures were excluded. The authors determined that to evaluate the effectiveness of ARIF techniques in comparison to open reduction and internal fixation, it is necessary to conduct trials with sufficient power and include long-term follow-up studies [61].

4.9 Complications

4.9.1 Osteoarthritis

Osteoarthritis (OA), particularly affecting the subtalar joint, is the most prevalent complication following fractures of the talar neck and body [62]. Fractures of the talar neck and body accompanied by lateral process fractures and fragmentation of the inferior articular surface further elevate the risk of developing subtalar arthritis [63].

Tibiotalar arthritis occurs about half as often as subtalar arthritis and usually appears alongside rather than on its own. Nonetheless, isolated tibiotalar arthritis can arise from talar body fractures. Symptomatic posttraumatic arthritis can be managed conservatively through bracing and medication [31, 45].

Treatment options for tibiotalar arthritis include arthrodesis and total ankle arthroplasty. Some studies have shown a preference for total ankle arthroplasty over arthrodesis, citing better functional outcomes and an enhanced ability to restore optimal gait mechanics [64]. However, the likelihood of additional surgeries may be more significant after arthroplasty than arthrodesis. Arthrodesis is the favored treatment for subtalar arthritis [31, 65].

4.9.2 Osteonecrosis

Osteonecrosis (ON) frequently arises as a complication following fractures and dislocations of the talar neck and body, historically being the most feared outcome of talus fractures. The likelihood of osteonecrosis post-talar fracture is heightened with increased initial fracture displacement and dislocation, and it is more prevalent in open injuries [31]. Hawkins found no cases of osteonecrosis in type I fractures, while Canale and Kelly observed a 13% occurrence in type I fractures [17, 18]. Hawkins reported a 42% incidence in type II fractures and a 91% incidence in 27 type III fractures [17].

However, advancements in treatment protocols and a better understanding of the injury have reduced osteonecrosis rates [37].

The Hawkins sign, visible 6–8 weeks post-injury, is a positive indicator of talar revascularization. It appears as patchy subchondral osteopenia or lucency at the talar dome on AP and mortise ankle views, serving as a useful prognostic tool. The presence of the Hawkins sign reliably suggests that osteonecrosis is unlikely, though its absence is not as predictive of osteonecrosis development [8].

Magnetic resonance imaging is highly effective in detecting osteonecrosis and assessing the extent of talar involvement. The primary diagnostic criterion for osteonecrosis is increased radiodensity of the talus compared to adjacent osseous structures [8].

Managing patients with osteonecrosis can be complex, as many are asymptomatic, and about half experience revascularization without talar body collapse. After an initial osteonecrosis diagnosis, many patients may eventually show revascularization without collapse, and many with radiographic osteonecrosis may not exhibit symptoms [8, 37].

Initial treatment for osteonecrosis is conservative. It is crucial to recognize that talar fractures can heal even with osteonecrosis development. The main factor determining a patient's progress in weight-bearing on the injured limb is fracture healing. Once radiographic healing is evident, the patient may begin weight-bearing. Although prolonged non-weight bearing was historically recommended, it did not prevent progression or collapse and is now largely discouraged [31, 66].

Additionally, revascularization of the talus may take up to 36 months, making extended non-weight-bearing impractical until the risk of collapse is non-practical. There is no conclusive evidence that weight-bearing on an avascular talus contributes to collapse. Hawkins noted that talus collapse occurred despite enforced non-weight-bearing for several years [31].

Persistent symptomatic osteonecrosis may require surgical intervention. Three general categories of procedures exist: joint-sparing (core decompression and vascularized bone grafting), joint-sacrificing (talar replacement), and salvage (arthrodesis) procedures. Joint-sparing procedures aim to preserve the native talus anatomy by promoting the healing of the devascularized area. Ultimately, the choice of procedure should be based on the surgeon's expertise, patient factors, and the severity of ON [31, 66].

4.10 Nonunion and malunion

Talar neck nonunion is rare, less than 5%. Talar neck malunion is more common, 20–37%. The malunion rate may be underestimated as it is hard to detect and measure misalignment on X-rays. There is no standardized radiographic definition or criteria for malunion. Preoperative planning is key to preventing malunion and ensuring proper fracture fixation during the initial surgery [15, 47].

Varus talar neck malunion is the most common deformity in the literature and can alter the biomechanics of the subtalar and talonavicular joints. Several factors, such as severity of malunion, presence and extent of arthrosis, and bone stock, will influence treatment. Malunion may require a medial opening wedge, corrective osteotomy and bone grafting. Arthrodesis of the affected joints is another option if osteotomy is not suitable [47].

5. Conclusion

Talar fractures are complex injuries with a high risk of complications due to the bone's anatomy and blood supply. Accurate diagnosis with CT and timely and anatomical reduction are key to success. Modern surgical techniques like dual incisions, plating, and arthroscopic assistance have improved the management of these injuries. Understanding fracture patterns and accurate planning is crucial to avoid complications such as osteonecrosis, malunion, and arthritis and to regain function.

Author details

Sedeek M. Mosaid*, Khaled Elawady, Ashok Marudanayagam and Rohit Rambani
Department of Trauma and Orthopaedics, United Lincolnshire Hospitals NHS Trust, Lincoln, United Kingdom

*Address all correspondence to: sedeeko2000@hotmail.com

References

[1] Li Y, Lai L, Wu X. Talar Fractures and Fracture Dislocations. New York, USA: Springer eBooks; 2020. pp. 403-416

[2] Fleming JJ, Kwaadu KY, Downey MW. Talar Fractures: The Injury, the Management, and the Aftermath. New York, USA: Springer eBooks; 2017. pp. 245-261

[3] Al-Jabri T, Muthian S, Wong K, Charalambides C. Talus fractures: All I need to know. Injury. 2021;**52**(11):3192-3199

[4] Alton T, Patton DJ, Gee AO. Classifications in brief: The Hawkins classification for talus fractures. Clinical Orthopaedics and Related Research. 2015;**473**(9):3046-3049

[5] Wang Y, Wang Z, Zhu Y, Fu L, Deng X, Chen W, et al. New classification based on CT and its value evaluation for fractures of the lateral process of the talus. The Journal of Foot and Ankle Surgery. 2023;**62**(4):644-650. Available from: https://www.sciencedirect.com/science/article/abs/pii/S1067251623000169?via%3Dihub

[6] Khan IA, Varacallo M. Anatomy, bony pelvis and lower limb, foot talus. In: StatPearls [Internet]. Treasure Island (FL): StatPearls Publishing; 2020. Available from: https://www.ncbi.nlm.nih.gov/books/NBK541086/

[7] MacGregor R, Byerly DW. Anatomy, bony pelvis and lower limb: Foot bones. In: StatPearls [Internet]. Treasure Island, FL, USA: StatPearls Publishing; 2023. Available from: https://pubmed.ncbi.nlm.nih.gov/32491379/

[8] Fortin PT, Balazsy JE. Talus fractures: Evaluation and treatment. The Journal of the American Academy of Orthopaedic Surgeons. 2001;**9**(2):114-127

[9] Hubbard D, Richman J. General Principles of Talus Fractures. New York, USA: Springer eBooks; 2020. pp. 29-35

[10] Schwartz AM, Runge WO, Hsu AR, Bariteau JT. Fractures of the talus: Current concepts. Foot & Ankle Orthopaedics. 2020;**5**(1):247301141990076

[11] Buza JA, Leucht P. Fractures of the talus: Current concepts and new developments. Foot and Ankle Surgery. 2018;**24**(4):282-290

[12] Miller AN, Prasarn ML, Dyke JP, Helfet DL, Lorich DG. Quantitative assessment of the vascularity of the talus with gadolinium-enhanced magnetic resonance imaging. Journal of Bone and Joint Surgery. 2011;**93**(12):1116-1121

[13] Mulfinger GL, Trueta J. The blood supply of the talus. The Journal of Bone and Joint Surgery British Volume. 1970;**52-B**(1):160-167

[14] Prasarn ML, Miller AN, Dyke JP, Helfet DL, Lorich DG. Arterial anatomy of the talus: A cadaver and gadolinium-enhanced MRI study. Foot and Ankle International. 2010;**31**(11):987-993

[15] Vallier HA. Fractures of the talus. Journal of Orthopaedic Trauma. 2015;**29**(9):385-392

[16] Perera A, Baker JF, Lui DF, Stephens MM. The management and outcome of lateral process fracture of the talus. Foot and Ankle Surgery. 2010;**16**(1):15-20

[17] Hawkins LG. Fractures of the neck of the talus. The Journal of Bone

and Joint Surgery. American Volume. 1970;**52**(5):991-1002

[18] Canale ST, Kelly FB. Fractures of the neck of the talus. Long-term evaluation of seventy-one cases. Journal of Bone and Joint Surgery. 1978;**60**(2):143-156

[19] Halvorson JJ, Winter SB, Teasdall RD, Scott AT. Talar neck fractures: A systematic review of the literature. The Journal of Foot and Ankle Surgery. 2013;**52**(1):56-61

[20] Sneppen O, Christensen SB, Krogsøe O, Lorentzen J. Fracture of the body of the talus. Acta Orthopaedica Scandinavica. 1977;**48**(3):317-324

[21] Buckley R, Sands A. Body. In: AO Surgery Reference. Davos (CH): AO Foundation. Available from: https://surgeryreference.aofoundation.org/orthopedic-trauma/adult-trauma/talus/body/definition

[22] LaMothe JM, Buckley R. Talus fractures: A current concepts review of diagnoses, treatments, and outcomes. Acta Chirurgiae Orthopaedicae et Traumatologiae Cechoslovaca. 2012;**79**(2):97-106

[23] Inokuchi S, Ogawa K, Usami N. Classification of fractures of the talus: Clear differentiation between neck and body fractures. Foot and Ankle International. 1996;**17**(12):748-750

[24] Marsh JL, Slongo TF, Agel J, Broderick JS, Creevey W, DeCoster TA, et al. Fracture and dislocation classification compendium—2007. Journal of Orthopaedic Trauma. 2007;**21**(Suppl.):S1-S6

[25] Barnett JR, Ma A, Khan W, O'Gorman A. The diagnosis, management and complications associated with fractures of the talus. The Open Orthopaedics Journal. 2017;**11**(1):460-466

[26] Hawkins LG. Fracture of the lateral process of the talus. The Journal of Bone and Joint Surgery. American Volume. 1965;**47**(6):1170-1175

[27] Sproule JA, Glazebrook MA, Younger AS. Varus Hindfoot deformity after talar fracture. Foot and Ankle Clinics. 2012;**17**(1):117-125

[28] Elgafy H, Ebraheim NA, Tile M, Stephen D, Kase J. Fractures of the talus: Experience of two level 1 trauma centers. Foot and Ankle International. 2000;**21**(12):1023-1029

[29] Peterson L, Romanus B, Dahlberg E. Fracture of the collum tali—An experimental study. Journal of Biomechanics. 1976;**9**(4):277-279

[30] Sundararajan S, Badurudeen A, Ramakanth R, Rajasekaran S. Management of talar body fractures. Indian Journal of Orthopaedics. 2018;**52**(3):258

[31] Lee C, Brodke D, Perdue PW, Patel T. Talus fractures: Evaluation and treatment. The Journal of the American Academy of Orthopaedic Surgeons. 2020;**28**(20):e878-e887

[32] Dale JD, Ha AS, Chew FS. Update on talar fracture patterns: A large level I trauma center study. AJR American Journal of Roentgenology. 2013;**201**(5):1087-1092. Available from: https://pubmed.ncbi.nlm.nih.gov/24147480/

[33] Young KW, Park YU, Kim JS, Cho HK, Choo HS, Park JH. Misdiagnosis of talar body or neck fractures as ankle sprains in low energy traumas. Clinics in Orthopedic Surgery. 2016;**8**(3):303

[34] Shakked RJ, Tejwani NC. Surgical treatment of talus fractures. The

Orthopedic Clinics of North America. 2013;**44**(4):521-528

[35] Grear BJ. Review of talus fractures and surgical timing. The Orthopedic Clinics of North America. 2016;**47**(3):625-637

[36] Banerjee R, Nickisch F, Coughlin MJ. Fractures and fracture-dislocations of the talus. In: Mann's Surgery of the Foot and Ankle. 9th ed. Philadelphia: Elsevier; 2014. pp. 2101-2153

[37] Githens M, Tangtiphaiboontana J, Carlock K, Campbell ST. Talus fractures: An update on current concepts in surgical management. The Journal of the American Academy of Orthopaedic Surgeons. 2022;**30**(15):e1015-e1024

[38] Anderson MR, Ketz JP, Flemister AS. Operative treatment of talar head fractures: Surgical technique. Journal of Orthopaedic Trauma. 2018;**32**(8):e334-e338

[39] Sangeorzan BJ, Wagner UA, Harrington RM, Tencer AF. Contact characteristics of the subtalar joint: The effect of talar neck misalignment. Journal of Orthopaedic Research. 1992;**10**(4):544-551

[40] Daniels TR, Smith JW, Ross TI. Varus malalignment of the talar neck. Its effect on the position of the foot and on subtalar motion. Journal of Bone and Joint Surgery. 1996;**78**(10):1559-1567. DOI:10.2106/00004623-199610000-00015

[41] Willms S, Fruson L, Buckley R. Nondisplaced talus neck fracture—Operative or nonoperative care? Injury. 2023;**54**(4):1027-1029

[42] Sanders R. Fractures and fracture dislocations of the talus. In: Coughlin MJ, Mann RA, editors. Surgery of the Foot and Ankle. 7th ed. St Louis: Mosby Year Book; 1999. pp. 1465-1518

[43] Beltran MJ, Mitchell PM, Collinge CA. Posterior to anteriorly directed screws for management of talar neck fractures. Foot and Ankle International. 2016;**37**(10):1130-1136

[44] Chateau F, Brokaw DS, Jelen BA, Scheid DK, Weber TG. Plate fixation of talar neck fractures: Preliminary review of a new technique in twenty-three patients. Journal of Orthopaedic Trauma. 2002;**16**(4):213-219

[45] Sanders DW, Busam M, Hattwick E, Edwards JR, MP MA, Johnson KD. Functional outcomes following displaced talar neck fractures. Journal of Orthopaedic Trauma. 2004;**18**(5):265-270

[46] Segura FP, Eslava S. Talar neck fractures: Single or double approach? Foot and Ankle Clinics. 2020;**25**(4):653-665

[47] Whitaker C, Turvey B, Illical EM. Current concepts in talar neck fracture management. Current Reviews in Musculoskeletal Medicine. 2018;**11**(3):456-474

[48] Swanson TV, Bray TJ, Holmes GB. Fractures of the talar neck. A mechanical study of fixation. The Journal of Bone and Joint Surgery. 1992;**74**(4):544-551

[49] Attiah M, Sanders DW, Valdivia G, Cooper I, Ferreira L, MacLeod MD, et al. Comminuted talar neck fractures: A mechanical comparison of fixation techniques. Journal of Orthopaedic Trauma. 2007;**21**(1):47-51. Available from: https://journals.lww.com/jorthotrauma/Fulltext/2007/01000/Plate_Fixation_of_Talar_Neck_Fractures_.9.aspx

[50] Charlson MD, Parks BG, Weber TG, Guyton GP. Comparison of plate and screw fixation and screw fixation alone in a comminuted talar neck fracture model. Foot and Ankle International. 2006;**27**(5):340-343

[51] Maceroli MA, Wong C, Sanders RW, Ketz JP. Treatment of comminuted talar neck fractures with use of minifragment plating. Journal of Orthopaedic Trauma. 2016;**30**(10):572-578

[52] Patel R, Van Bergeyk A, Pinney S. Are displaced talar neck fractures surgical emergencies? A survey of orthopaedic trauma experts. Foot and Ankle International. 2005;**26**(5):378-381

[53] Buckwalter JA, Westermann R, Mooers B, Karam M, Wolf B. Timing of surgical reduction and stabilization of talus fracture-dislocations. American Journal of Orthopedics (Belle Mead, N.J.). 2018;**46**(6):E408-E413

[54] Swords M, Shank J, Benirschke S. Surgical treatment of posteromedial talus fractures: Technique description and results of 10 cases. Indian Journal of Orthopaedics. 2018;**52**(3):269-275

[55] Shank JR, Benirschke SK, Swords MP. Treatment of peripheral talus fractures. Foot and Ankle Clinics. 2017;**22**(1):181-192

[56] Seil R, Rupp S, Pape D, Dienst M, Kohn D. Surgical approaches to osteochondral lesions of the talus. Der Orthopäde. 2001;**30**(1):47-52

[57] van Bergen CJ, Tuijthof GJ, Sierevelt IN, van Dijk CN. Direction of the oblique medial malleolar osteotomy for exposure of the talus. Archives of Orthopaedic and Trauma Surgery. 2011;**131**(7):893-901. DOI: 10.1007/s00402-010-1227-8

[58] Rammelt S, Zwipp H. Talar neck and body fractures. Injury. 2009;**40**(2):120-135

[59] Hamilton GA, Doyle MD, Castellucci-Garza FM. Arthroscopic-assisted open reduction internal fixation. Clinics in Podiatric Medicine and Surgery. 2018;**35**(2):199-221

[60] Bonasia DE, Rossi R, Saltzman CL, Amendola A. The role of arthroscopy in the management of fractures about the ankle. American Academy of Orthopaedic Surgeons. 2011;**19**(4):226-235

[61] Cellier N, Sleth C, Bauzou F, Kouyoumdjian P, Coulomb R. Arthroscopic reduction and internal fixation (ARIF) for talar body fractures: Systematic review. SICOT-J. 2023;**9**:20

[62] Dodd A, Lefaivre KA. Outcomes of talar neck fractures. Journal of Orthopaedic Trauma. 2015;**29**(5):210-215

[63] Romeo NM, Hirschfeld AG, Githens M, Benirschke SK, Firoozabadi R. Significance of lateral process fractures associated with talar neck and body fractures. Journal of Orthopaedic Trauma. 2018;**32**(12):601-606

[64] Norvell DC, Ledoux WR, Shofer JB, Hansen ST, Davitt J, Anderson JG, et al. Effectiveness and safety of ankle arthrodesis versus arthroplasty. The Journal of Bone and Joint Surgery. American Volume. 2019;**101**(16):1485-1494. DOI: 10.2106/JBJS.18.01257

[65] Veljkovic AN, Daniels TR, Glazebrook MA, Dryden PJ, Penner MJ, Wing KJ, et al. Outcomes of total ankle replacement, arthroscopic ankle arthrodesis, and open ankle arthrodesis for isolated non-deformed end-stage ankle arthritis. Journal of Bone and Joint Surgery. 2019;**101**(17):1523-1529. DOI: 10.2106/jbjs.18.01012

[66] Gross CE, Sershon RA, Frank JM, Easley ME, Holmes GB. Treatment of osteonecrosis of the talus. JBJS Reviews. 2016;**4**(7):1-9

Chapter 9

Perspective Chapter: Calcaneus Fracture

Jamal Al-Asiri

Abstract

Calcaneus fractures, the most common tarsal fractures, present significant challenges due to their complex anatomy and high-energy mechanisms. Historically, advancements from Böhler's foundational work on open reduction to modern minimally invasive techniques have transformed management. Key classification systems, such as Essex-Lopresti (tongue-type vs. joint depression) and Sanders CT-based classification (Types I–IV), guide treatment decisions by correlating fracture patterns with prognosis. Displaced intra-articular fractures (Sanders II–IV) typically require surgical intervention, while non-operative management is reserved for non-displaced fractures or high-risk patients. Surgical approaches like the extensile lateral approach (ELA) offer anatomical reduction but carry risks of wound complications, whereas minimally invasive techniques, including the sinus tarsi approach (STA), reduce soft tissue damage and infection rates. Emerging technologies, such as 3D printing, computer-assisted surgery, and biodegradable implants, enhance precision and patient-specific care. Complications, including wound dehiscence, infection, post-traumatic arthritis, and malunion, remain prevalent, necessitating strategies like delayed surgery, patient optimization, and meticulous tissue handling. Rehabilitation protocols emphasize early mobilization and progressive weight-bearing to restore function. Despite advancements, challenges persist in balancing anatomical restoration with minimizing morbidity, particularly in severe fractures. Multidisciplinary collaboration and evidence-based practices are critical to optimizing outcomes, underscoring the need for personalized treatment aligned with patient-specific factors and evolving technologies.

Keywords: calcaneus fractures, sanders classification, sinus tarsi approach, postoperative complications, minimally invasive surgery

1. Introduction

The treatment of calcaneus fractures has undergone substantial advancements over the past century, transitioning from rudimentary methods to more sophisticated surgical approaches. Initially, limited understanding of calcaneal anatomy and fracture mechanics resulted in poor functional outcomes. In 1931, Böhler emphasized the importance of restoring calcaneal height and alignment through open reduction and internal fixation (ORIF), marking a pivotal moment in calcaneal fracture management [1]. However, the absence of advanced diagnostic tools and surgical implants at the time often led to complications such as infections and malunions [2].

In the mid-twentieth century, Gissane highlighted the role of anatomical alignment, particularly the "critical angle of Gissane," in achieving better recovery outcomes [2]. Essex-Lopresti's classification system, introduced in 1952, categorized calcaneal fractures into tongue-type and joint depression fractures, offering a framework that continues to influence clinical practice [3, 4]. This classification significantly improved the understanding and treatment strategies for calcaneal fractures.

Advancements in imaging technology and surgical techniques during the latter half of the twentiethth century further enhanced patient outcomes. For instance, Palmer's introduction of the sinus tarsi approach in 1948 provided a less invasive surgical method with reduced soft tissue complications compared to extensive exposures [5]. In 1998, Tornetta demonstrated the effectiveness of minimally invasive techniques, which enabled sufficient fracture reduction while minimizing wound complications [6]. These historical milestones underscore the progression of calcaneal fracture management, balancing the need for precise fracture alignment with reducing patient morbidity.

2. Anatomy of the calcaneus

The calcaneus, commonly referred to as the heel bone, is the largest tarsal bone in the foot and is fundamental to weight-bearing and locomotion. It forms the posterior base of the foot, articulating superiorly with the talus at the subtalar joint and anteriorly with the cuboid bone to contribute to the calcaneocuboid joint [7]. Its complex structure and strategic location make it critical in force transmission and mobility. Key anatomical features include the following:

- *Posterior facet*: The posterior facet is the largest of the three articular surfaces located on the superior aspect of the calcaneus. It plays a crucial role in force transmission through the subtalar joint, enabling smooth interaction between the calcaneus and talus during gait and other weight-bearing activities [8] Damage to this facet is often associated with compromised joint function.

- *Sustentaculum tali*: This medial bony projection supports the talus, providing a stabilizing platform for its articulation. Additionally, it serves as an attachment site for the deltoid ligament, a critical structure in maintaining medial ankle stability [7]. Its location and function are integral in balancing forces exerted during movement.

- *Calcaneal tuberosity*: The posterior prominence of the calcaneus is where the Achilles tendon inserts. This feature is essential for plantarflexion and propulsion during activities like walking, running, and jumping. The integrity of the tuberosity is crucial for maintaining lower limb biomechanics, and injuries in this area often result in functional deficits [8].

- *Peroneal tubercle*: Located on the lateral surface of the calcaneus, this small protrusion guides the peroneal tendons, preventing them from displacing. It is

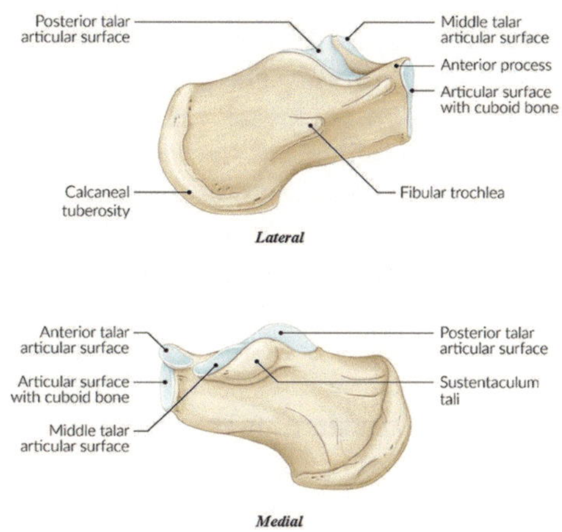

Figure 1.
Illustrations show calcaneal osteology. (Reproduced with permission from Amboss: The Leg, Ankle, and Foot. Updated February 23, 2021. Available at: https://images.app.goo.gl/Pf8xhw4sZb2qjFWg6.

a key landmark in understanding lateral calcaneal fractures and their impact on tendon function [7].

- *Anterior process*: The anterior portion of the calcaneus articulates with the cuboid bone, forming a component of the calcaneocuboid joint. This joint is essential in stabilizing the lateral column of the foot and contributing to its flexibility and strength during gait [7, 8].

- Understanding the intricate anatomy of the calcaneus is paramount in diagnosing injuries and planning surgical interventions. Knowledge of its structure not only aids in restoring alignment and function after fractures but also minimizes complications, optimizing patient outcomes (**Figure 1**) [8, 9].

3. Epidemiology and mechanisms of injury

Calcaneus fractures are the most frequently occurring fractures of the tarsal bones, representing approximately 1–2% of all fractures. Notably, around 75% of these injuries involve the posterior facet of the subtalar joint, highlighting the significance of this anatomical feature in calcaneal injuries (10). These fractures typically arise from high-energy trauma, with mechanisms such as falls from significant heights or motor vehicle accidents being the most common causes. The axial loading of the heel during these incidents generates substantial force, often leading to severe fracture patterns [3, 10].

The demographic most affected by calcaneus fractures comprises individuals in their prime working years, generally between 20 and 40 years of age. This age group not only faces the immediate challenges of the injury but also experiences significant socioeconomic impacts due to extended recovery periods and the potential for lasting disabilities. The high prevalence of these fractures among manual laborers is particularly concerning, as it underscores the need for effective treatment strategies to support timely recovery, facilitate return to work, and mitigate the economic burden associated with prolonged disability [11].

Additionally, calcaneus fractures are frequently accompanied by other injuries, complicating both treatment and rehabilitation. Associated injuries often include lumbar spine fractures, caused by the same axial loading mechanism, and other lower extremity fractures, further contributing to the complexity of patient management [12]. This multifaceted nature of calcaneus fractures necessitates a comprehensive approach to care, addressing both the fracture and its associated injuries to optimize patient outcomes [4].

4. Classification systems and fracture patterns

The classification of calcaneus fractures is a cornerstone in their effective management, as it guides treatment decisions and aids in predicting patient outcomes [13]. Two primary classification systems are widely used to describe these fractures: the Essex-Lopresti classification and the Sanders classification.

4.1 Essex-Lopresti classification

Introduced in 1952, the Essex-Lopresti classification focuses on intra-articular calcaneus fractures and divides them into two main types based on the fracture pattern and mechanism of injury [3]:

- *Tongue-type fractures*: These fractures are characterized by a vertical fracture line that extends posteriorly. The pull of the Achilles tendon on the posterior segment often causes displacement, which can lead to significant functional impairment if not properly addressed.

- *Joint depression fractures*: These fractures involve a horizontal primary fracture line. The posterior facet of the subtalar joint is typically displaced downward into the body of the calcaneus, disrupting the normal joint alignment and biomechanics.

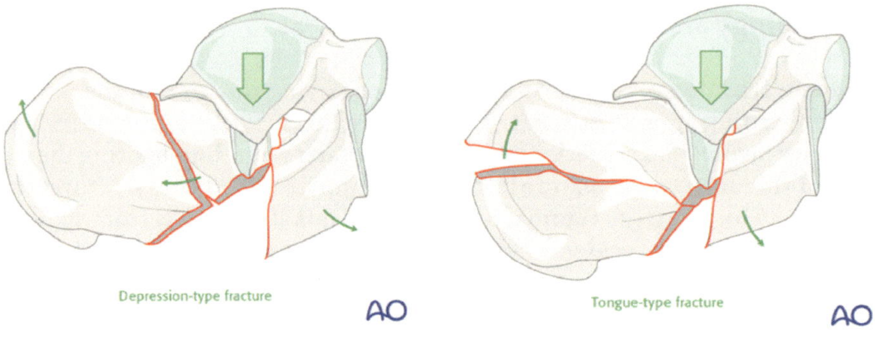

Figure 2.
Essex-Lopresti classification: We see first an example of a "joint depression" and, in the lower image, a "tongue type." The joint depression is notorious for the degree of joint involvement and displacement. Note that, in the tongue-type fracture, the fracture exits posteriorly, splitting the posterior portion into two. Different fixation techniques are required to reduce and stabilize this deformity. Available at https://surgeryreference.aofoundation.org/orthopedic-trauma/adult-trauma/calcaneous/displaced-body-fractures/definition#m-ller-ao-ota-classification.

This classification provides a straightforward framework for identifying fracture patterns and guiding initial treatment approaches (**Figure 2**).

5. Sanders classification

The Sanders classification, developed in 1993, is based on computed tomography (CT) imaging and is currently the most widely used system for intra-articular calcaneus fractures. It categorizes fractures based on the number and location of fracture lines through the posterior facet of the calcaneus, with prognostic and surgical planning implications [14, 15]:

- *Type I*: Nondisplaced fractures with less than 2 mm displacement.
- *Type II*: Two-part fractures involving a single fracture line.
- *Type III*: Three-part fractures with two fracture lines, resulting in multiple fragments.
- *Type IV*: Comminuted fractures with more than three fragments, often associated with significant joint disruption and poor outcomes.

The Sanders classification is particularly valuable for surgical planning and predicting outcomes. Studies have shown that higher types (type III and type IV) are associated with worse functional results due to the increased complexity of the fracture and the greater likelihood of joint malalignment (**Figure 3**) [13].

5.1 Clinical relevance

Both classification systems complement each other and are critical in understanding the nature of calcaneus fractures. The Essex-Lopresti classification provides a simple and effective way to categorize fractures based on their gross morphology, while the Sanders classification offers a detailed assessment using CT imaging, facilitating precise surgical intervention and enabling more accurate prognostication.

5.2 Diagnostic and imaging advancements

The effective diagnosis and management of calcaneus fractures depend on a thorough understanding of calcaneal anatomy and precise characterization of fracture patterns. Advances in imaging modalities have significantly enhanced diagnostic accuracy and surgical planning, ensuring better outcomes for patients [16].

5.3 Conventional radiographs

Conventional radiographs remain the initial step in evaluating calcaneus fractures. Standard views, including lateral and axial projections, provide essential information about fracture alignment, displacement, and overall calcaneal structure. Key angular measurements obtained from these radiographs aid in assessing fracture severity and structural disruption:

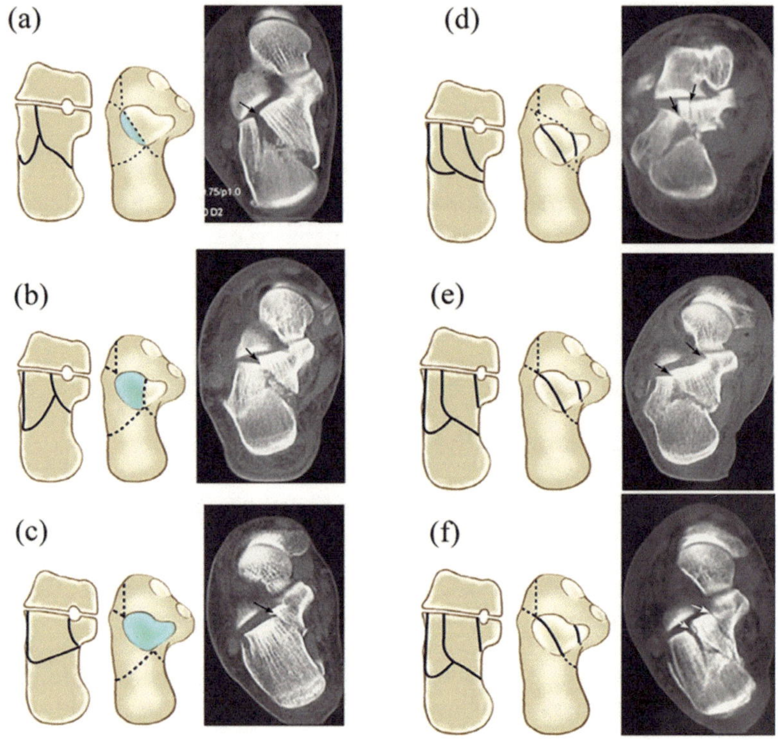

Figure 3.
The CT images of Sanders type II and type III calcaneal fractures. a: IIa: fracture line lateral to the fracture line; b IIb: fracture line medial; c IIc: fracture line adjacent to the sustentaculum tali; and d, e and f: three-part fracture of the posterior talar articular surface of type III: IIIab, IIIac, IIIbc. Available at: https://josr-online.biomedcentral.com/articles/10.1186/s13018-024-04606-1.

- *Böhler's angle*: This angle is formed by lines drawn from the highest point of the anterior process to the highest point of the posterior facet and from there to the highest point of the calcaneal tuberosity. A decreased Böhler's angle, typically below 25 degrees, is a reliable indicator of fracture collapse and loss of calcaneal height. Its measurement is crucial in evaluating the extent of injury and planning reconstruction [10, 17]

- *Gissane's angle*: Formed by the intersection of the downward and upward slopes of the calcaneal superior surface, alterations in this angle suggest significant disruption of the calcaneal structure. This parameter is particularly useful for assessing the involvement of the subtalar joint [18].

While radiographs are invaluable for initial assessments, their limitations in visualizing complex fracture patterns necessitate advanced imaging techniques (**Figure 4**).

5.4 Computed tomography (CT)

CT imaging has revolutionized the evaluation of calcaneus fractures by offering detailed three-dimensional views of the fracture anatomy. It allows precise

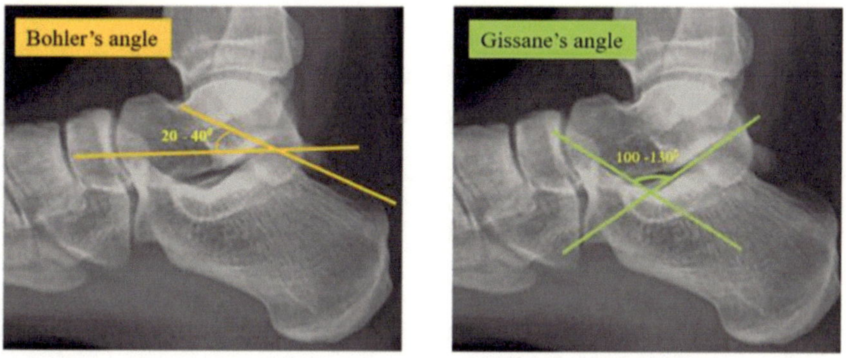

Figure 4.
Bohler's and Gissane's angles are drawn in lateral view. Bohler's angle is the intersection of a line drawn from the highest point of the calcaneal tuberosity to the highest point of the posterior facet and a line between the anterior and posterior articulating facets. A Bohler's angle of 20° or less is a sign of a calcaneal fracture. Gissane angle is the intersection of two lines drawn parallel to the anterior and posterior facets of the subtalar joint. A normal angle of Gissane is 100 to 130. Available at: Ömeroğlu [19].

identification of fracture lines, fragment displacement, and joint involvement, facilitating accurate classification using the Sanders system. The multiplanar reconstructions provided by CT are essential for understanding the spatial relationships of fracture fragments, aiding in surgical planning and outcome prediction [14, 20, 21].

5.5 Magnetic resonance imaging (MRI)

Although not routinely used in the evaluation of calcaneus fractures, MRI may be employed in specific cases to assess associated soft tissue injuries. This includes damage to ligaments, tendons, and other surrounding structures that may influence treatment strategies [22]. Its role is primarily adjunctive, as CT remains the gold standard for bony injury assessment.

5.6 Clinical implications

Integrating advanced imaging modalities into the diagnostic process has dramatically improved the ability to classify and manage calcaneus fractures. Radiographic measurements such as Böhler's and Gissane's angles provide critical initial insights, while CT imaging offers comprehensive details for surgical planning. MRI serves a supplementary role in cases with suspected soft tissue involvement, ensuring a holistic approach to patient care.

6. Operative vs. non-operative management of calcaneus fractures

Choosing between operative and non-operative management of calcaneus fractures is a topic of ongoing debate in orthopedic practice [23–26]. This decision is influenced by several factors, including the type of fracture, patient-specific factors (e.g., comorbidities, age, and activity level), and potential risks associated with surgical intervention. Each approach has distinct indications, benefits, and limitations.

6.1 Non-operative management

Non-operative management is generally recommended for selecting patient populations and specific fracture patterns. The main indications include the following:

- *Nondisplaced fractures*: These include Sanders Type I fractures with minimal or no displacement. These fractures typically maintain articular congruity and do not require surgical intervention [14].

- *Patients with significant comorbidities or poor skin conditions*: Individuals with severe systemic illnesses, such as diabetes or peripheral vascular disease, or those with compromised skin integrity around the fracture site, are at a higher risk of postoperative complications [27].

- *Patients unable or unwilling to undergo surgery*: In such cases, conservative management avoids the risks associated with anesthesia and surgery.

Non-operative treatment typically includes a combination of immobilization with a cast or boot, early initiation of range-of-motion exercises to prevent joint stiffness, and progressive weight bearing as tolerated. While this approach minimizes the risks of surgical complications, it may result in suboptimal anatomical alignment of the calcaneus. This misalignment can lead to long-term functional limitations, including chronic pain, gait abnormalities, and an increased risk of subtalar arthritis [4, 10].

7. Operative management

Operative management is indicated for fractures with significant displacement or associated complications. The primary goals of surgical intervention are to restore articular congruity, realign the calcaneus to its original height and width, and re-establish normal foot biomechanics. Specific indications for surgery include the following:

- *Displaced intra-articular fractures*: Fractures with more than 2 mm of articular displacement (typically Sanders type II, III, and IV fractures) benefit from surgical reduction and fixation to restore joint integrity [14].

- *Open fractures*: Surgical intervention is mandatory to manage open fractures, as these injuries carry a high risk of infection and require immediate debridement and stabilization [28, 29].

- *Tongue-type fractures with posterior skin compromise*: These fractures, where the displaced fragment threatens or damages the overlying skin, require urgent surgical intervention to reduce the fracture and alleviate soft tissue tension [30].

Surgical techniques, including open reduction and internal fixation (ORIF) and minimally invasive approaches, aim to achieve anatomical reduction while minimizing soft tissue complications. Operative management has been associated with improved functional outcomes, particularly in younger patients and those with less severe fracture patterns [12]. However, surgical intervention carries risks, including infection, wound dehiscence, and hardware-related complications [31, 32]. Careful patient selection is essential to maximize the benefits of surgery.

7.1 Comparative outcomes and considerations

Calcaneus fractures remain challenging injuries despite advancements in both surgical and nonsurgical treatments. These fractures often affect young, active individuals and are associated with long-term complications, including permanent disability, reduced quality of life, and significant socioeconomic costs [33]. The Buckley trial identified subgroups of patients who could benefit more from surgical management, such as women, individuals under 29 years of age, and those not receiving worker's compensation. In contrast, male patients, heavy laborers, those on worker's compensation, and patients with more severe radiographic abnormalities were more likely to require arthrodesis [12]. The association may reflect that men are more prone to sustaining high-energy trauma, such as work-related injuries, while heavy laborers are more susceptible to post-malunion pain. Furthermore, severe radiographic findings likely compromise foot and ankle biomechanics, while worker's compensation may influence the perception of symptoms. These factors should inform the surgeon's decision-making process, as surgical restoration of hindfoot anatomy and biomechanics may provide better outcomes for certain patients with displaced intra-articular calcaneal fractures (DIAFCs).

The UK Heel Fracture Trial [23] underscored the critical role of patient preferences in choosing a treatment strategy. Some fractures, particularly those with lateral wall displacement causing impingement, are often severe enough to necessitate surgery. Investigators noted that including such severe fractures in the trial, with randomization between surgical and nonsurgical management, might have significantly altered its findings. As a result, the broad conclusion that "patients with calcaneal fractures do not benefit from surgery" appears overly simplistic. While the trial highlights issues such as potential selection bias and challenges in result interpretation, it emphasizes that surgery carries inherent risks and does not guarantee excellent outcomes. Surgeons must remain cautious in balancing these considerations.

When planning treatment, surgeons must anticipate potential long-term consequences of their management choices. They need to evaluate the likelihood of specific outcomes and how complications can be addressed. Current evidence offers limited certainty and cannot fully predict results. Therefore, decision-making should integrate statistical evidence with the surgeon's clinical expertise, judgment, and experience. Patient preferences must also be factored in, with surgeons presenting unbiased and comprehensive information to facilitate informed choices [4, 34].

8. Surgical techniques and comparative studies in calcaneal fractures

Surgical management of displaced intra-articular calcaneal fractures (DIACFs) has evolved significantly, with various approaches being developed to optimize outcomes while minimizing complications. Among these, the extensile lateral approach (ELA) remains a traditional gold standard, while minimally invasive techniques (MIS) offer alternative strategies with reduced risks of soft tissue complications. Comparative studies highlight the strengths and limitations of these approaches [35].

8.1 Extensile lateral approach (ELA)

The extensile lateral approach (ELA) is a well-established method for treating complex and comminuted DIACFs. This approach utilizes a large L-shaped incision along the lateral calcaneal wall, providing extensive exposure for visualizing and manipulating fracture fragments. ELA enables the restoration of the posterior facet, calcaneal height, and alignment with internal fixation devices, such as plates and screws [36, 37].

Despite its advantages in achieving anatomical reduction, the extensive soft tissue dissection inherent in ELA contributes to a higher risk of wound complications. Reported complication rates range from 10 to 25%, including wound dehiscence, infection, hematoma, and sural nerve injury [12, 38, 39]. Risk factors such as smoking, diabetes, peripheral vascular disease, and prolonged operative times exacerbate these complications [40–42]. These risks have prompted the development of less invasive techniques (**Figure 5**).

8.2 Minimally invasive surgical (MIS) techniques

Minimally invasive techniques aim to reduce soft tissue disruption while achieving effective fracture reduction and fixation. These approaches are associated with reduced wound complications, shorter operative times, and quicker recoveries [43–45].

8.3 Sinus tarsi approach

The sinus tarsi approach (STA) involves a small incision, typically 3–5 cm, over the sinus tarsi to access the subtalar joint and posterior facet, facilitating direct visualization and reduction of the posterior facet fragment with fixation using screws or miniplates [46, 47]. As a minimally invasive alternative to the extensile lateral approach (ELA), STA has gained significant popularity for managing displaced intra-articular calcaneal fractures. Numerous studies have emphasized its advantages, including a notable reduction in wound complications and a decrease in surgical duration, making it a preferred approach in appropriate clinical settings.

The meta-analysis by Mehta et al. provides robust evidence supporting the sinus tarsi approach (STA) for treating displaced intra-articular calcaneal fractures,

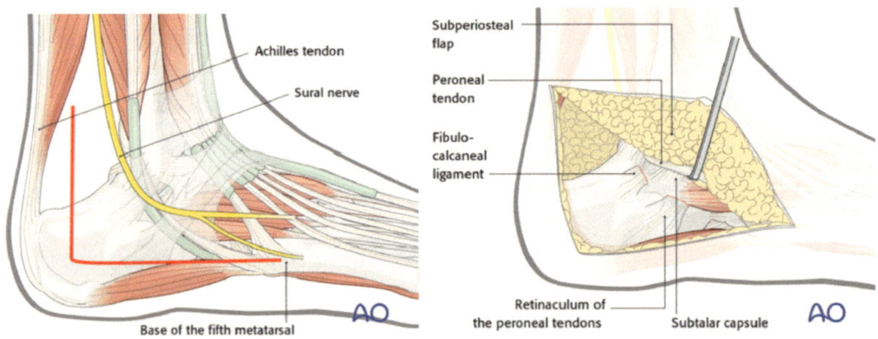

Figure 5.
Extensile lateral approach for intra-articular displaced calcaneus fracture. Available at: https://surgeryreference.aofoundation.org/orthopedic-trauma/adult-trauma/calcaneous/approach/extended-lateral-approach-to-the-calcaneus.

particularly in reducing wound complications compared to the extensile lateral approach (ELA). STA is associated with a significantly lower odds ratio for wound complications (0.20, 95% CI 0.11–0.36), demonstrating a substantially reduced risk [46]. This finding is corroborated by additional studies highlighting STA's benefits: lower incidences of wound healing complications and postoperative sural nerve injuries ($p < 0.000$) [47], and a trend toward fewer wound complications, although not always statistically significant ($p \geq 0.05$) [48]. STA also offers a shorter operative time, with studies reporting significantly faster procedures compared to ELA ($p < 0.001$ and $p \leq 0.05$) [48, 49]. Despite less extensive surgical exposure, STA achieves comparable functional outcomes to ELA, with no significant differences in American Orthopedic Foot and Ankle Society (AOFAS) scores [46]. Basile et al. [48] further noted similar clinical and radiographic outcomes between the two approaches. Collectively, these findings establish STA as a minimally invasive, efficient, and effective alternative to ELA, with reduced wound complications and surgical durations (**Figure 6**).

8.4 Percutaneous fixation

Percutaneous fixation uses small incisions and fluoroscopic guidance to achieve fracture reduction and stabilization with screws, pins, or wires. This technique is particularly effective for less comminuted fractures (e.g., Sanders Type II) and in patients with elevated risk for wound healing complications [46, 47].

Hsu et al. reviewed the outcomes of percutaneous fixation, reporting low wound complication rates (2–4%) and satisfactory functional results [47]. However, this technique may be less effective in achieving precise anatomical reduction in complex, comminuted fractures [46].

8.5 Arthroscopic-assisted reduction

Arthroscopic-assisted reduction combines MIS with arthroscopy, enabling direct visualization of the subtalar joint during fracture reduction. This technique is designed to improve articular surface restoration while maintaining the benefits of minimally invasive approaches [48, 49].

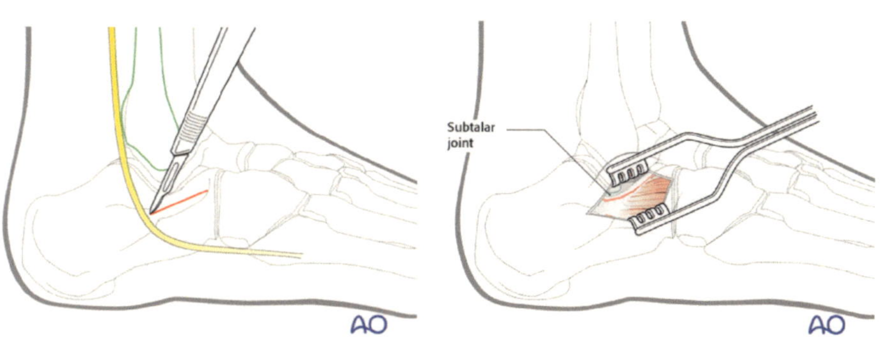

Figure 6.
Sinus tarsi approach to the intra-articular calcaneus fracture. Available at: https://surgeryreference.aofoundation.org/orthopedic-trauma/adult-trauma/calcaneous/approach/sinus-tarsi-approach-to-the-calcaneus?searchurl=/searchresults.

Yeap et al., compares outcomes between open reduction internal fixation (ORIF) and arthroscopic-assisted percutaneous screw fixation (APSF) for displaced intra-articular calcaneal fractures. Both approaches resulted in similar radiographic reductions and functional outcomes based on AOFAS and SF-36 scores. However, APSF demonstrated advantages, including significantly shorter preoperative and postoperative durations, earlier return to work (2.9 vs. 6.2 months), and no wound complications in either group. One study involving percutaneous fixation of Sanders type IIA and IIB fractures noted an excellent mean AOFAS score of 92 with 0% wound dehiscence and infection rate when reductions were confirmed with subtalar arthroscopy [50].

While APSF's minimally invasive nature offers reduced hospital stays and faster recovery, the study highlights its limitations, such as a small sample size and lack of randomization, which may affect the generalizability of the findings. Further research with larger cohorts is recommended to confirm these outcomes [51].

9. Comparative insights and future directions

The choice of surgical technique depends on fracture complexity, patient-specific factors, and the surgeon's expertise. While ELA provides excellent access for complex fractures, its risks make MIS techniques increasingly appealing. Comparative studies emphasize the efficacy of MIS approaches like the sinus tarsi and percutaneous techniques in reducing soft tissue complications while preserving functional outcomes. Emerging methods, such as arthroscopic-assisted reduction, offer promising results in improving anatomical restoration and minimizing long-term sequelae, warranting further exploration. Clinicians are still working to identify the specific fracture patterns that are best suited for these approaches. However, these techniques are generally considered beneficial for patients with soft tissue compromise, elevated risk factors for wound healing complications, and fractures with minimal comminution [47].

9.1 Advanced fixation methods and future technologies in calcaneal fracture management

The management of displaced calcaneal fractures continues to benefit from advances in surgical technology, which aim to improve outcomes by enhancing precision, reducing complications, and tailoring treatments to individual patients. Emerging methods and technologies are transforming the landscape of fracture fixation, offering innovative solutions to longstanding challenges.

9.2 Computer-assisted surgery (CAS)

Computer-assisted surgery (CAS) integrates imaging technologies with navigation systems to optimize intraoperative precision. CAS allows surgeons to achieve three-dimensional (3D) visualization of the calcaneus, facilitating accurate reduction of fracture fragments and precise placement of fixation devices. This technology ensures restoration of the calcaneal anatomy and alignment, critical for functional outcomes [52–54].

Based on the current evidence, the advantages of CAS over traditional fixation are clear. The long-term clinical effects of the two methods are also good, and the short-term effect of robot assistance is better. However, the quality of some studies is low, and more high-quality randomized controlled trials (RCTs) are needed for further verification [54].

These advantages make CAS particularly valuable in managing complex and comminuted fractures, where anatomical landmarks may be distorted.

9.3 Three-dimensional (3D) printing and patient-specific implants

Three-dimensional printing technology has revolutionized surgical planning and implant customization. By using patient-specific CT data, 3D printing enables the creation of anatomical models and custom implants tailored to the unique geometry of the calcaneus. This approach enhances preoperative planning and ensures a better fit for fixation devices [55].

Compared to the conventional group, when comparted to the conventional surgery, the 3D model-assisted group provide successful intervention and reduce operation, instrumentation time and the fluoroscopy usage with less blood loss. Performing 3D-assisted surgery helps the quality of reduction during the surgery and stability of internal fixation to protect achieved reduction at follow-up more successfully [53, 55].

9.4 Biodegradable implants

Metallic screws are commonly utilized in the treatment of calcaneal fractures due to their low risk of infection and minimal incidence of skin irritation. Current evidence indicates that metallic screw fixation performed via the sinus tarsi approach yields comparable outcomes to plate fixation. Postoperative evaluations, including the American Orthopedic Foot & Ankle Society (AOFAS) score, Böhler's and Gissane's angles, and the maintenance of reduction, show no significant differences between these two fixation methods [56, 57].

Biodegradable fixation devices, including screws and plates made from materials such as polylactic acid (PLA), offer an alternative to traditional metal implants. These devices are designed to degrade within the body over time, eliminating the need for subsequent hardware removal surgeries. Additionally, biodegradable implants reduce long-term risks associated with metallic hardware, such as irritation, infection, and allergic reactions [58–61].

Biodegradable implants are increasingly important in eliminating the need for painful and inconvenient secondary surgeries required for implant removal or replacement. To ensure successful healing fractures with biodegradable implants, a comprehensive approach must be adopted. This includes selecting appropriate raw materials, designing and manufacturing implants with compatible features, planning for the implantation phase, and addressing the remodeling and degradation stages as the healing process concludes [59].

Understanding the behavior of the bone-implant interface is critical, requiring an analysis of mechanical properties, degradation dynamics, and biological interactions. This combined analysis informs the development of effective and optimized implant designs tailored to support bone healing. An ideal biodegradable implant must provide sufficient mechanical strength during recovery while gradually losing integrity at the bone-implant interface as healing progresses, ensuring seamless integration and support throughout the recovery period [61].

9.5 Augmented reality (AR) in surgery

Augmented reality (AR) is an emerging technology that overlays digital information onto the surgeon's field of view during an operation. AR enhances anatomical visualization and orientation, aiding in real-time decision-making and improving surgical accuracy [62–64]. This technology is particularly advantageous in cases of complex calcaneal fractures, where traditional visualization methods may be insufficient due to severe anatomical distortion.

The potential applications of AR in fracture management, highlighting its ability to reduce surgical errors and improve precision [65]. While AR is still in the experimental stages, its integration with other technologies such as CAS and 3D printing could revolutionize the surgical treatment of calcaneal fractures [53].

10. Future directions

The integration of advanced technologies such as CAS, 3D printing, biodegradable implants, and AR represents a paradigm shift in calcaneal fracture management. As these technologies become more widely adopted, they promise to enhance patient-specific care, improve functional outcomes, and reduce complications. Continued research and development are essential to refine these methods and assess their long-term efficacy [4].

11. Orthobiologics and bone grafts in calcaneal fracture management

Orthobiologics, including bone morphogenetic proteins (BMPs) and mesenchymal stem cells (MSCs), are emerging as promising adjuncts in the management of calcaneal fractures, particularly in cases with bone loss or compromised healing potential [66]. These biological agents stimulate osteogenesis and enhance bone repair by promoting cellular activity and differentiation at the fracture site [66–68].

Bone morphogenetic proteins, such as BMP-2 and BMP-7, have demonstrated efficacy in augmenting bone healing, especially in challenging cases involving non-union or significant bone loss [69]. Additionally, MSCs, derived from sources such as bone marrow or adipose tissue, can differentiate into osteoblasts, thereby contributing to bone regeneration [70]. However, while initial studies suggest positive outcomes, the efficacy and safety profiles of these agents require further validation through rigorous clinical trials.

The existing evidence is of low quality, largely due to study designs prone to significant selection bias, small sample sizes, insufficient reporting of patient and surgical risk factors for non-union, and variability in study populations, orthobiologic materials, surgical techniques, and outcome assessments. Consequently, there is limited guidance for surgeons on identifying patients who might benefit most from orthobiologics or selecting the appropriate orthobiologic. The lack of evidence supporting the superiority of orthobiologics over their absence underscores the importance of thoroughly evaluating individual patient risk factors for non-union before considering orthobiologic use [68]. Additionally, patients and clinicians should be aware that using orthobiologics for foot and ankle arthrodesis is classified as "off-label."

11.1 Challenges and future directions

The integration of orthobiologics into routine clinical practice faces challenges, including cost, regulatory approval, and potential complications such as ectopic bone formation. There is insufficient evidence to assess costs or cost-effectiveness of orthobiologics. Two studies reported operation time, finding longer times for procedures involving graft harvest but no difference in operation time when non-graft orthobiologic products were used [71, 72].

Future research should prioritize optimizing delivery methods, determining appropriate dosages, and assessing long-term outcomes to potentially establish these therapies as a standard approach in managing calcaneal fractures. Based on current evidence, we recommend implementing utilization reviews and approval processes prior to orthobiologic use. This approach would help target orthobiologic application and any subsequent surgical interventions to patients or arthrodesis sites at the highest risk of non-union. Providers and policymakers should remain mindful of the costs and potential morbidity associated with the widespread adoption of orthobiologics, particularly given the insufficient to low-quality evidence supporting their benefits, which are largely based on radiographic rather than clinical outcomes.

11.2 Primary subtalar fusion: Indications, outcomes, and comparative studies

Primary subtalar arthrodesis, or fusion of the subtalar joint during the initial surgical intervention, is a targeted approach for managing severely comminuted calcaneal fractures, particularly Sanders Type IV fractures where articular reconstruction is deemed unfeasible [73–75]. This procedure stabilizes the hindfoot, reduces pain, and facilitates early weight-bearing, making it a valuable option in specific clinical scenarios.

11.2.1 Indications

Primary subtalar fusion is indicated in the following cases:

- *Severely comminuted fractures (e.g., Sanders Type IV):* When joint restoration is impractical due to extensive damage [74–76].

- *Elderly patients with poor bone quality:* Patients with osteoporosis or compromised healing capacity.

- *Pre-existing subtalar arthritis:* Cases where arthritic changes preclude effective reconstruction [75, 77].

11.2.2 Outcomes

Studies indicate that primary subtalar arthrodesis can lead to favorable outcomes in patients with severe calcaneal fractures. A retrospective analysis involving 12 patients showed a mean American Orthopedic Foot and Ankle Society (AOFAS) score of 82.25, indicating satisfactory functional recovery [77]. A case series by Buckley et al. examined 14 patients with comminuted intra-articular calcaneal fractures treated with primary subtalar arthrodesis. After a 26-month follow-up, the mean AOFAS score was 72.4 points. The authors concluded that primary subtalar fusion is the treatment of choice for Sanders type IV fractures [78]. A meta-analysis was done to compare the functional outcome of ORIF vs. primary subtalar arthrodesis (PSA) for Sanders type II and type III calcaneal fractures according to American Orthopedic Foot and Ankle Score (AOFAS) hindfoot-ankle scores. They concluded that while high-quality randomized controlled trials comparing ORIF to primary subtalar arthrodesis for type II and type III fractures would further elucidate superior treatment outcomes, this meta-analysis of available data shows a tendency for ORIF of type II and type III Sanders calcaneal fractures to have a better functional outcome at approximately 2 years postoperatively compared to primary subtalar arthrodesis [76].

11.2.3 Considerations

While primary subtalar fusion sacrifices subtalar motion, this limitation is often outweighed by the benefits of pain reduction and enhanced stability. Patient selection is critical to optimizing outcomes. The procedure is reserved for cases where joint salvage is unlikely to yield satisfactory results, such as in the elderly or those with severe comminution [73].

Additionally, counseling patients about the functional trade-offs, such as reduced ankle mobility, is essential for setting realistic postoperative expectations.

11.3 Complications in calcaneal fracture management

Complications are a significant concern in the management of calcaneal fractures and vary depending on the treatment modality and surgical approach used. Recent studies have shed light on the frequency, nature, and contributing factors of complications, providing insights into strategies for their prevention and management.

11.4 Wound complications and reoperations

In a recent meta-analysis [79] that include a total of 21 articles (4 randomized control trials, 17 cohort studies) comprising of 2086 patients with calcaneal fractures, treated with either ELA (n = 1129) or STA (n = 957) met inclusion criteria. It finds the risk of postoperative wound-related complications (RR 2.82, 95% CI: 2.00–3.98, I2 = 27%) and the risk of reoperation (RR 1.85, 95% CI: 0.69–5.00, I2 = 67%) was higher in ELA patients comparted to STA patients. However, the increased risk of postoperative wound-related complications with an ELA vs. STA was shown to be trending downward in recent publications.

11.4.1 Infections

Managing calcaneus fractures poses a significant challenge for trauma surgeons due to the bone's unique anatomical structure and the limited soft-tissue coverage. While operative treatment offers potential benefits, these can be outweighed by complications. Among the most serious is wound infection, which may result in implant removal, non-union, or even amputation. The overall prevalence of Surgical site infections (SSI) in reported data is between 0 and 20% for closed and 19–33% for open calcaneal fractures [79–83].

In a systematic review by Attenasio et al., including 2086 patients (1129 ELA vs. 957 STA), the studies included all four Sanders fracture types (88.8% of which were type II and III). They reported significantly higher (2.82 times) wound complications (necrosis, infection, and dehiscence) in the ELA compared to STA [79].

11.4.2 Nerve injuries

Sural nerve injury is a potential complication of lateral approaches, particularly ELA, resulting in sensory deficits, neuromas, or neuropathic pain. Rates of sural nerve injury with ELA have been reported to be between (9.1–25%) [36, 40, 84–86]. Careful dissection, precise anatomical identification, and avoidance of excessive tension on nerve structures are critical to minimizing these injuries.

11.4.3 Non-union and malunion

Non-union is rare in calcaneal fractures but can occur due to factors such as poor vascular supply, infection, or inadequate fixation. Malunion, on the other hand, is more common, particularly in non-operatively managed fractures or cases with inadequate reduction [87, 88]. Malunions often manifest as various deformities or loss of calcaneal height, leading to altered gait mechanics and chronic pain [89].

Patients treated non-operatively will require surgical intervention to avoid functional impairment and long-term disability. This is particularly important as these fractures frequently occur in young to middle-aged industrial workers. Without surgical treatment, displaced fractures can lead to severely disabling malunions characterized by distinct clinical and radiographic feature [90].

11.4.4 Post-traumatic arthritis

Damage to the subtalar joint cartilage during the initial injury often leads to post-traumatic arthritis, which is characterized by chronic pain and stiffness. The severity of arthritis is closely related to the fracture type and the precision of articular surface restoration [91–95]. A study indicated that up to 33% of patients with displaced intra-articular fractures developed subtalar arthritis severe enough to warrant arthrodesis [96].

11.4.5 Venous thromboembolism (VTE)

Venous thromboembolism (VTE) is an uncommon occurrence following isolated foot and ankle fractures. Current guidelines do not support the routine use of VTE prophylaxis after these types of fractures or related surgeries. Preventative strategies, such as prophylactic anticoagulation, are tailored to the identification of underlying patient risk factors—both acquired and inherited—that increase the likelihood of developing VTE [97].

Patients with calcaneal fractures are at risk of deep vein thrombosis (DVT) and pulmonary embolism (PE) due to prolonged immobilization and the hypercoagulable state induced by trauma. There is 1.5% incidence of symptomatic VTE in surgically managed patients, so routine chemoprophylaxis is not indicated [97].

11.4.6 Compartment syndrome

Although rare, compartment syndrome of the foot can occur due to swelling within the calcaneal compartments, leading to ischemia and tissue necrosis if not promptly recognized and treated [98]. Treatment of compartment syndrome in the acute phase includes emergency fasciotomy to release pressure from the compartment to prevent additional tissue damage [91, 98–101].

11.4.7 Complex regional pain syndrome (CRPS)

Hyperalgesia and allodynia are key features of complex regional pain syndrome (CRPS), a chronic pain condition that typically affects the limbs and often arises after a traumatic event or surgical procedure involving an extremity. To date, most research on the incidence of CRPS has focused on wrist fractures, with limited studies examining its occurrence after foot and ankle surgeries and none specifically addressing its prevalence following calcaneal fractures. Retrospective analysis of patients with calcaneal fractures has identified male gender, shorter immobilization periods, and vitamin C supplementation as significant factors in reducing the risk of developing CRPS. Prospective studies with larger patient populations and comparisons of various treatment protocols would provide more valuable insights [102].

12. Strategies to reduce complications in calcaneal fracture management

Effective management of calcaneal fractures includes implementing strategies to minimize complications, which can significantly impact patient outcomes. These strategies focus on patient optimization, precise surgical timing, meticulous surgical techniques, and the application of prophylactic measures.

12.1 Patient optimization

Optimizing patient health prior to surgery can significantly reduce the risk of complications, particularly wound-related issues.

- *Controlling comorbidities:* Addressing conditions such as diabetes, which impairs wound healing, is critical. Glycemic control reduces the risk of infection and promotes better tissue repair [103, 104].

- *Smoking cessation:* Smoking is a well-known risk factor for delayed wound healing and increases the likelihood of infection. Preoperative smoking cessation has been shown to improve surgical outcomes [105].

12.1.1 Surgical timing

Timing of surgery plays a crucial role in reducing complications, especially wound-related issues.

- *Delayed surgery:* Waiting until soft tissue swelling subsides is a widely accepted strategy. The presence of the "wrinkle sign," which indicates subsidence of edema and improved skin condition, serves as a reliable marker for safe surgical timing. Buckley et al. emphasized that delayed surgery reduces tension on soft tissues, thereby minimizing wound complications [78].

12.1.2 Surgical technique

Meticulous surgical technique is essential to avoid unnecessary complications and ensure optimal outcomes.

- *Minimizing soft tissue dissection:* Minimally invasive approaches, such as the sinus tarsi approach, are increasingly favored to reduce soft tissue disruption and the associated risk of wound complications [4, 10].

- *Tissue handling:* Careful and meticulous handling of soft tissues during surgery helps preserve vascular supply and prevent necrosis.

- *Selecting the appropriate approach:* The choice of surgical approach should be tailored to the fracture pattern and patient-specific factors, balancing the need for adequate exposure with minimizing soft tissue damage [79, 94, 106].

13. Prophylactic measures

Prophylactic interventions are critical in reducing the incidence of complications related to infection, venous thromboembolism (VTE), and delayed detection of issues (**Figure** 7).

- *Antibiotics:* The routine use of prophylactic antibiotics has been proven effective in reducing the risk of surgical site infections [107–109].

- *VTE prophylaxis:* Trauma and immobility predispose patients to venous thromboembolism. Prophylactic anticoagulation for high-risk patients, along with mechanical measures such as compression devices, significantly reduces this risk [97, 110].

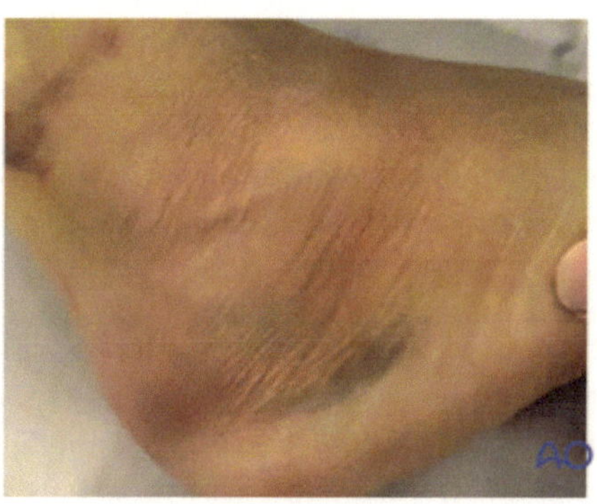

Figure 7.
The image shows a foot 14 days after injury appropriate for surgery, with the "wrinkle sign" present. Available at: https://surgeryreference.aofoundation.org/orthopedic-trauma/adult-trauma/calcaneous/approach/sinus-tarsi-approach-to-the-calcaneus?searchurl=/searchresults.

- *Close postoperative monitoring:* Early detection of complications through vigilant postoperative monitoring allows timely intervention, potentially preventing progression to more severe issues [111, 112].

14. Outcomes in calcaneal fracture management

Functional outcomes following calcaneal fracture treatment are influenced by numerous factors, including fracture severity, accuracy of fracture reduction, choice of surgical approach, and the presence or absence of complications. Advances in treatment modalities and evidence from recent studies have provided deeper insights into long-term functional and quality-of-life outcomes.

The outcomes of displaced intra-articular calcaneal fractures vary significantly and are influenced by multiple factors. To date, large randomized controlled trials have not established clear advantages of open reduction and internal fixation (ORIF) over nonsurgical management. Key determinants of patient outcomes include the precision of reduction, the severity of the initial injury, and the number of articular fragments involved. For instance, the Sanders classification system plays a crucial role in predicting outcomes, with patients sustaining Sanders type I or type II injuries experiencing significantly better results compared to those with Sanders type IV fractures [36, 113]. While anatomic reduction is typically achievable for most Sanders type II and type III fractures, it is rarely possible for Sanders type IV injuries.

A level II study published in 2013 compared ORIF to nonsurgical treatment for displaced intra-articular calcaneal fractures. The findings revealed no superiority of ORIF at 1 year postoperatively, though longer-term benefits were observed 8 to 12 years after surgery. Despite the advantages of ORIF in reducing subtalar arthritis, it was associated with a higher complication rate. Among the fractures, 57% were reduced to within 2 mm, while 19% of patients experienced infections [114]. Notably, one patient required transtibial amputation due to methicillin-resistant *Staphylococcus aureus* infection, and another underwent removal of instrumentation followed by intravenous antibiotic therapy.

Complications profoundly affect outcomes, prompting many surgeons to explore minimally invasive techniques for managing complex calcaneal fractures. These approaches may yield better outcomes compared to the traditional extensile lateral approach, provided they achieve comparable anatomic reductions and stable fixation [115]. Poor outcomes are often linked to surgical fixation with inadequate reduction or significant complications. The choice of surgical technique significantly influences wound complication rates, with studies showing lower rates of wound issues using the sinus tarsi or other minimally invasive methods compared to the extensile approach. Wound complication rates with the extensile lateral approach range from 30 to 40%, compared to 8 to 15% with a sinus tarsi approach [113, 116–119]. However, delayed surgery using minimally invasive methods—typically 7 to 10 days post-injury—can increase the risk of wound complications due to the challenges of indirect techniques.

Another key predictor of outcomes is the Bohler angle at the time of injury. Patients with a Bohler angle between 15 and 36°, moderate tongue-type fracture patterns, and non-work-related injuries generally experience favorable outcomes. Surgical restoration of the Bohler angle within this range, without requiring arthrodesis, in cases of unilateral, non-work-related injuries also correlates with better results [119].

The largest study to date on open calcaneal fractures analyzed 127 cases over 12 years, reporting an overall complication rate of 23.5%. Of these fractures, 12.2% resulted in deep wound infections, and 2.5% led to amputations [120]. A systematic review of 616 open calcaneal fractures found an average time to surgical repair of 9.8 days, with a complication rate of 21% [121].

14.1 Return to work and quality of life

Surgical restoration of angles can positively influence the functional outcomes of patients, but this is not the only variable and thus should not be exclusively used to analyze the functional outcome and time to return to work of patients [122]. Patients with calcaneal fractures experience significantly lower health-related quality of life (HRQoL) compared to the general population and often face chronic disabilities. Factors such as comorbidities, psychiatric history, or female gender are associated with even lower HRQoL scores [123].

14.2 Rehabilitation and physiotherapy

Postoperative rehabilitation plays a pivotal role in optimizing recovery after calcaneal fracture management. Structured rehabilitation programs emphasizing early mobilization, joint range of motion, and strength training have been shown to improve functional outcomes and reduce stiffness.

Rehabilitation following calcaneal fractures begins with managing edema and preventing Achilles tendon contracture. For all types of calcaneal fractures, immediate application of a splint with compression bandages and elevation is recommended to control swelling. In surgically treated fractures, a non-removable splint should be placed over the surgical dressings until the wound heals, which typically occurs within 2 to 3 weeks, at which point range of motion exercises can begin. For nonsurgically managed fractures, range of motion exercises may be initiated as soon as soft tissue swelling subsides.

Bony union generally takes 6 to 12 weeks, at which time progressive weight-bearing activities can start. Partial weight bearing is traditionally introduced between 6 and 8 weeks, followed by full weight bearing between 3 and 4 months, with brace removal typically occurring between 4 and 6 months. Studies have shown that early weight bearing—starting as soon as 4 to 5 weeks postoperatively—does not increase the subsidence of the subtalar joint when treated with locking plates and 4.0 mm screws. In fact, a multicenter randomized study indicated that weight-bearing initiation at 3 weeks postoperatively improved joint congruence, fracture reduction, and patient outcome scores.

Patients can generally expect to return to their preinjury occupation within 6 to 9 months. By this time, most regain near-full dorsiflexion and plantar flexion of the ankle, along with 50 to 75% of subtalar joint inversion and eversion.

15. Conclusion

The management of calcaneus fractures has undergone transformative advancements over the past century, marked by significant progress in anatomical understanding, diagnostic imaging, classification systems, surgical techniques, and the integration of emerging technologies. Historical milestones, such as Böhler's emphasis on restoring calcaneal height and Essex-Lopresti's classification system, laid the groundwork for modern treatment paradigms that prioritize anatomical restoration and functional recovery.

Technological advancements, including computed tomography (CT) imaging, have revolutionized the precision of fracture assessment, enabling the application of refined classification systems such as the Sanders classification. These tools have guided the development of both traditional and minimally invasive surgical techniques, enhanced surgical outcomes while mitigating complications.

Operative management remains the gold standard for displaced intra-articular calcaneal fractures, with open reduction and internal fixation (ORIF) providing superior functional outcomes. Minimally invasive surgical approaches, such as the sinus tarsi approach, have gained traction by reducing soft tissue complications without compromising functional recovery. The advent of cutting-edge techniques, including computer-assisted surgery, three-dimensional printing, and orthobiologics, has further improved fracture fixation and healing, offering patient-specific solutions to complex cases.

Despite these advancements, challenges persist, including high rates of wound complications, post-traumatic arthritis, and long-term functional limitations in severe fractures. Patient selection, optimized surgical timing, and meticulous surgical technique remain critical to minimizing these risks. Additionally, the role of postoperative rehabilitation is increasingly recognized as a cornerstone of recovery, emphasizing the need for structured physiotherapy programs to maximize functional outcomes.

The future of calcaneus fracture management lies in the continued integration of innovative technologies, improved biological therapies, and evidence-based practices to enhance patient care. With ongoing research and development, clinicians are better equipped than ever to deliver personalized and effective treatments, balancing the dual goals of anatomical restoration and functional rehabilitation.

This evolution underscores the importance of multidisciplinary collaboration in achieving optimal outcomes for patients with calcaneus fractures, as orthopedic surgeons continue to refine their approaches based on emerging evidence and technological advances.

Author details

Jamal Al-Asiri
Department of Surgery, Orthopedic Division, McMaster University, Canada

*Address all correspondence to: alasirja@mcmaster.ca

References

[1] Böhler L, Hey Groves EW. The treatment of fractures. The American Journal of the Medical Sciences. 1935;**190**(2):276. DOI: 10.1097/00000441-193508000-00034

[2] Guerado E, Bertrand ML, Cano JR. Management of calcaneal fractures: What have we learnt over the years? Injury. 2012;**43**(10):1640-1650. DOI: 10.1016/j.injury.2012.05.011

[3] Essex-Lopresti P. The mechanism, reduction technique, and results in fractures of the OS calcis. British Journal of Surgery. 1952;**39**(157):395-419. DOI: 10.1002/bjs.18003915704

[4] Chirayath A, Dhaniwala N, Kawde K. A comprehensive review on managing fracture calcaneum by surgical and non-surgical modalities. Curēus (Palo Alto, CA). 2024;**16**(2):e54786. DOI: 10.7759/cureus.54786

[5] Palmer I. The mechanism and treatment of fractures of the calcaneus: Open reduction with the use of cancellous grafts. Journal of Bone and Joint Surgery American Volume. 1948;**30**(1):2-8. DOI: 10.2106/00004623-194830010-00002

[6] Tornetta P. Percutaneous treatment of calcaneal fractures. Clinical Orthopaedics and Related Research. 2000;**375**(375):91-96. DOI: 10.1097/00003086-200006000-00011

[7] Standring S. In: Standring S, editor. Gray's Anatomy : The Anatomical Basis of Clinical Practice. 42nd ed. New York: Elsevier; 2021

[8] Brockett CL, Chapman GJ. Biomechanics of the ankle. Orthopaedics and Trauma. 2016;**30**(3):232-238. DOI: 10.1016/j.mporth.2016.04.015

[9] Keener BJ, Sizensky JA. The anatomy of the calcaneus and surrounding structures. Foot and Ankle Clinics. 2005;**10**(3):413-424. DOI: 10.1016/j.fcl.2005.04.003

[10] Allegra PR, Rivera S, Desai SS, Aiyer A, Kaplan J, Gross CE. Intra-articular calcaneus fractures: Current concepts review. Foot & Ankle Orthopaedics. 2020;**5**(3):2473011420927334. DOI: 10.1177/2473011420927334

[11] Brauer CA, Manns BJ, Ko M, Donaldson C, Buckley R. An economic evaluation of operative compared with nonoperative management of displaced intra-articular calcaneal fractures. Journal of Bone and Joint Surgery American volume. 2005;**87**(12):2741-2749. DOI: 10.2106/JBJS.E.00166

[12] Buckley R, Tough S, McCormack R, Pate G, Leighton R, Petrie D, et al. Operative compared with nonoperative treatment of displaced intra-articular calcaneal fractures: A prospective, randomized, controlled multicenter trial. Journal of Bone and Joint Surgery American Volume. 2002;**84**(10):1733-1744. DOI: 10.2106/00004623-200210000-00001

[13] Jiménez-Almonte JH, King JD, Luo TD, Aneja A, Moghadamian E. Classifications in brief: Sanders classification of intraarticular fractures of the calcaneus. Clinical Orthopaedics and Related Research. 2019;**477**(2):467-471. DOI: 10.1097/CORR.0000000000000539

[14] Sanders R. Intra-articular fractures of the calcaneus: Present

state of the art. Journal of Orthopaedic Trauma. 1992;**6**(2):252-265. DOI: 10.1097/00005131-199206000-00022

[15] Meinberg EG, Agel J, Roberts CS, Karam MD, Kellam JF. Fracture and dislocation classification compendium-2018. Journal of Orthopaedic Trauma. 2018;**32**(1):S1-S170. DOI: 10.1097/BOT.0000000000001063

[16] Aghnia Farda N, Lai J-Y, Wang J-C, Lee P-Y, Liu J-W, Hsieh I-H. Sanders classification of calcaneal fractures in CT images with deep learning and differential data augmentation techniques. Injury. 2021;**52**(3):616-624. DOI: 10.1016/j.injury.2020.09.010

[17] Isaacs JD, Baba M, Huang P, Symes M, Guzman M, Nandapalan H, et al. The diagnostic accuracy of Böhler's angle in fractures of the calcaneus. The Journal of Emergency Medicine. 2013;**45**(6):879-884. DOI: 10.1016/j.jemermed.2013.04.055

[18] Lau BC, Allahabadi S, Palanca A, Oji DE. Understanding radiographic measurements used in foot and ankle surgery. Journal of the American Academy of Orthopaedic Surgeons. 2022;**30**(2):e139-e154. DOI: 10.5435/JAAOS-D-20-00189

[19] Ömeroğlu M. First step evaluation of patient with foot and ankle injury. Arşiv Kaynak Tarama Dergisi. 2021;**30**(4):185-208. DOI: 10.17827/etd.905091

[20] Moussa KM, Hassaan MAE, Moharram AN, Elmahdi MD. The role of multidetector CT in evaluation of calcaneal fractures. Egyptian Journal of Radiology and Nuclear Medicine. 2015;**46**(2):413-421. DOI: 10.1016/j.ejrnm.2015.02.013

[21] Janzen D, Connell D, Munk P, Buckley R, Meek R, Schechter M. Intraarticular fractures of the calcaneus: Value of CT findings in determining prognosis. American Journal of Roentgenology. 1992;**158**(6):1271-1274. DOI: 10.2214/ajr.158.6.1590122

[22] Zeiss J, Ebraheim N, Rusin J, Coombs RJ. Magnetic resonance imaging of the calcaneus: Normal anatomy and application in calcaneal fractures. Foot & Ankle. 1991;**11**(5):264-273. DOI: 10.1177/107110079101100503

[23] Griffin D, Parsons N, Shaw E, Kulikov Y, Hutchinson C, Thorogood M, et al. Operative versus non-operative treatment for closed, displaced, intra-articular fractures of the calcaneus: Randomised controlled trial. BMJ (Online). 2014;**349**(5):g4483. DOI: 10.1136/bmj.g4483

[24] Meena S, Hooda A, Sharma P, Mittal S, Sharma J, Chowdhury B. Operative versus non operative treatment of displaced intraarticular fracture of calcaneum: A meta-analysis of randomized controlled trials. Acta Orthopaedica Belgica. 2017;**83**(1):161-169

[25] Baertl S, Alt V, Rupp M. Surgical enhancement of fracture healing – Operative vs. nonoperative treatment. Injury. 2021;**52**:S12-S17. DOI: 10.1016/j.injury.2020.11.049

[26] Lewis SR, Lewis SR, Pritchard MW, Solomon JL, Griffin XL, Bruce J. Surgical versus non-surgical interventions for displaced intra-articular calcaneal fractures. Cochrane Database of Systematic Reviews. 2023;**2023**(11):CD008628. DOI: 10.1002/14651858.CD008628.pub3

[27] Zhang W, Chen E, Xue D, Yin H, Pan Z. Risk factors for wound complications of closed calcaneal

fractures after surgery: A systematic review and meta-analysis. Scandinavian Journal of Trauma, Resuscitation and Emergency Medicine. 2015;**23**(1):18. DOI: 10.1186/s13049-015-0092-4

[28] Worsham JR, Elliott MR, Harris AM. Open calcaneus fractures and associated injuries. The Journal of Foot and Ankle Surgery. 2016;**55**(1):68-71. DOI: 10.1053/j.jfas.2015.06.015

[29] Lopas LA, Counihan MM, Donegan DJ, Benirschke SK, Adams MR. Open Calcaneus Fractures. In: Fractures and Dislocations of the Talus and Calcaneus. Cham: Springer International Publishing; 2020. pp. 239-250. DOI: 10.1007/978-3-030-37363-4_17

[30] Gardner MJ, Nork SE, Barei DP, Kramer PA, Sangeorzan BJ, Benirschke SK. Secondary soft tissue compromise in tongue-type calcaneus fractures. Journal of Orthopaedic Trauma. 2008;**22**(7):439-445. DOI: 10.1097/BOT.0b013e31817ace7e

[31] Larose G, Tufescu T, Vidal R, Laxdal I. Soft tissue complications following extensile lateral compared with minimally invasive surgical approaches in the operative treatment of calcaneus fractures. Canadian Journal of Surgery. 2022;**65**(6):E792-E797. DOI: 10.1503/cjs.021221

[32] Al-Mudhaffar M, Prasad CVR, Mofidi A. Wound complications following operative fixation of calcaneal fractures. Injury. 2000;**31**(6):461-464. DOI: 10.1016/S0020-1383(00)00026-7

[33] Bruce J, Sutherland A, Bruce J. Surgical versus conservative interventions for displaced intra-articular calcaneal fractures. Cochrane Database of Systematic Reviews. 2013;**2013**(1):CD008628. DOI: 10.1002/14651858.CD008628.pub2

[34] Kwon JY, Diwan A, Susarla S, Chacko AT, Rodriguez EK. Effect of surgeon training, fracture, and patient variables on calcaneal fracture management. Foot & Ankle International. 2011;**32**(3):262-271. DOI: 10.3113/FAI.2011.0262

[35] Zeng Z, Yuan L, Zheng S, Sun Y, Huang F. Minimally invasive versus extensile lateral approach for sanders type II and III calcaneal fractures: A meta-analysis of randomized controlled trials. International Journal of Surgery. 2018;**50**:146-153. DOI: 10.1016/j.ijsu.2017.12.034

[36] Sanders R. Displaced intra-articular fractures of the calcaneus. Journal of Bone and Joint Surgery American volume. 2000;**82**(2):225-250. DOI: 10.2106/00004623-200002000-00009

[37] Rammelt S, Zwipp H. Calcaneus fractures: Facts, controversies and recent developments. Injury. 2004;**35**(5):443-461. DOI: 10.1016/j.injury.2003.10.006

[38] Li Y, Bao RH, Jiang ZQ, Wu HY. Complications in operative fixation of calcaneal fractures. Pakistan Journal of Medical Sciences. 2016;**32**(4):857-862. DOI: 10.12669/pjms.324.10225

[39] Koutserimpas C, Magarakis G, Kastanis G, Kontakis G, Alpantaki K. Complications of intra-articular calcaneal fractures in adults: Key points for diagnosis, prevention, and treatment. Foot & Ankle Specialist. 2016;**9**(6):534-542. DOI: 10.1177/1938640016668030

[40] Folk JW, Starr AJ, Early JS. Early wound complications of operative treatment of calcaneus fractures: Analysis of 190 fractures. Journal of Orthopaedic Trauma. 1999;**13**(5):369-372. DOI: 10.1097/00005131-199906000-00008

[41] Schepers T, Den Hartog D, Vogels LMM, Van Lieshout EMM. Extended lateral approach for intra-articular calcaneal fractures: An inverse relationship between surgeon experience and wound complications. The Journal of Foot and Ankle Surgery. 2013;**52**(2):167-171. DOI: 10.1053/j.jfas.2012.11.009

[42] Backes M, Schepers T, Beerekamp MSH, Luitse JSK, Goslings JC, Schep NWL. Wound infections following open reduction and internal fixation of calcaneal fractures with an extended lateral approach. International Orthopaedics. 2014;**38**(4):767-773. DOI: 10.1007/s00264-013-2181-1

[43] Levine DS, Helfet DL. An introduction to the minimally invasive osteosynthesis of intra-articular calcaneal fractures. Injury. 2001;**32**(1):51-54. DOI: 10.1016/S0020-1383(01)00061-4

[44] Giannini S, Cadossi M, Mosca M, Tedesco G, Sambri A, Terrando S, et al. Minimally-invasive treatment of calcaneal fractures: A review of the literature and our experience. Injury. 2016;**47**:S138-S146. DOI: 10.1016/j.injury.2016.07.050

[45] Rodemund C, Krenn R, Kihm C, Leister I, Ortmaier R, Litzlbauer W, et al. Minimally invasive surgery for intra-articular calcaneus fractures: A 9-year, single-center, retrospective study of a standardized technique using a 2-point distractor. BMC Musculoskeletal Disorders. 2020;**21**(1):753. DOI: 10.1186/s12891-020-03762-9

[46] Weber M, Lehmann O, Sägesser D, Krause F. Limited open reduction and internal fixation of displaced intra-articular fractures of the calcaneum. Journal of Bone and Joint Surgery British Volume. 2008;**90**(12):1608-1616. DOI: 10.1302/0301-620X.90B12.20638

[47] Hsu AR, Anderson RB, Cohen BE. Advances in surgical management of intra-articular calcaneus fractures. Journal of the American Academy of Orthopaedic Surgeons. 2015;**23**(7):399-407. DOI: 10.5435/JAAOS-D-14-00287

[48] Schuberth JM, Cobb MD, Talarico RH. Minimally invasive arthroscopic-assisted reduction with percutaneous fixation in the management of intra-articular calcaneal fractures: A review of 24 cases. The Journal of Foot and Ankle Surgery. 2009;**48**(3):315-322. DOI: 10.1053/j.jfas.2009.01.002

[49] Gao D, Wong TM, Fang C, Leung FK, Li X, Jia B, et al. Arthroscopic-assisted percutaneous fixation of intra-articular calcaneal fractures using an intraoperative distraction device. Journal of Orthopaedic Surgery (Hong Kong). 2021;**29**(1):2309499020979095. DOI: 10.1177/2309499020979095

[50] Rammelt S, Amlang M, Barthel S, Gavlik J-M, Zwipp H. Percutaneous treatment of less severe intraarticular calcaneal fractures. Clinical Orthopaedics and Related Research. 2010;**468**(4):983-990. DOI: 10.1007/s11999-009-0964-x

[51] Yeap EJ, Rao J, Pan CH, Soelar SA, Younger ASE. Is arthroscopic assisted percutaneous screw fixation as good as open reduction and internal fixation for the treatment of displaced intra-articular calcaneal fractures? Foot and Ankle Surgery. 2016;**22**(3):164-169. DOI: 10.1016/j.fas.2015.06.008

[52] Kutaish H, Acker A, Drittenbass L, Stern R, Assal M. Computer-assisted surgery and navigation in foot and ankle: State of the art and fields of application. EFORT Open Reviews. 2021;**6**(7):531-538. DOI: 10.1302/2058-5241.6.200024

[53] Park H-J, You K-H, Huang B, Yoon JH, Kim HN. Can 3-dimensional printing for calcaneal fracture surgery decrease operation time and improve quality of fracture reduction? The Journal of Foot and Ankle Surgery. 2023;**62**(1):21-26. DOI: 10.1053/j.jfas.2022.03.004

[54] Shi J, Shen J, Guo W, Zhang C. Robot-assisted versus traditional fixation for the treatment of calcaneal fractures: A meta-analysis. BMC Musculoskeletal Disorders. 2024;**25**(1):591-599. DOI: 10.1186/s12891-024-07726-1

[55] Ozturk AM, Ozer MA, Suer O, Derin O, Govsa F, Aktuglu K. Evaluation of the effects of using 3D - patient specific models of displaced intra - Articular calcaneal fractures in surgery. Injury. 2022;**53**:S40-S51. DOI: 10.1016/j.injury.2020.04.057

[56] Pitts CC, Almaguer A, Wilson JT, Quade JH, Johnson MD. Radiographic and postoperative outcomes of plate versus screw constructs in open reduction and internal fixation of calcaneus fractures via the sinus tarsi. Foot & Ankle International. 2019;**40**(8):929-935. DOI: 10.1177/1071100719848063

[57] Fan B, Zhou X, Wei Z, Ren Y, Lin W, Hao Y, et al. Cannulated screw fixation and plate fixation for displaced intra-articular calcaneus fracture: A meta-analysis of randomized controlled trials. International Journal of Surgery. 2016;**34**:64-72. DOI: 10.1016/j.ijsu.2016.08.234

[58] Daghino W, Bistolfi A, Aprato A, Massè A. Bioabsorbable implants in foot trauma surgery. Injury. 2019;**50**:S47-S55. DOI: 10.1016/j.injury.2019.01.016

[59] Usami T, Takada N, Nishida K, Sakai H, Iwata H, Yonezu H, et al. Fixation of intra-articular calcaneal fractures: A comparative study of the postoperative outcome between HA/PPLA screws and locking plates. Heliyon. 2023;**9**(3):e14046. DOI: 10.1016/j.heliyon.2023.e14046

[60] Zhang J, Xiao B, Wu Z. Surgical treatment of calcaneal fractures with bioabsorbable screws. International Orthopaedics. 2011;**35**(4):529-533. DOI: 10.1007/s00264-010-1183-5

[61] Chandra G, Pandey A. Biodegradable bone implants in orthopedic applications: A review. Biocybernetics and Biomedical Engineering. 2020;**40**(2):596-610. DOI: 10.1016/j.bbe.2020.02.003

[62] Jud L, Fotouhi J, Andronic O, Aichmair A, Osgood G, Navab N, et al. Applicability of augmented reality in orthopedic surgery - A systematic review. BMC Musculoskeletal Disorders. 2020;**21**(1):103. DOI: 10.1186/s12891-020-3110-2

[63] Bagwe S, Singh K, Kashyap A, Arora S, Maini L. Evolution of augmented reality applications in orthopaedics: A systematic review. Journal of Arthroscopy and Joint Surgery. 2021;**8**(1):84-90. DOI: 10.1016/j.jajs.2021.02.006

[64] Longo UG, De Salvatore S, Candela V, Zollo G, Calabrese G, Fioravanti S, et al. Augmented reality, virtual reality and artificial intelligence in orthopedic surgery: A systematic review. Applied Sciences. 2021;**11**(7):3253. DOI: 10.3390/app11073253

[65] Gupta A, Ambade R. From diagnosis to therapy: The role of virtual and augmented reality in orthopaedic trauma surgery. Curēus (Palo Alto, CA). 2022;**14**(9):e29099. DOI: 10.7759/cureus.29099

[66] Begam H, Roy S, Mukherjee P, Chanda A, Kundu B, Nandi SK, et al. Bone morphogenic proteins and bioceramic scaffolds in orthopedics. In: Innovative Bioceramics in Translational Medicine II, Springer Series in Biomaterials Science and Engineering. Vol. 18. Singapore: Springer Singapore Pte. Limited; 2022. pp. 187-207. DOI: 10.1007/978-981-16-7439-6_9

[67] Peterson JR, Chen F, Nwankwo E, Dekker TJ, Adams SB. The use of bone grafts, bone graft substitutes, and orthobiologics for osseous healing in foot and ankle surgery. Foot and Ankle Orthopaedics. 2019;**4**(3):2473011419849019. DOI: 10.1177/2473011419849019

[68] Greer N, Yoon P, Majeski B, Wilt TJ. Orthobiologics in foot and ankle arthrodesis: A systematic review. The Journal of Foot and Ankle Surgery. 2021;**60**(5):1029-1037. DOI: 10.1053/j.jfas.2020.09.022

[69] Fuchs T, Stolberg-stolberg J, Michel PA, Garcia P, Amler S, Wähnert D, et al. Effect of bone morphogenetic protein-2 in the treatment of long bone non-unions. Journal of Clinical Medicine. 2021;**10**(19):4597. DOI: 10.3390/jcm10194597

[70] Kangari P, Talaei-Khozani T, Razeghian-Jahromi I, Razmkhah M. Mesenchymal stem cells: Amazing remedies for bone and cartilage defects. Stem Cell Research & Therapy. 2020;**11**(1):492. DOI: 10.1186/s13287-020-02001-1

[71] Weinraub GM, Schuberth JM, Lee M, Rush S, Ford L, Neufeld J, et al. Isolated medial incisional approach to subtalar and talonavicular arthrodesis. The Journal of Foot and Ankle Surgery. 2010;**49**(4):326-330. DOI: 10.1053/j.jfas.2010.04.015

[72] Sun L, Kong Z, Xu M. Minimally invasive subtalar arthrodesis for traumatic subtalar arthritis. Journal of International Medical Research. 2019;**47**(12):6129-6138. DOI: 10.1177/0300060519847814

[73] Buch BD, Myerson MS, Miller SD. Primary subtaler arthrodesis for the treatment of comminuted calcaneal fractures. Foot & Ankle International. 1996;**17**(2):61-70

[74] Huefner T, Thermann H, Geerling J, Pape HC, Pohlemann T. Primary subtalar arthrodesis of calcaneal fractures. Foot & Ankle International. 2001;**22**(1):9-14. DOI: 10.1177/107110070102200102

[75] Radnay CS, Clare MP, Sanders RW. Subtalar fusion after displaced intra-articular calcaneal fractures: Does initial operative treatment matter?: Surgical technique. Journal of Bone and Joint Surgery American Volume. 2010;**92**(Supplement_1_Part_1):32-43. DOI: 10.2106/JBJS.I.01267

[76] Patel TK, Gainer J, Lamba C, Adil SA, Singh V, Emmer T. Meta-analysis: Functional outcome of ORIF versus primary subtalar arthrodesis of Sanders type II and type III calcaneal fractures. The Journal of Foot and Ankle Surgery. 2021;**60**(5):1038-1043. DOI: 10.1053/j.jfas.2021.04.009

[77] Lawall A, RN, Soares Martins J, Machado da Silva BA, Freire de Moura Júnior A, Miguel da Silva MH, Ferreira Magalhães W, et al. Primary subtalar arthrodesis in the treatment of comminuted calcaneal fractures: a functional and quality of life analysis. Journal of the Foot & Ankle (Online). 2022;**16**(2):157-162

[78] Buckley R, Leighton R, Sanders D, Poon J, Coles CP, Stephen D, et al. Open reduction and internal fixation compared with ORIF and primary subtalar arthrodesis for treatment of Sanders type IV calcaneal fractures: A randomized Multicenter trial. Journal of Orthopaedic Trauma. 2014;**28**(10):577-583. DOI: 10.1097/BOT.0000000000000191

[79] Attenasio A, Heiman E, Hong IS, Bhalla AP, Jankowski JM, Yoon RS, et al. Postoperative wound complications in extensile lateral approach versus sinus tarsi approach for calcaneal fractures: Are we improving? Updated meta-analysis of recent literature. Injury. 2024;**55**(6):111560. DOI: 10.1016/j.injury.2024.111560

[80] Benirschke SK, Kramer PA. Wound healing complications in closed and open calcaneal fractures. Journal of Orthopaedic Trauma. 2004;**18**(1):1-6. DOI:10.1097/00005131-200401000-00001

[81] Folk JW, Starr AJ, Early JS, Carr JB. Early wound complications of operative treatment of calcaneus fractures: Analysis of 190 fractures. Journal of Orthopaedic Trauma. 1999;**13**(5):369-372

[82] Ding L, He Z, Xiao H, Chai L, Xue F. Risk factors for postoperative wound complications of calcaneal fractures following plate fixation. Foot & Ankle International. 2013;**34**(9):1238-1244. DOI: 10.1177/1071100713484718

[83] Koski A, Kuokkanen H, Tukiainen E. Postoperative wound complications after internal fixation of closed calcaneal fractures: A retrospective analysis of 126 consecutive patients with 148 fractures. Scandinavian Journal of Surgery. 2005;**94**(3):243-245. DOI: 10.1177/145749690509400313

[84] Abidi NA, Dhawan S, Gruen GS, Vogt MT, Conti SF. Wound-healing risk factors after open reduction and internal fixation of calcaneal fractures. Foot & Ankle International. 1998;**19**(12):856-861. DOI: 10.1177/107110079801901211

[85] Buckley RE, Meek RN. Comparison of open versus closed reduction of Intraarticular calcaneal fractures: A matched cohort in workmen. Journal of Orthopaedic Trauma. 1992;**6**(2):216-222. DOI: 10.1097/00005131-199206000-00014

[86] Paley D, Fischgrund J. Open reduction and circular external fixation of intraarticular calcaneal fractures. Clinical Orthopaedics and Related Research. 1993;**290**(290):125-131. DOI: 10.1097/00003086-199305000-00016

[87] Kumar N. Non-union of calcaneum – A rare complication of calcaneal fracture – A case report with brief review of literature. Journal of Clinical Orthopaedics and Trauma. 2015;**6**(3):187-189. DOI: 10.1016/j.jcot.2015.02.005

[88] Schepers T, Patka P. Calcaneal nonunion: Three cases and a review of the literature. Archives of Orthopaedic and Trauma Surgery. 2008;**128**(7):735-738. DOI: 10.1007/s00402-007-0516-3

[89] Banerjee R, Saltzman C, Anderson RB, Nickisch F. Management of calcaneal malunion. Journal of the American Academy of Orthopaedic Surgeons. 2011;**19**(1):27-36. DOI: 10.5435/00124635-201101000-00004

[90] Buckley RE, Tough S. Displaced intra-articular calcaneal fractures. Journal of the American Academy of Orthopaedic Surgeons. 2004;**12**(3):172-178. DOI: 10.5435/00124635-200405000-00005

[91] Lim EVA, Leung JPF. Complications of intraarticular calcaneal fractures. Clinical Orthopaedics and Related Research. 2001;**391**(391):7-16. DOI: 10.1097/00003086-200110000-00003

[92] Giannoudis PV, Tzioupis C, Papathanassopoulos A, Obakponovwe O, Roberts C. Articular step-off and risk of post-traumatic osteoarthritis. Evidence today. Injury. 2010;**41**(10):986-995. DOI: 10.1016/j.injury.2010.08.003

[93] Maskill JD, Bohay DR, Anderson JG. Calcaneus fractures: A review article. Foot and Ankle Clinics. 2005;**10**(3):463-489. DOI: 10.1016/j.fcl.2005.03.002

[94] Gougoulias N, McBride D, Maffulli N. Outcomes of management of displaced intra-articular calcaneal fractures. The Surgeon (Edinburgh). 2021;**19**(5):e222-e229. DOI: 10.1016/j.surge.2020.10.003

[95] Sanders R, Fortin P, DiPasquale T, Walling A. Operative treatment in 120 displaced intraarticular calcaneal fractures: Results using a prognostic computed tomography scan classification. Clinical Orthopaedics and Related Research. 1993;**290**(290):87-95. DOI: 10.1097/00003086-199305000-00012

[96] Sanders R, Vaupel ZM, Erdogan M, Downes K. Operative treatment of displaced intraarticular calcaneal fractures: Long-term (10-20 years) results in 108 fractures using a prognostic CT classification. Journal of Orthopaedic Trauma. 2014;**28**(10):551-563. DOI: 10.1097/BOT.0000000000000169

[97] Calder JDF, Freeman R, Domeij-Arverud E, van Dijk CN, Ackermann PW. Meta-analysis and suggested guidelines for prevention of venous thromboembolism (VTE) in foot and ankle surgery. Knee Surgery, Sports Traumatology, Arthroscopy. 2016;**24**(4):1409-1420. DOI: 10.1007/s00167-015-3976-y

[98] Myerson M, Manoli A. Compartment syndromes of the foot after calcaneal fractures: Calcaneal fractures. Clinical Orthopaedics and Related Research. 1993;**290**:142-150

[99] Ojike NI, Roberts CS, Giannoudis PV. Foot compartment syndrome: A systematic review of the literature. Acta Orthopaedica Belgica. 2009;**75**(5):573-580

[100] Perry MD, Manoli A. Foot compartment syndrome. The Orthopedic Clinics of North America. 2001;**32**(1):103-111. DOI: 10.1016/S0030-5898(05)70197-8

[101] Frink M, Hildebrand F, Krettek C, Brand J, Hankemeier S. Compartment syndrome of the lower leg and foot. Clinical Orthopaedics and Related Research. 2010;**468**(4):940-950. DOI: 10.1007/s11999-009-0891-x

[102] Kazez M, Yalin M, Agar A. Chronic regional pain syndrome following calcaneal fractures: What causes it and how may vitamin C aid? Acta Orthopaedica Belgica. 2024;**90**(2):271-277. DOI: 10.52628/90.2.11928

[103] Morisaki S, Yoshii K, Tsuchida S, Oda R, Fuke T, Takahashi K. The role of preoperative glycemic control in decreasing surgical site infections in lower extremity fractures. Journal of Orthopaedic Surgery and Research. 2023;**18**(1):1-700. DOI: 10.1186/s13018-023-04204-7

[104] Hao S, Liu Y, Yu M, Sun F, Wang D, Xi X, et al. The efficacy of targeted perioperative management for diabetic patients with traumatic

calcaneal fractures. Evidence-based Complementary and Alternative Medicine. 2022;**2022**:1294416-1294417. DOI: 10.1155/2022/1294416

[105] Liu D, Zhu L, Yang C. The effect of preoperative smoking and smoke cessation on wound healing and infection in post-surgery subjects: A meta-analysis. International Wound Journal. 2022;**19**(8):2101-2106. DOI: 10.1111/iwj.13815

[106] Luo L, Chen J, An Z, Sun W, Li M, Ouyang C, et al. Efficacy and postoperative complication rates of different surgical approaches for calcaneal fractures: A network meta-analysis. Alternative Therapies in Health and Medicine. 2024;**30**(7):207-213

[107] Backes M, Dingemans SA, Dijkgraaf MGW, van den Berg HR, van Dijkman B, Hoogendoorn JM, et al. Effect of antibiotic prophylaxis on surgical site infections following removal of orthopedic implants used for treatment of foot, ankle, and lower leg fractures: A randomized clinical trial. JAMA : The Journal of the American Medical Association. 2017;**318**(24):2438-2445. DOI: 10.1001/jama.2017.19343

[108] Classen DC, Evans RS, Pestotnik SL, Horn SD, Menlove RL, Burke JP. The timing of prophylactic administration of antibiotics and the risk of surgical-wound infection. The New England Journal of Medicine. 1992;**326**(5):281-286. DOI: 10.1056/NEJM199201303260501

[109] Upadhyyaya GK, Tewari S. Enhancing surgical outcomes: A critical review of antibiotic prophylaxis in orthopedic surgery. Curēus (Palo Alto, CA). 2023;**15**(10):e47828. DOI: 10.7759/cureus.47828

[110] Zheng X, Li D-Y, Wangyang Y, Zhang X-C, Guo K-J, Zhao F-C, et al. Effect of chemical thromboprophylaxis on the rate of venous thromboembolism after treatment of foot and ankle fractures. Foot & Ankle International. 2016;**37**(11):1218-1224. DOI: 10.1177/1071100716658953

[111] Wynne R, Botti M, Stedman H, Holsworth L, Harinos M, Flavell O, et al. Effect of three wound dressings on infection, healing comfort, and cost in patients with sternotomy wounds: A randomized trial. Chest. 2004;**125**(1):43-49. DOI: 10.1378/chest.125.1.43

[112] Uçkay I, Hoffmeyer P, Lew D, Pittet D. Prevention of surgical site infections in orthopaedic surgery and bone trauma: State-of-the-art update. The Journal of Hospital Infection. 2013;**84**(1):5-12. DOI: 10.1016/j.jhin.2012.12.014

[113] Gougoulias N, Khanna A, McBride DJ, Maffulli N. Management of calcaneal fractures: Systematic review of randomized trials. British Medical Bulletin. 2009;**92**(1):153-167. DOI: 10.1093/bmb/ldp030

[114] Ågren P-H, Wretenberg P, Sayed-Noor AS. Operative versus nonoperative treatment of displaced intra-articular calcaneal fractures: A prospective, randomized, controlled multicenter trial. Journal of bone and joint surgery American volume. 2013;**95**(15):1351-1357. DOI: 10.2106/JBJS.L.00759

[115] Kwon JY, Williams C. Do we have to walk before we can run? surgical management of calcaneus fractures. Foot & Ankle International. 2020;**41**(2):244-245. DOI: 10.1177/1071100719891957

[116] Sharr PJ, Mangupli MM, Winson IG, Buckley RE. Current management options for displaced intra-articular calcaneal fractures: Non-operative, ORIF, minimally invasive reduction and

fixation or primary ORIF and subtalar arthrodesis. A contemporary review. Foot and Ankle Surgery. 2016;**22**(1):1-8. DOI: 10.1016/j.fas.2015.10.003

[117] DeWall M, Henderson CE, McKinley TO, Phelps T, Dolan L, Marsh JL. Percutaneous reduction and fixation of displaced intra-articular calcaneus fractures. Journal of Orthopaedic Trauma. 2010;**24**(8):466-472. DOI: 10.1097/BOT.0b013e3181defd74

[118] Zhang T, Su Y, Chen W, Zhang Q, Wu Z, Zhang Y. Displaced intra-articular calcaneal fractures treated in a minimally invasive fashion: Longitudinal approach versus sinus tarsi approach. Journal of Bone and Joint Surgery American Volume. 2014;**96**(4):302-309. DOI: 10.2106/JBJS.L.01215

[119] Kwon JY, Guss D, Lin DE, Abousayed M, Jeng C, Kang S, et al. Effect of delay to definitive surgical fixation on wound complications in the treatment of closed, intra-articular calcaneus fractures. Foot and Ankle International. 2015;**36**(5):508-517. DOI: 10.1177/1071100714565178

[120] Wiersema B, Brokaw D, Weber T, Psaradellis T, Panero C, Weber C, et al. Complications associated with open calcaneus fractures. Foot & Ankle International. 2011;**32**(11):1052-1057. DOI: 10.3113/FAI.2011.1052

[121] Spierings KE, Min M, Nooijen LE, Swords MP, Schepers T. Managing the open calcaneal fracture: A systematic review. Foot and Ankle Surgery. 2019;**25**(6):707-713. DOI: 10.1016/j.fas.2018.10.005

[122] Alexandridis G, Gunning AC, Leenen LPH. Health-related quality of life in trauma patients who sustained a calcaneal fracture. Injury. 2016;**47**(7):1586-1591. DOI: 10.1016/j.injury.2016.04.008

[123] Motizuki FPZ, Martynetz JR, Polati MF, de Paula SS, Klein Júnior A, Suzuki GYK. Correlation between the quality of calcaneal fracture reduction and time to return to work. Scientific Journal of the Foot & Ankle (Online). 2018;**12**(4):304-309. DOI: 10.30795/scijfootankle.2018.v12.837